Understanding Overdiagnosis

Understanding Overdiagnosis

Medical and Social Science Perspectives

Alexandra Brandt Ryborg Jønsson

Associate Professor of Health and Society, Roskilde University, Denmark
Associate Professor of Medical Anthropology, UiT, The Arctic University of Norway, Tromsø

John Brandt Brodersen

General Practitioner, Zealand University Hospital, Denmark
Professor of General Medicine, Roskilde University, Denmark
Professor of General Medicine, UiT—The Arctic University of Norway, Tromsø

OXFORD
UNIVERSITY PRESS

OXFORD
UNIVERSITY PRESS

Great Clarendon Street, Oxford, OX2 6DP,
United Kingdom

Oxford University Press is a department of the University of Oxford.
It furthers the University's objective of excellence in research, scholarship,
and education by publishing worldwide. Oxford is a registered trade mark of
Oxford University Press in the UK and in certain other countries.

Originally published in Danish in 2022 by Samsfundslitteratur.
Updated and first published in English in 2026 by Oxford University Press.

Published in the United States of America by Oxford University Press
546 Fifth Avenue, New York, NY 10036, United States of America

British Library Cataloguing in Publication Data
Data available

Library of Congress Control Number: 2026940048

ISBN 978–0–19–895601–3

DOI: 10.1093/med/9780198956013.001.0001

Contents

Preface

The success of modern healthcare is undeniable. Advances in diagnostics, pharmaceuticals, and medical technologies have transformed once-fatal diseases into manageable conditions, extended life expectancy, and alleviated suffering on an unprecedented scale. These achievements have reinforced a powerful narrative of progress: that more medicine, earlier detection, and more sensitive diagnostics are not only desirable but inherently beneficial. Within this narrative, health is something to be secured through vigilance, monitoring, and timely intervention.

Yet this logic has a blind spot. In the pursuit of doing good by preventing disease, reducing risk, and improving lives, medicine can, in some cases, do too much. It is this paradox that lies at the heart of this book. Here, Jules Romains' satirical play *Doctor Knock* (1923) appears less like a historical curiosity and more like a disquieting mirror of contemporary medicine. In the play, a doctor famously declares that 'healthy people are simply patients who do not yet know it'. What was intended as satire now resonates uncomfortably with a medical landscape characterised by expanding diagnostic categories, lowering thresholds, and an ever-growing population of what has been described as patients-in-waiting (Timmermans & Buchbinder, 2010).

Each year, large numbers of individuals are diagnosed with somatic conditions that would never have caused symptoms or led to death. Others find ordinary life challenges redefined as mental disorders, often without sufficient attention to the social, relational, and biographical circumstances in which these experiences arise. These processes are increasingly described under the heading of *overdiagnosis*. It is estimated that in for instance Australia, approximately one-in-five women and one-in-four men with a cancer diagnosis are overdiagnosed. While the term may sound technical, its consequences are anything but abstract. Overdiagnosis can lead to unnecessary treatments, anxiety, stigma, and a reorientation of lives around identities of illness and risk. At the same time, it places growing demands on healthcare systems already under strain, diverting resources from those who are genuinely ill, and increases CO_2 emissions exacerbating the climate crisis.

It may seem counterintuitive that healthcare grounded in clinical expertise and good intentions could become harmful through excess. But overdiagnosis is not the result of individual error or professional negligence. Rather, it emerges from deeply embedded assumptions about health, risk, responsibility, and the moral value of action. It is produced at the intersection of technological possibility, institutional incentives, cultural expectations, and political priorities. To understand overdiagnosis, therefore, requires more than clinical and epidemiological analysis alone.

There has been growing scholarly attention to overdiagnosis in recent years. A number of influential books have raised the issue, including Gilbert Welch's *Should*

I be tested for cancer? (2004), Gilbert Welch, Lisa Schwartz, and Steven Woloshin's *Overdiagnosed: Making people sick in the pursuit of health* (2011), and Susan O'Sullivan's *The age of diagnosis* (2025). Overdiagnosis in mental health has likewise been examined in works such as Allan Frances' *Saving normal* (2013) and Joel Paris's *Overdiagnosis in psychiatry* (2015).

This book is written out of a shared concern, but with a conviction that overdiagnosis cannot be adequately understood or addressed within a single disciplinary frame. We address this topic from different professional backgrounds, rooted in medicine and anthropology, respectively. From medicine, we draw on clinical experiences and epidemiological research documenting the scope and mechanisms of overdiagnosis. From anthropology and the social sciences, we bring analytical tools for understanding how medical knowledge travels, how diagnoses acquire meaning, and how healthcare practices are shaped by social norms, institutional logics, and moral economies of care.

We do not to argue against prevention, early detection, or diagnostics as such. These remain essential pillars of modern healthcare. Nor is this book intended as a denunciation of medical professionals, who operate within systems that reward action, vigilance, and intervention. We seek to create space for reflection: to examine when, how, and why medical interventions cease to be beneficial, and how well-intentioned practices may generate unintended harm. As such, we aim to illuminate the social conditions under which harm from too much medicine is produced, normalised, or rendered invisible. This does not entail promoting a particular position on screening programmes, diagnostic technologies, or healthcare policies. Instead, this book equips readers with conceptual and analytical tools that enable them to critically assess evidence, interrogate assumptions, and recognise overdiagnosis as a phenomenon that is simultaneously medical, social, and cultural.

Drawing on more than twenty years of research on overdiagnosis, we introduce and discuss a substantial body of international scholarship on the topic. We are grateful to the many colleagues whose work has informed and inspired this field. Unless otherwise cited, the empirical cases presented are based on our own research. Where necessary, cases have been fictionalised to protect anonymity and to enhance analytical clarity.

Ultimately, this book begins from a simple but unsettling question: what happens when medicine's capacity to detect, label, and intervene outpaces its ability to benefit those it seeks to help? By taking this question seriously, we hope to contribute to a more reflective, equitable, sustainable, and humane practice of healthcare.

Alexandra Brandt Ryborg Jønsson
John Brandt Brodersen
Copenhagen
2026

This book is an altered version of the Danish book *Snart er vi alle patienter. Overdiagnostik i medicinske og samfundsfaglige perspektiver.* Copenhagen: Samfundslitteratur, 2022. The content has been reworked and updated to address an international audience. Some similarities with the Danish book are to be expected. All rights to the Danish edition are held by the authors.

1
Overdiagnosis

Jim's prostate cancer

A few weeks following his 65th birthday, Jim went to the doctor's office for a general health check-up, spurred by his wife. She had read in the newspaper that men of their generation had high risk of diseases but did not go to the doctor as often as needed. Recalling the situation for a research interview, Jim said he had felt the consultation was unnecessary because he felt fine, but his wife, sitting next to him, remarked that it was not at all unnecessary, because they had discovered that he had cancer. As part of the check-up the doctor had done a PSA test, a blood test that measures prostate-specific antigen (PSA) levels, which can indicate the presence of prostate cancer. And Jim's had been slightly elevated, so he was diagnosed. Still, due to the cancer's indolent nature, it did not require treatment, and Jim was instead placed in a watchful-waiting programme where he was carefully monitored through biannual check-ups at the urology clinic.

Jim and his wife were part of an anthropological research project on ageing that Alexandra conducted, and this incident was narrated as a reply to when and why they would consult their doctor. Jim was one of several participants in Alexandra's study diagnosed with prostate cancer via opportunistic PSA screening without experiencing any symptoms. Two have since passed away from other diseases, having lived with prostate cancer for decades that never caused them any harm.

The recounts of living with prostate cancer that was found by coincidence and had not spread or caused any symptoms mirror the epidemiological evidence. According to the American Cancer Society, more than 3.3 million men in the United States are living with prostate cancer. Yet, only 1 in 30 men diagnosed with prostate cancer will die from it (Jacklin et al., 2021), supporting the saying that 'more men die *with* prostate cancer than *because* of it'. However, a diagnosis of prostate cancer should not be trivialised. Prostate cancer can in some cases follow an aggressive course and be a life-threatening disease. It may generate embarrassment, anxiety about treatment, concerns about sexual function, and fear of disease progression (Bekele & Martínez-Hernáez, 2025). Even men who are successfully treated often report persistent worry about cancer for the remainder of their lives (van der Kamp et al., 2022).

Globally, millions or possibly billions of people receive diagnoses for conditions that will never cause symptoms or contribute to death. Like Jim, they undergo increasingly highly sensitive examinations capable of detecting ever smaller biological changes that would otherwise remain unnoticed. Others are diagnosed because diagnostic thresholds are adjusted, or normal ranges are redefined. For example, blood pressure values derived from middle-aged populations may be applied to older adults resulting in more people diagnosed with high blood pressure. In mental health, diagnostic categories may be broadened to such an extent that ordinary variation in behaviour or emotion is medicalised.

When a diagnosis does not provide benefit, and the condition diagnosed will never cause the person symptoms or death, it is defined as *overdiagnosis*. Overdiagnosis is increasing across both somatic and mental health conditions (Frances, 2013; Paris, 2015; Glaziou et al., 2020; Sanders et al., 2024). It affects individuals through unnecessary treatment, anxiety, and labelling, and it burdens healthcare systems by diverting limited resources. Still, the idea of overdiagnosis is often met with resistance in the broader public because it appears counterintuitive to suggest that detecting abnormalities may be harmful. A common response is that it is 'better to be safe than sorry'. But the challenge when it comes to overdiagnosis is that no latent risk has been prevented, so you are no safer with than without the diagnosis. Instead, a naturally occurring condition or abnormality that would never have caused harm is reclassified as disease.

Was Jim overdiagnosed? Neither he nor his doctor can know. Although Jim and his wife are grateful that the cancer was detected at an indolent localised stage, epidemiological evidence suggests that it is highly unlikely his tumour will ever cause symptoms or death. And if that does not happen, Jim will have been overdiagnosed. But once a diagnosis is made, ignoring it is neither ethically nor clinically acceptable. Overdiagnosis must therefore be addressed upstream by examining its drivers. Medical evidence shows, for example, that restricting PSA testing to men with specific symptoms rather than testing asymptomatic ageing men with common lower urinary tract symptoms can substantially reduce overdiagnosis (Østerø & Brodersen, 2018). Such an approach allows healthcare resources to be directed towards diagnostics of patients with potentially progressive disease and towards palliative care for those who ultimately die from prostate cancer.

What overdiagnosis is

Diagnosis is the process through which medicine distinguishes disease from non-disease. A diagnosis is conventionally based on coherence between three elements: the patient's medical history (anamnesis), findings from the clinical examination, and results from diagnostic tests or imaging. In practice, however, this coherence is often imperfect. Some patients report symptoms that are not reflected in clinical findings or paraclinical tests. Others have no symptoms at all but receive a diagnosis based on abnormalities detected through examinations or screening tests. Diagnosis is therefore not an exact science. As a result, several unintended outcomes may occur, including misdiagnosis, underdiagnosis, and overdiagnosis.

Broadly, *overdiagnosis* means making people into patients unnecessarily (Brodersen et al., 2018a). In somatic conditions, overdiagnosis arises when a test, screening

Box 1.1 Definition: Overdiagnosis in somatic conditions

Overdiagnosis is the outcome of processes or mechanisms that lead to the detection and identification of deviations, abnormalities, risk factors, or pathophysiological and/or pathoanatomical conditions that will never in themselves cause the person's symptoms (except for deviations and abnormalities), morbidity, or death. (Brodersen, 2017a).

procedure, examination, or change in diagnostic thresholds leads to a technically correct diagnosis, but the diagnosed condition would never have caused symptoms, morbidity, or death. A more detailed definition is provided in Box 1.1. The absence of symptoms creates an important distinction between overdiagnosis in somatic and mental conditions. In somatic conditions, overdiagnosis occurs when a person never experiences symptoms attributable to the diagnosed condition. In mental health, symptoms are often fluid, contextual, and widely distributed in the population. Many people experience psychological symptoms without having a psychiatric disorder. In this context, overdiagnosis is best understood as situations in which individuals are unnecessarily turned into patients, that is, cases where a diagnosis does not provide the person any benefit. This definition raises difficult questions. Who determines what constitutes benefit? A diagnosis may provide access to educational support, social services, or workplace accommodations, and may therefore be experienced as helpful. Nevertheless, such benefits do not resolve the underlying problem of unnecessary medicalisation and do not provide any clinical prognostic benefits.

In this book, our primary focus is on overdiagnosis in somatic diagnosis. Overdiagnosis in mental health is addressed selectively where it illuminates broader mechanisms. Readers with a particular interest in psychiatric overdiagnosis should orient themselves in *Overdiagnosis in psychiatry* (Paris 2015) and *Saving normal* (Frances 2013).

Overdiagnosis is not a property of the individual or the diagnosis alone. It is the result of a practice; diagnostic testing, screening, lowering thresholds, that makes overdiagnosis possible. Overdiagnosis occurs through two main mechanisms:

1. **Identification of abnormalities** that will never cause harm during a person's lifetime. For example, malignant cells are detected in a man's prostate gland and classified as prostate cancer, even though these cells would never result in symptoms or death.
2. **Medicalisation of normal variation or life challenges**, through the expansion of disease definitions or the lowering of diagnostic or treatment thresholds. For example, a person is diagnosed with hypertension because their blood pressure exceeds a fixed threshold, even though this level would never have affected their health.

<table>
<tr><th>Reasons for overdetection</th><th>Reasons for overdefinition</th></tr>
<tr><td>The body: a reservoir for indolent pathological conditions
Short remaining lifespan
New technology: higher resolution and sensitivity</td><td>Reduction of thresholds for risk factors
Reduction of treatment thresholds
Expansion of disease definitions</td></tr>
<tr><td colspan="2">Same consequences:
Labelling
Overtreatment
Psychosocial burden
Overuse and unjust allocation of healthcare services</td></tr>
</table>

Figure 1.1 Two types of overdiagnosis: causes and consequences (Brodersen et al., 2018a).

Reproduced with permission from Samfundslitteratur.

Definitional complexity and overlapping concepts

Defining overdiagnosis becomes more complex because it overlaps conceptually with related phenomena, including incidental findings, false positives, overtreatment, overuse, misdiagnosis, clinical variation, undiagnosis, and underdiagnosis. This overlap contributes to the absence of a single, unambiguous definition in the literature (Welch et al., 2011; Hofmann, 2014; S.M. Carter et al., 2015b; Rogers & Mintzker, 2016; Brodersen et al., 2018a; Woloshin & Kramer, 2021). To understand overdiagnosis as an independent phenomenon, it is therefore essential to distinguish clearly between these concepts and to identify when overlap occurs and when it does not. These distinctions are developed throughout the chapter.

There are two principal forms of overdiagnosis: *overdetection* and *overdefinition*. Although the mechanisms that produce them differ, their consequences are the same. Both result in unnecessary diagnoses, where individuals are made patients without deriving clinical benefit and may instead experience harm (see Figure 1.1).

Overdetection

Overdetection is, in simple terms, about finding too much. It refers to the identification of pathological findings that fulfil diagnostic criteria but will never cause symptoms, morbidity, or death. In such cases, something is identified in the body and classified as disease even though the person would never have noticed it or experienced harm. More precisely, overdetection occurs when deviations, abnormalities, risk factors, or pathophysiological or pathoanatomical conditions are identified, and these findings will never become clinically manifest later in life (Brodersen et al., 2014). For brevity, we refer to these collectively as pathological conditions and, when referring specifically to cells, as neoplastic cells, unless otherwise specified. But even the terminology is linguistically misleading. Both *pathophysiological* and *pathoanatomical* contain the word 'pathology', meaning the study of disease. Physiology concerns the function of organs and systems, while anatomy concerns their structure. Pathophysiology therefore refers to functional changes associated with disease, whereas pathoanatomy refers to structural changes observable in tissues or organs.

Many pathological conditions detected in healthy individuals are harmless. A tissue alteration may meet histological criteria for cancer without ever progressing to symptomatic or fatal disease. In genetics, this is a well-known distinction: we all have unique sequences of DNA, which is referred to as our genotype. Since we have two forms inherited from both our parents, we also talk about phenotype. This is the observable expression of a person's genotype. So, you may have a genetic disposition for a particular disease, which is your genotype, but you will not necessarily experience that disease, because your phenotype does not express that disease. In the same way, we all have natural reservoirs of biological deviations, that will never be expressed and turn into disease. Evidence for this can for example be seen in studies of lung nodules, which are common across age groups in non-smoking populations (Cai et al., 2024). This may help explain the high degree of lung cancer overdiagnosis observed among non-smoking Asian women undergoing low-dose computed tomography (CT) screening (Gao et al., 2022).

One problem is that the evidence on which these results are based comes from group-level research. At the individual level at the time of diagnosis, it will not be possible to determine in a person without symptoms whether the diagnosed pathological condition will lead to morbidity and/or death later in life (Brodersen et al., 2014). Understanding what happens at the individual level is only possible in retrospect after the person has died. As Danish philosopher Søren Kierkegaard (1813–1855) famously said, *Life can only be understood backwards, but it must be lived forwards.* This captures the core dilemma of overdetection: we can only know whether someone was overdiagnosed at the end of their life. At the population level, however, overdetection can be inferred epidemiologically. An increase in disease incidence without a corresponding increase in morbidity or mortality strongly suggests overdiagnosis.

Historical roots of overdetection

The concepts of pathophysiology and pathoanatomy emerged during the rise of modern medicine between approximately 1880 and 1950. In *Doctors and their patients: A social history*, medical historian Edward Shorter describes this period as one in which diagnostic thinking shifted fundamentally (Shorter, 1985). Shorter outlines how people's ideas about when they could or should go to the doctor and what they could expect from these visits have changed from the mid-eighteenth century to the present, distinguishing between three phases: the traditional, modern, and post-modern periods:

In the *traditional period* (1750–1880), disease was primarily understood as imbalance in bodily fluids. Diagnoses were broad and often based on causes of death rather than on systematic clinical examination.

In the *modern period* (1880–1950), medicine began to classify and categorise symptoms and illnesses in a more systematic way. This development coincided with advances in microscopy and bacteriology. Disease came to be understood as a visible pathological condition located in specific tissues or organs. It was during this period that the diagnostic logic familiar today was established: coherence between anamnesis, clinical examination, and abnormal test findings.

The *postmodern period* (from around 1950 onwards) is characterised by an increasing focus on early detection, risk factors, and predisease states, as well as a marked expansion of psychiatric diagnoses. Healthcare systems have become pro-active rather than reactive, for example by actively inviting citizens to screening and encouraging medical consultations for defined symptoms. The underlying logic is that early detection of pathological conditions can prevent disease and prolong life (Damhus et al., 2024). This logic rests on an implicit assumption inherited from the modern period: that pathological conditions detected in asymptomatic individuals will eventually progress to disease.

Reservoirs of disease and evidence from autopsy studies

The last three decades of research have given us another insight, namely that far from all early identified pathological conditions in healthy people turn into disease later in life (Welch et al., 2011). Autopsy studies provide particularly clear evidence of overdetection. When pathological conditions are found post-mortem in individuals who never experienced symptoms and did not die from the condition, this demonstrates that the human body can harbour disease-like cells and conditions without clinical relevance and that the person was never aware of (Bell et al., 2015; Furuya-Kanamori et al., 2016; Thomas et al., 2017). A frequently cited example comes from a Danish autopsy study conducted at Frederiksberg Hospital in 1987. Pathologists performed medicolegal autopsies on 110 women aged 20–54 years who had died from accidents or other causes permitting forensic examination (Nielsen et al., 1987). The study found that 22 women had neoplastic cells or tissue in at least one breast. Ten of the 22 women had neoplastic cells in multiple locations in the breast, while nine of the 22 women had neoplastic cells in both breasts. Only one of these women had been diagnosed with breast cancer during her lifetime, while the other 21 did not know about their pathologic cells. If these neoplastic cells had been detected while the women were alive, 21 of the 22 cases would have constituted overdiagnosis. However, if the neoplastic cells had developed and caused *symptoms* at a later stage, and the women then would have been diagnosed, they would not have been overdiagnosed. As the 110 deceased women were relatively young, many of them could have had a long remaining lifespan during which the neoplastic cells could have developed and caused symptoms, if they had not died in an accident. In contrast, the lifetime risk of developing breast cancer in 1987 was about 10 percent for women in Denmark. In other words, the observed prevalence of neoplastic cells far exceeded the expected lifetime risk of developing breast cancer.

The example of the autopsy study from Denmark demonstrates that many women worldwide might have neoplastic cells in their breasts that they never develop symptoms from or die from. A systematic review by Thomas and colleagues identified 13 autopsy studies from multiple countries examining the prevalence of breast cancer and precursor lesions (Thomas et al., 2017). The mean prevalence of pathological findings was 19.5 percent, including 0.85 percent invasive cancer, 8.9 percent carcinoma in situ, and 9.8 percent atypical hyperplasia. These findings suggest a substantial global reservoir of indolent pathological conditions in women's breasts. However, it is important to note that there might be variation in prevalence between countries of such indolent pathological malignant cells in women's breasts due to different cultures, living conditions, smoking habits, race, and other factors. Similar autopsy studies of prostate and thyroid cancer show even larger reservoirs of pathological findings that never grew to cause symptoms or death (Bell et al., 2015; Furuya-Kanamori et al., 2016).

How does overdetection occur?

Overdetection is an unintended consequence of diagnostic interventions, including tests, imaging, examinations, and screening. It arises primarily from three interacting factors: biology, competing risk, and technology (Box 1.2).

Box 1.2 Three reasons for overdetection

1. *Biology*: The human body is full of harmless pathological conditions.
2. *Competing risk*: Individuals may die from other causes before a detected condition becomes clinically relevant.
3. *Technology*: Increasing test sensitivity allows detection of ever-smaller abnormalities.

Biology: The human body is full of harmless pathological conditions

Throughout life and with increasing probability as the body ages, pathological conditions occur in the human body. Some regress spontaneously, others remain dormant, and some progress rapidly to symptomatic disease. A common metaphor distinguishes between 'turtle', 'bird' and 'bear' cancers to describe differences in growth rates (Figure 1.2).

Turtle cancer is so slow that it is not dangerous and not worth finding or treating. Bird cancer is so fast and 'flies' in unpredictable patterns that it cannot be caught. Here, the aim of treatment is often palliative and not curative. Bear cancer is dangerous, but it can be caught with caution. Only bear cancer can benefit from being caught early and treated earlier. Since some cancers are 'turtles' growing so slowly that they will never become a problem, a pathological condition can be found too early (Brodersen et al., 2014). This variability makes it impossible in clinical practice to

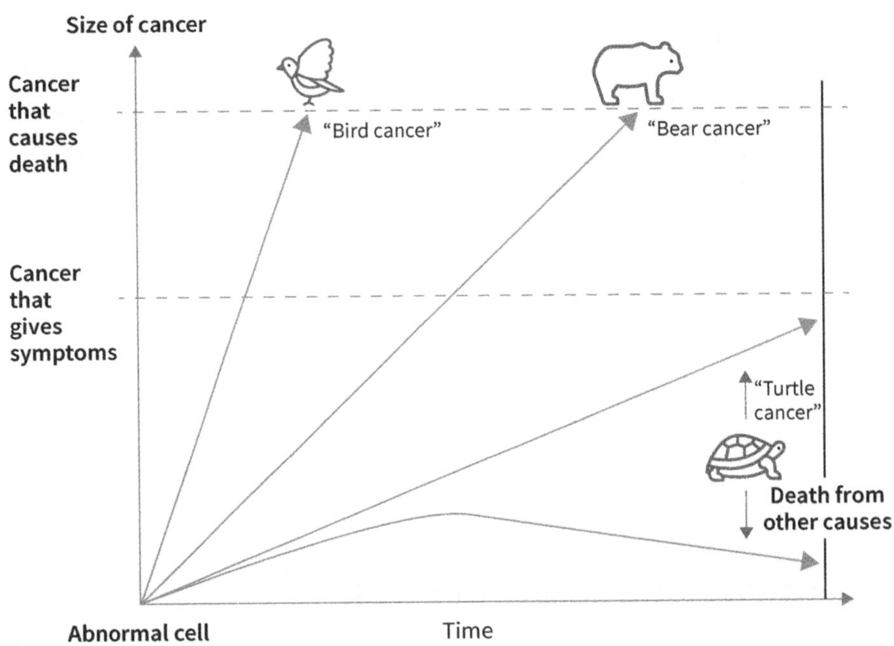

Figure 1.2 A model using animal analogies to illustrate that cancer has different growth rates.

'Bird cancer' grows rapidly and becomes lethal quickly, 'bear cancer' grows more slowly but can still cause death, while slow-growing 'turtle cancer' may never cause symptoms before death from other causes.

Reproduced with permission from Samfundslitteratur.

distinguish harmless from harmful pathological conditions at the time of diagnosis. Figure 1.3 shows a generic and hypothetical model of cancer growth rates; individuals with identical screening findings may have radically different disease trajectories.

In Figure 1.3, person A receives a *false negative* screening result: A is told at the first screening round that no cancer can be found, but there is actually a cancer growing so fast that A experiences symptoms before the second screening round. In addition, person A's cancer is highly malignant. Because of its rapid progression and malignant nature, A ultimately dies from it, despite participating in screening. Persons B, C, D, and E have neoplastic cells that are not yet detectable in the first and second screening rounds but may be detected in the third or fourth screening rounds. They develop symptoms from their cancers before they would die from other causes. Person F's pathologic cells grows so slowly that it can only be detected in the fifth round of screening, but F never experiences symptoms from the condition, before dying from another cause. Person G's and H's pathologic cells are not detected in the screening programmes, and they do not cause symptoms and do not affect their mortality. They are not diagnosed and die from other causes without ever knowing that they have had neoplastic cells. Person I's neoplastic cells may be detected in the second and third screening rounds; however, the condition has a spontaneous regression before person I gets symptoms. While hypothetically, we can conclude that persons F and I are overdiagnosed: person F dies before developing symptoms of cancer, while person I has a pathological condition with spontaneous regression. Figure 1.3 illustrates the dilemma that if you test, examine, or screen for pathological conditions that in many

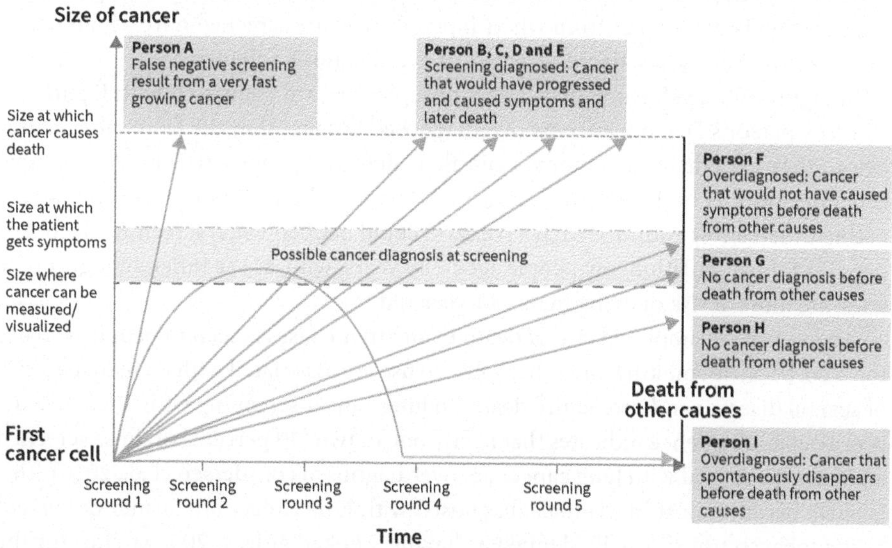

Figure 1.3 What happens at cancer screening. Modified version from Brodersen et al. (2014).

Reproduced with permission from Samfundslitteratur.

cases regress spontaneously, grow very slowly, or do not grow at all, overdiagnosis can occur.

Prostate cancer provides a paradigmatic example. Autopsy studies show that pathological prostate cancer is extremely common in older men. A systematic review of 29 autopsy studies found that prevalence increased from 5 percent in men aged <30 years to 59 percent in men aged ≥79 years (Bell et al., 2015). Most of these cancers never cause symptoms. When screening is introduced, prostate cancer incidence increases by at least 40 percent, but mortality remains unchanged (Ilic et al., 2018; Vaccarella et al., 2024). Modelling studies suggest that more than 40 percent of prostate cancer diagnoses represent overdiagnosis (Glasziou et al., 2020).

Comparable patterns are seen in cervical cancer screening (Östör, 1993). Mild dysplasia or low-grade intraepithelial lesion, composed of the mildest type of neoplastic cells that can be identified in women during cervical cancer screening, is suggested to cause overdiagnosis of cervical cancer. Most of these mild dysplasia cells regress spontaneously to normal cells or do not progress to moderate or severe dysplasia.

Competing risk: Individuals may die from other causes before a detected condition becomes clinically relevant

Overdetection is amplified when individuals have a high risk of dying from causes other than the detected condition. This is particularly relevant in older populations with a competing risk of age-related death, because everyone dies at some point. The key question is: When and from what? If people who are screened have a high risk of dying from other causes, then the degree of overdiagnosis will increase.

In Figure 1.4, death from all causes is brought forward compared with Figure 1.3, whereby persons D and E are now overdiagnosed because they die from other causes before they experience symptoms from their detected neoplastic cells. At the same time, person F is no longer overdiagnosed, because the person dies before participating in screening round 5. Such a scenario could happen when screening the oldest people of the population, say people aged ≥80 years, who, as the inherent logic of life goes, are more at risk of dying than a 40-year-old.

An example of amplified risk of death from other causes is seen in people who use tobacco, because smoking and other tobacco use are associated with an increased risk of several diseases and premature death. In lung cancer screening with CT scans, the best available evidence indicates that nearly one in two (49 percent) of those screened and later diagnosed with lung cancer are overdiagnosed (Brodersen et al., 2020). This is likely because most individuals diagnosed with lung cancer are former or current heavy tobacco users, usually defined as having smoked at least 20 cigarettes (or the equivalent) per day for 20 years. These individuals face a substantially higher risk of dying from cardiovascular diseases. Many individuals diagnosed with screening-detected lung cancer simply do not have enough lifetime remaining to develop

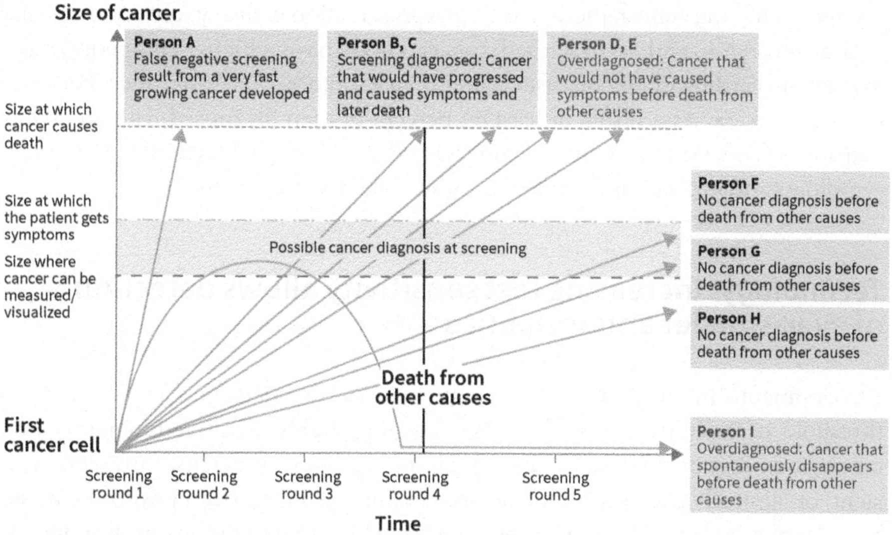

Figure 1.4 Shortened expected life-time (Brodersen et al., 2014): how age and competing mortality affect overdiagnosis.
When death occurs sooner, some screen-detected cancers become overdiagnosed because symptoms would never appear, while others are never detected because the person dies before later screening rounds.
Reproduced with permission from Samfundslitteratur.

symptoms or die from lung cancer before they pass away from other causes associated with tobacco use. It is crucial to understand that the pathological diagnosis of 'lung cancer' is not an error; rather, overdiagnosis occurs because the person dies from causes other than lung cancer before they experience symptoms of the cancer itself.

Whether a person is overdiagnosed with lung cancer depends on biology, particularly the tumour's growth rate and potential to metastasise, and the competing risk of dying from other conditions, such as the severity of cardiovascular disease or other risk factors. For example, if there were a breakthrough in preventive treatments for cardiovascular disease, the rate of overdiagnosis in lung cancer CT screening would decrease. This is because the lung cancer screening participants would then be less likely to die from cardiovascular disease, increasing the chances of experiencing symptoms and potentially dying from their lung cancer.

Similar dynamics apply to screening for abdominal aortic aneurysm (AAA), a swelling or bagging out of the main blood vessel (artery) that leads away from the heart, down through the abdomen to the rest of the body. AAA can be detected via an ultrasound examination and a CT scan, but many individuals diagnosed through screening will die from other causes before the aneurysm causes symptoms, leading to substantial overdiagnosis (Johansson et al., 2015). Two factors influence the results here. First, the pathological condition itself may either not grow or grow very slowly.

Second, as in lung cancer, there is an overrepresentation of heavy tobacco users diagnosed with AAA, and, as described, tobacco users have a higher competing risk of dying from cardiovascular diseases (other than a ruptured AAA) or cancer compared to non-smokers. As a result, at least 44 percent of men diagnosed with an abdominal aortic aneurysm through screening will be overdiagnosed, as they do not develop symptoms and instead die from other causes (Johansson et al., 2015).

Technology: Increasing test sensitivity allows detection of ever-smaller abnormalities

Developments in diagnostic technology increase overdetection by lowering the threshold of visibility. High-resolution imaging, highly sensitive biomarkers, and continuous monitoring detect abnormalities that were previously invisible, transient, or clinically irrelevant. One notable example is the Quadra positron emission tomography–computed tomography scanner, which represents a giant leap forward in scanning technology. This device not only offers a lower radiation dose and shorter scan times compared to previous models, but its higher resolution also enables non-invasive measurement of blood flow, providing insights into organ function (Prenosil et al., 2022). Meanwhile, blood test assays are evolving to detect and measure increasingly smaller subcomponents of biomarkers such as proteins or vitamins, which can reflect the biological state of the body. For instance, the Grail blood test uses various biomarkers to screen for 50 different types of cancer from a single blood sample (Carr et al., 2021). At the same time, the use of what we refer to as *paraclinical examinations*, an umbrella term encompassing imaging, blood tests, and other diagnostic tests, has been steadily increasing. This trend is evident within the established healthcare system and in the growing availability of self-testing, which can be easily accessed and performed on computers, wearables, and smartphone apps. As a result, an increasing number of biological and mental functions can be measured more often, leading to a greater probability of identifying conditions that might otherwise remain unnoticed.

Figure 1.5 illustrates how increasing technological development amplifies overdiagnosis through detecting and categorising neoplastic cells at even smaller stages. In Figure 1.5, person G is overdiagnosed because the technology detects changes that would previously have remained invisible. Hypothetically, a subset of conditions that were previously undetectable, unmeasurable, or invisible will also now be classified as abnormal findings, as illustrated in person H's case. Continuous monitoring further increases overdetection by capturing abnormalities that would otherwise resolve spontaneously or only appear in a short time interval (Haase et al., 2026).

In epidemiology, *The Will Rogers phenomenon* is used to describe a statistical illusion in which improvements in diagnostic precision create the appearance of better outcomes without any real change in individual prognosis. When more sensitive tests reclassify patients from one diagnostic category to another, most often from a less severe to a more severe group, the average outcomes in both groups can appear to

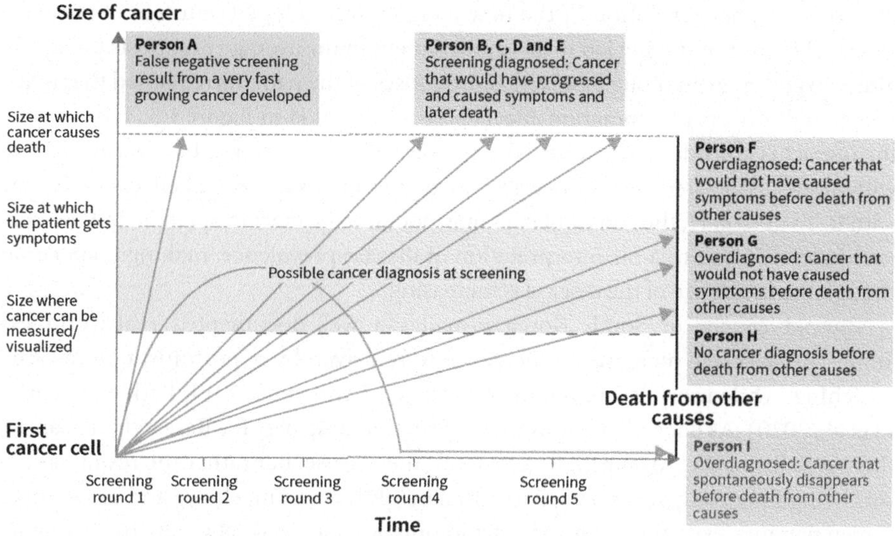

Figure 1.5 Lowered threshold for when cancer can be detected by more sensitive diagnostic technology, increasing overdiagnosis.
When cancers can be detected at smaller sizes, additional slow-growing or harmless abnormalities are identified. Some individuals are therefore diagnosed with cancers that would never have caused symptoms before death from other causes.
Reproduced with permission from Samfundslitteratur.

improve. This occurs because patients with relatively better prognoses are moved into the more severe category, while those remaining in the less severe category are, on average, healthier. Importantly, no individual patient benefits from this reclassification; the apparent improvement is entirely an artefact of categorisation rather than a true therapeutic gain. Relating to overdiagnosis, the Will Rogers phenomenon describes a situation where a change in cancer prognosis is not a result of improved treatment, but rather due to the introduction of new technology with higher resolution. For example, Feinstein and colleagues explain how developments in diagnostic technology, such as CT and ultrasound scans, have led to changes in the staging of patients diagnosed with lung cancer, which in turn has altered the prognosis for patients in different stage groups (Feinstein et al., 1984, 1985). In a cohort of patients with lung cancer diagnosed between 1953 and 1964, a variety of diagnostic tests was used. The same diagnostic tests were applied to a 1977 cohort, but this time, all patients were also examined using CT scans and/or ultrasound, both of which have higher resolution than the previous diagnostic methods. Feinstein et al. found that the newer technology uncovered previously unrecognised metastases that could not be detected by the older diagnostic battery. Therefore, patients who were originally classified as having localised lung cancer were reclassified as having cancer that had spread to lymph nodes or other organs, not because their disease had progressed, but simply due to the higher resolution of the new imaging technology (Feinstein et al., 1984, 1985). This shift in staging led to an improvement in the average prognosis for all staging categories, even though the actual prognoses of the patients remained the same.

The Will Rogers phenomenon affects persons G and H in Figure 1.5. To person G, the impact is considerable because the person will live the rest of life overdiagnosed, with all the associated risks of overtreatment and the psychosocial effects that come with it. To person H, the consequences may not directly affect the person, but the phenomenon can lead to a misinterpretation of disease prevalence, making it appear as though the incidence of the disease is increasing.

Thyroid cancer in South Korea provides a well-documented real-world example. Remarkable increases in incidence were driven by opportunistic ultrasound screening, while mortality remained unchanged (Ahn et al., 2014; Park et al., 2016; Li et al., 2020). As flagged by the WHO International Agency for Research on Cancer, this surge is not due to an actual increase in the disease, but rather the result of doctors being financially incentivised to purchase ultrasound machines and use them to screen patients, even those who are asymptomatic (Vaccarella et al., 2016). This practice, known as opportunistic screening (see Chapter 4), has led to a vast increase in the detection of thyroid cancer. Between 1999 and 2008, the incidence of thyroid cancer in South Korea increased 6.4-fold (Park et al., 2016). However, thyroid cancer mortality rates during the same period remained virtually unchanged (Ahn et al., 2014; Park et al., 2016). This was not due to improvements in treatment, but because the majority of the newly identified thyroid cancer cases would never have caused symptoms or harm. Thus, the individuals diagnosed would have survived regardless of treatment. In other words, the number of people who died from thyroid cancer remained the same before and after 1999, and the effectiveness of treatment was just as high in 1999 as it was in 2008. However, more people were unnecessarily categorised as sick and overdiagnosed with thyroid cancer. The International Agency for Research on Cancer has investigated the global trends in overdiagnosis of thyroid cancer and concluded 'that overdiagnosis of thyroid cancer is increasing rapidly worldwide and has now become a major global public health challenge (Li et al., 2020).

Box 1.3 The Will Rogers Phenomenon

The term *Will Rogers phenomenon* takes its name from a quip attributed to Will Rogers, who joked that when people moved from Oklahoma to California, they *raised the average intelligence of both states*. The humour lies in the absurdity: individuals of below-average intelligence in California could still be above average in Oklahoma, so their relocation would simultaneously improve the mean in both populations.

Over time, this joke has become a metaphor for a mathematical phenomenon that describes a situation where, by transferring an element from one set to another, the average value of both sets increases. This occurs when the element being moved is below the average in its original set but above the average in the new set.

Overdefinition

Overdiagnosis through *overdefinition* occurs when disease categories are expanded, or diagnostic and treatment thresholds are lowered without evidence that this improves patient outcomes. Overdefinition operates through two closely related mechanisms:

1. *Lowering thresholds* for treatment or risk factors without evidence that this leads to a better prognosis for people.
2. *Expanding disease definitions* so that individuals with milder, ambiguous, or transient symptoms are classified as sick (Brodersen et al., 2018a).

Lowering thresholds for risk factors and treatment

In practice, the thresholds for risk factors and treatment are often co-dependent. When thresholds for risk factors are lowered, treatment thresholds are typically lowered at the same time. Lowering diagnostic thresholds increases the number of individuals classified as ill, even though only a small proportion will ever develop symptoms or die from the disease in question. Hypertension provides a paradigmatic example. Over time, the diagnostic threshold for high blood pressure has been repeatedly lowered, with variation across countries and guidelines. Treatment recommendations have followed these definitional changes, and increasing numbers of asymptomatic individuals are labelled with hypertension, despite having a low absolute risk of adverse outcomes.

A population-based study from Nord-Trøndelag County in Norway illustrates this dynamic (Box 1.4). Using contemporary European guideline thresholds, 95 percent of the population had at least one elevated cardiovascular risk factor. Yet, far from all will develop cardiovascular disease or die from it.

There is no robust evidence of high quality to show that clinicians are benefiting the population by treating individuals with mildly elevated blood pressure (between 140/90 and 165/100 mmHg) (Wang et al., 2025). Studies have shown that systematically inviting a healthy adult population group for general health checks, informing them about any increased risk of cardiovascular disease, and offering lifestyle conversations or medications to lower blood pressure and cholesterol resulted in no reduction in either mortality or morbidity (Krogsbøll et al., 2019). The Danish Inter99 study, known for its large-scale, multiple follow-ups over several years, and high validity of the Danish registries, revealed that most individuals who later die from cardiovascular disease do not have elevated risk factors for the condition (Vinther et al., 2013). WHO has investigated in a Health Evidence Network Synthesis Report the effectiveness of systematic population-level screening programmes for reducing the burden of cardiovascular diseases. The conclusion is clear: screening for cardiovascular risk

Box 1.4 Case: Nord-Trøndelag County, Norway

The population of Nord-Trøndelag County in Norway is among the longest-living in Europe. Yet, using guideline thresholds from the European Society of Cardiology:

- blood pressure >140/90 mmHg
- cholesterol >8 mmol/L
- body mass index >25 kg/m^2

95 percent of the population has at least one elevated risk factor (Petursson et al., 2009).

Despite this, there is no excess mortality among individuals with untreated elevated blood pressure (Jørgensen et al., 2017). Moreover, labelling individuals with high blood pressure is associated with poorer self-rated health (Jørgensen et al., 2015).

factors does not lower cardiovascular-related morbidity and mortality or healthcare expenses (Jørgensen et al., 2024).

Thresholds as political and geographical constructs

Thresholds for disease are not fixed biological truths. They are negotiated and historically contingent. For many years, systolic blood pressure was considered acceptable if it did not exceed '100 plus age'. In the mid-1980s, this was standardised to 165/95 mmHg. Later, it was lowered to 140/90 mmHg for all adults, regardless of age or sex.

In 2017, the American College of Cardiology and the American Heart Association proposed lowering the hypertension threshold to 130/80 mmHg (Muntner et al., 2017). More recently, the European Society of Cardiology suggested lowering treatment thresholds for selected subgroups. This means that people with a blood pressure of 135/85 mmHg would be considered healthy in some parts of the world but would be considered patients in the US and Europe. These changes would classify even more asymptomatic individuals as patients, increasing overdiagnosis and overtreatment (Haase et al., 2019).

Such proposals have faced substantial criticism regarding their evidentiary basis (Bell et al., 2018). Importantly, individuals with blood pressure values just above a newly lowered threshold have a much lower risk than those with markedly elevated levels, even though both groups receive the same diagnosis. Lowering a threshold does not automatically constitute overdiagnosis. However, when definitional expansion is not accompanied by improved prognosis (decreased mortality or morbidity, or increased quality of life), it is a strong signal of overdefinition (Moynihan et al., 2019).

Every time a threshold for a risk factor is lowered, new 'patients' may be included who were not considered patients before the threshold change. This adjustment means that the new 'patients' have a lower risk of developing the disease or dying from it compared to those who were previously diagnosed. In other words, there is a significant difference in risk, even though both groups are placed in the same category. For example, there is a considerable difference between having a blood pressure of 145/95 and 220/120 mmHg, yet both groups are equally diagnosed with high blood pressure.

Expansion of disease definitions

Overdefinition also occurs when disease categories are broadened to include individuals with milder, ambiguous, or transient symptoms. This process medicalises normal variation and everyday life challenges. Examples include difficulties with sleep, concentration, mood, grief, and age-related physical decline. While some individuals with severe or persistent symptoms may benefit from diagnosis and treatment, many others do not. In these cases, diagnosis may cause harm through labelling, unnecessary treatment, and psychosocial impact. Support for such individuals can often be provided through social, educational, or community-based interventions, but, in many places, this access to such help would require a formal medical diagnosis. A specific and controversial form of disease definition is *disease mongering*; promoting diseases in order to expand markets for medical treatments.

Disease mongering

Disease mongering refers to the practice of 'selling' diagnoses. In this context, normal conditions are transformed into medical problems due to the potential financial gain for pharmaceutical companies, leading to an overdefinition of what constitutes an illness. The conditions in question are often common discomforts or malaise that many people experience at various points in their lives. For example, many of us occasionally struggle with sleeping problems, feeling sad or depressed particularly in response to major life challenges and have difficulty focusing on our studies, work, or daily tasks. Disease mongering emerges when such everyday experiences are categorised as pathological, thus destabilising the understanding of what constitutes the basic conditions of human life. People who struggle with sleep, feel sad or upset, or have trouble concentrating on daily tasks may indeed be ill and in need of help. The same applies to conditions such as long-lasting mourning, where the sorrow becomes so overwhelming that it limits the bereaved in their daily functioning. Another example is the natural age-related decline in muscle mass, which can make it difficult for elderly people to manage everyday tasks, as they become dependent on assistance, something most older people would prefer to avoid. Of course, these individuals should be supported if effective interventions are available, such as bereavement support groups or exercise classes at a senior centre. However, from a medical point of view, access to such support does not have to be justified through a diagnosis, such as prolonged grief disorder or sarcopenia (Petersen et al., 2021; Haase et al., 2022). However, when the definition of symptoms is expanded by commercial interests and these symptoms are actively diagnosed and suggested, disease mongering results in overdiagnosis.

Disease mongering has primarily been associated with dubious conditions where there is an opportunity to sell medical treatments. A key strategy in marketing campaigns for medications involves overselling common life circumstances and life events as medical problems, for instance, 'low T' (low testosterone in older men), 'restless legs syndrome', 'overeating', 'dry eyes symptom', 'baldness', and 'social phobia' (social anxiety disorder). There are even more absurd cases of medicalisation, such as the pathologising of 'short eyelashes' and 'road rage disorder' (Moynihan et al., 2002).

It may be true that diagnosis and treatment can benefit people with very severe cases of some of these conditions. However, it is with great concern that researchers have pointed out how these 'diseases' are often invented by the pharmaceutical industry, which conveniently has a treatment ready for them. Disease mongering contributes to the overdiagnosis problem, particularly in societies with less restrictive health legislation. Those interested in exploring this issue further may find value in reading *Selling sickness* (Moynihan & Cassels, 2005) and also consulting the longstanding work of healthnewsreview.org, an American organisation that critically reviews advertising and news coverage of alleged medical conditions.

What overdiagnosis is NOT

Because there is no single, universally accepted definition of overdiagnosis, the concept is often conflated with related phenomena in both the literature and public debate. Terms such as misdiagnosis, false positives, overtreatment, and overuse are sometimes used interchangeably with overdiagnosis. While these phenomena may overlap in practice, they are analytically distinct. Clarifying these distinctions is necessary to understand overdiagnosis as a specific and independent problem.

Incidental findings

Overdiagnosis is not synonymous with incidental findings, although incidental findings may result in overdiagnosis. Incidental findings, also known as incidentalomas, are unexpected abnormalities that are identified during an examination, test, imaging, or other procedures performed for another purpose. A common example is a cyst or tumour on an adrenal gland detected through a CT scan of the lungs (the goal of the CT scan is to examine the lungs, but if the lower parts of the lungs are to be included in the scan images, the adrenal glands are also visualised). Many incidental findings will never cause symptoms or contribute to death. When such findings are labelled as disease and lead to follow-up, monitoring, or treatment without benefit to the individual, they constitute overdiagnosis (Doust & Glasziou, 2013). However, not all incidental findings are overdiagnosed. Some may be clinically relevant and require intervention.

False positives

Overdiagnosis should not be confused with false positive test results. A false positive occurs when a test suggests the presence of disease, but subsequent investigations show that no pathological condition exists. In contrast, overdiagnosis involves a diagnosis that fulfils the diagnostic criteria but is clinically unnecessary. False positives are common in screening programmes and in populations where the pre-test probability for disease is low, for example, in general practice. The critical period from when the screening participant receives the abnormal screening result to when further investigations confirm or dismiss the suspicion of cancer can vary from a few days to several months (Brodersen & Thorsen, 2008). During this time, screening participants having false positives may experience the same negative psychological and social consequences as people who have been (over)diagnosed with cancer (Brodersen & Siersma, 2013). In some cases, false positives may overlap with overdiagnosis or misdiagnosis. If a positive test result leads directly to a diagnosis without adequate confirmatory testing, individuals may be diagnosed with a condition they do not have. For example, among asymptomatic individuals undergoing rapid antigen testing for COVID-19, a substantial proportion of positive results may be false positives. If no confirmatory polymerase chain reaction (PCR) test is performed, these individuals may be overdiagnosed or misdiagnosed with infection (Schneider et al., 2022; Bell et al., 2023). Rarely, even the diagnostic work-up following a false positive result may itself be misleading. For example, there are cases where individuals have received a false positive mammogram screening result, and the subsequent needle biopsy (tissue sample) showed that they had breast cancer. But the breast cancer diagnosis could not be confirmed in the subsequent surgery where the person had a part, or all, of their breast removed. In this case, the person was not overdiagnosed, but they were overtested and overtreated.

Overtreatment

Overdiagnosis is not the same as overtreatment, although overdiagnosis often leads to overtreatment. Overtreatment occurs when interventions provide no benefit or cause more harm than good, regardless of whether the diagnosis is correct. Many cases of overtreatment are not preceded by overdiagnosis. *Acute otitis media* in children and *acute bronchitis* in adults are commonly and correctly diagnosed yet frequently treated with antibiotics despite strong evidence that antibiotics offer minimal to no benefit in these conditions (Venekamp et al., 2015; Smith et al., 2017). Such treatment exposes individuals to side-effects and contributes to antibiotic resistance at the societal level. Conversely, overdiagnosed individuals may avoid overtreatment, for example through active surveillance. However, they may still experience psycho-social harm and overuse through repeated follow-up examinations.

Overuse and overtesting

Overdiagnosis is also distinct from overuse and overtesting. Overuse refers broadly to unnecessary examinations, tests, treatments, etc. Overtesting refers specifically to the use of diagnostic tests such as blood tests, imaging, or screening (when people are asymptomatic) in situations where they are unlikely to improve outcomes. Overuse and overtesting does not inevitably lead to overdiagnosis, but it increases the likelihood that overdiagnosis will occur. Overtesting can occur in both symptomatic and asymptomatic individuals. For example, the frequency of PSA testing in general practice is strongly associated with the number of men diagnosed with prostate cancer: clinics that perform more PSA tests diagnose more men with prostate cancers, yet prostate cancer mortality remains unchanged (Mukai et al., 2010; Hjertholm et al., 2015). This pattern suggests that increased testing primarily identifies indolent conditions. Reducing overuse may therefore reduce overdiagnosis. Proposed strategies include removing low-value tests from electronic ordering systems, providing decision support at the point of care, and making the costs of tests visible to clinicians (Martins et al., 2017; Roedbro & Jervelund, 2025).

Misdiagnosis

Overdiagnosis and misdiagnosis are frequently confused, particularly in cancer care. A misdiagnosis is an incorrect diagnosis that can, in principle, be corrected with further information. Overdiagnosis is a correct diagnosis that later proves unnecessary because the condition never becomes clinically relevant. In cancer diagnostics, this distinction is difficult in practice. At the time of diagnosis, it is usually impossible to determine whether a detected cancer will progress or remain indolent. Pathological grading systems, such as the Gleason score in prostate cancer, estimate probabilities at the population level but cannot provide certainty for the individual. Most men with low Gleason scores will never experience symptoms, but a small minority will (Loeb et al., 2016). Research into biomarkers and predictive models aims to improve this distinction. There have been some, but not decisive, improvements. Hypothetically, a future prediction model might be able to deterministically distinguish between those who will get sick and/or die from cancer and those who will not. With such a prediction model, it will be possible to determine who is correctly diagnosed and who is misdiagnosed from an overdiagnosis.

Clinical variation

Clinical variation refers to differences in diagnostic practices, testing rates, or treatment patterns across regions, institutions, or clinicians. Such variation may reflect differences in population characteristics, access to services, or professional norms. Clinical variation can be mapped with *Health atlases*, which are maps, bar charts or other types of graphics that illustrate for example geographical variation, such as the spread of a population's health status across locations and institutions. Health atlases can stimulate fruitful discussions about appropriate care (DaSilva and Gray, 2016) but such data can also give rise to misleading interpretations and conclusions (Haase et al., 2024). Health atlases can also be used to illustrate clinical variation within a larger or smaller geographical area. This has for example been done in the US, Europe, Norway, and Denmark, where health atlases comparing the countries and variation within the countries show a great geographical variation in the prevalence and incidence of the ADHD (attention deficit hyperactivity disorder) diagnosis (Fulton et al., 2009; Madsen et al., 2015; Widding-Havneraas et al., 2023). One could generate hypotheses from such data about potential un-, under- and overdiagnosis in some of the countries or within certain geographical areas within one country (Zoega et al., 2011).

Figure 1.6 is an example from a Danish cluster of general practice clinics, showing large variation in how many PSA tests were taken in 2018. One clinic took zero PSA tests, and on the other end of the scale, another clinic took more than 250. However, when variation in diagnostic intensity is associated with increased detection of early

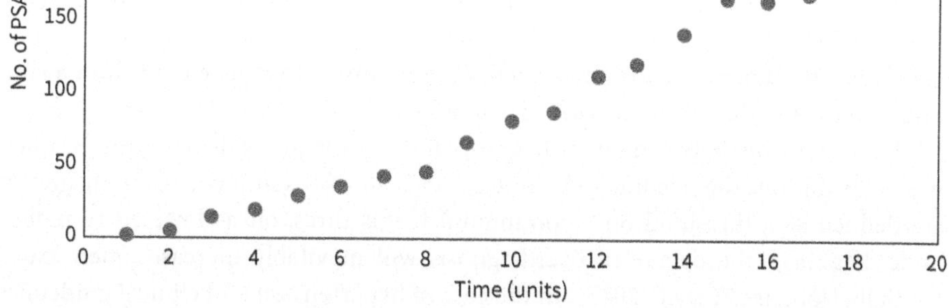

Figure 1.6 Number of prostate-specific antigen (PSA) tests prescribed via different general practice clinics in 2018. The clinics are from the same cluster (same local area). There is a strong upward trend across the measured observations.
Reproduced with permission from Samfundslitteratur.

or localised disease without corresponding reductions in morbidity or mortality, it may signal overdiagnosis. A study showed that with increased testing came higher rates of investigation, diagnosis, and treatment in high-testing practices without improved prognostic outcomes (Hjertholm et al., 2015). The participating clinics were divided into four groups based on their PSA test rates. Men in the highest-testing quartile of clinics were compared to men in the lowest quartile, showing increased risk of trans-rectal ultrasound, biopsy, getting a prostate cancer diagnosis, getting a localised diagnosis with no differences regarding advanced stages, having a prostatectomy and having radiotherapy. There were no differences in prostate cancer or overall mortality; however, the survival rate of prostate cancer increased. This study reveals strong signals of overdiagnosis and some of the potential harms related to the overinvestigation and overtreatment these men experienced (Hjertholm et al., 2015).

Yet, many factors can affect the distribution (Figure 1.6)—for instance, the number of doctors working in the clinic, and the age and gender distribution of patients. These factors, and the possible lack of other information, make it difficult to interpret the data and compare clinics, not least internationally. There is simply too much information missing to make such interpretations, and for data to be comparable it needs to be adjusted for other factors that may affect variation—this is often referred to as standardised data. Therefore, clinical variation alone cannot demonstrate overdiagnosis.

Undiagnosis and underdiagnosis

Overdiagnosis is not simply the opposite of undiagnosis. Undiagnosis refers to cases in which a condition is present but not detected, often because the person is not tested or due to test limitations, for example measurement error or false negative result (see also Chapter 3). In contrast, underdiagnosis refers to systematic failure to identify all disease at the population level and/or an aggressive disease biology. Underdiagnosis can be regarded as the opposite of overdiagnosis. An example might be a 65-year-old male being screened for AAA where the ultrasound examination shows a diameter of the aorta to be 29 mm. The current threshold for diagnosing an aneurysm is 30 mm. Ten years after taking part in the screening programme this male died from a ruptured aneurysm: the person was underdiagnosed.

The relationship between underdiagnosis and overdiagnosis depends on the diagnostic definition, the accuracy of the test, and who is examined. Some diagnoses are defined as a threshold on a continuum. If this threshold is lowered to reduce underdiagnosis, the degree of overdiagnosis will inevitably increase, often exponentially (Johansson et al., 2015). In the case of hypertension and clinical guidelines aforementioned, fewer people in the USA and Europe will be underdiagnosed if the thresholds are lowered for systolic and diastolic blood pressures; however, at the same time many more people will be overdiagnosed because of the distribution of cardiovascular events, which are much rarer for those being underdiagnosed compared to the numbers being overdiagnosed (Bell et al., 2017; Haase et al., 2019). Overdiagnosis, undiagnosis, and underdiagnosis should be understood as unintended adverse effects, with different mechanisms causing them. Addressing overdiagnosis does not mean neglecting undiagnosis and underdiagnosis. However, if thresholds are lowered and more screenings are done to mitigate underdiagnosis, it will inevitably lead to overdiagnosis, as shown.

Harms of overdiagnosis

Overdiagnosis offers no clinical benefit and entails harm. It is sometimes argued that individuals may feel relieved, reassured, or gain a better understanding of themselves through a diagnosis, even when the diagnosis is unnecessary. However, from a clinical and ethical perspective, turning people into patients without affecting their morbidity or mortality constitutes an iatrogenic effect of healthcare. It has also been argued that overdiagnosis leads to hermeneutical injustice (Nielsen, 2025). In the following chapters, we examine both the drivers and the harms of overdiagnosis in detail. Here, we provide a brief overview of the main ways in which overdiagnosis causes harm.

From a societal perspective, overdiagnosis leads to substantial waste of healthcare resources. Costs arise from unnecessary diagnostic tests, the overtreatment that often follows, and from the broader economic consequences of labelling healthy individuals as patients. These consequences include increased sick leave, loss of employment, reduced tax revenue, and early retirement. Taken together, these effects make overdiagnosis a substantial concern for healthcare systems and societies. Another consequence of overdiagnosis is the dilution of severe suffering. When large numbers of individuals with mild or transient symptoms are diagnosed, severe illness risks becoming normalised. This occurs at the expense of the smaller group of individuals whose symptoms are persistent, worsening, and potentially debilitating. In conditions such as insomnia, depression, and ADHD, individuals with severe symptoms are likely to benefit from diagnosis and treatment. By contrast, those with mild and fleeting symptoms such as occasional sleep problems, feeling sad or upset, or difficulties concentrating on everyday tasks are unlikely to benefit. In these cases, diagnosis and treatment may cause harm rather than help.

At the individual level, overdiagnosis is associated with a range of negative psychosocial consequences. Being diagnosed with a potentially life-threatening disease may lead to anxiety, sleep disturbances, feelings of dejection, depression, and behavioural changes (Brodersen et al., 2010b, 2018a, 2018b; Brodersen & Siersma, 2013; Friberg et al., 2021). For example, a study from Brazil showed that individuals diagnosed with mild hypertension experienced several adverse psychosocial effects (Gyuricza et al., 2019). It may be argued that such types of labelling effects or pathologisation are the price that individuals must pay to have their hypertension treated and thus reduce their risk of getting sick or dying from diseases triggered by high blood pressure. However, the medicalisation and label of high blood pressure may also lead to increased sick leave (Haynes et al., 1978), which can have major additional costs because an (over)diagnosis is accompanied by (over)treatment. Additionally, the labelling effect (Scheff, 1966) suggests that a diagnosis can influence or shape the self-identity and behaviour of those who are classified (or labelled) with that diagnosis.

Finally, overdiagnosis will inevitably lead to increased CO_2 emission and thus contribute to the global climate crisis (Barratt & McGain, 2021). A taxonomy of the unintended harm of too much medicine, including overdiagnosis, suggests that the harm should be investigated at four levels: Patient, Practitioner, Public and Planet, in eight different categories: Physical, Psychological, Social, Occupational, Financial burden, Opportunity costs, Inequity, Environmental (Gram et al., 2025).

2
Health culture

Health, it seems, has become a core value guiding our lives. Across the globe, media outlets regularly publish articles and features offering advice on maintaining personal health. Renowned platforms such as the BBC, *The Guardian* or *The Sydney Morning Herald* include sections dedicated to health, providing readers with tips on staying healthy during different times of the year. Researchers, politicians, and stakeholders consistently emphasise the importance of a healthy population and outline the steps needed to achieve it. Many countries monitor their populations' mental and physical health, as a means to improve public well-being, prevent disease, and ensure the efficient allocation of healthcare resources. At the same time, private clinics as well as self-proclaimed experts promote a variety of products and services to purchase in the name of health.

Indeed, the focus on health in every aspect of our lives is growing. As early as in the 1980s, political economist Robert Crawford highlighted how health had risen to the status of a meta-value, becoming an overarching concern that shapes the daily experience of individuals. Crawford coined this phenomenon 'healthism', describing it as an ideology that prioritises a lifestyle where health and physical activity are valued above all else, relying heavily on the individual's motivation to achieve optimal well-being. Engaging in healthism often involves abstaining from indulgent, lazy, or 'bad' personal habits (Crawford, 1980, p. 368). This, in turn, cultivates what sociologist Deborah Lupton describes as the 'rational, reflective self'; a self that is constantly monitoring, measuring, and evaluating its own health (Lupton, 1997; see Chapter 5).

Healthism goes hand in hand with an increased political emphasis on individual responsibility and freedom (Kristensen, 2016, p. 84), affected by, but also adding to, a desire to live well and long, and to present oneself as healthy. Combined with this political focus on individuals' responsibility for themselves, a notion that good population health benefits the societal economy can be traced in public discourses as well as in policies. A report made by consulting firm McKinsey states that 'the economic benefits from the health improvements … add 8 percent to global GDP in 2040, that translates into 0.4 percent faster growth every year. These benefits arise through … fewer early deaths, fewer health conditions' (Remes et al., 2020).

But healthism and its underlying ideology can become a socially divisive force. By placing the burden of health on individual responsibility, this ideology creates polarisation: some people successfully conform to the self-discipline and norms promoted by healthism, while others cannot, or choose not to, leading to their exclusion from certain social circles (Kristensen et al., 2016). Put simply, some individuals manage to maintain healthy lifestyles through, for example, exercise and diet, while others do not. What might otherwise be viewed as a personal choice becomes a visible marker of social distinction. Picture a fit runner, who, on the tracks of the park, passes by a smoking obese person—seeming to display 'good' and 'bad' health behaviour; this stereotypical and judgemental example unfortunately captures the underlying societal divide and understanding that health is a matter of personal choice, while overlooking the fundamental conditions and structures that form human life and health. This becomes particularly problematic when different types of behaviours are moralised. People who smoke or are obese, despite society's awareness campaigns about the health risks of these factors, are contrasted with people who follow dietary advice and exercise; they become the 'irresponsible' versus the 'responsible'. However, it is overly simplistic to understand smoking and obesity as the consequences of individual choices. Health behaviours, such as smoking, are linked to culture, upbringing, education, living conditions, and various other factors; and the threshold between normal weight and obesity is more about aesthetics than being at risk of becoming sick (see also Chapter 3). Nevertheless, an individual's health behaviour is increasingly seen as a target for political intervention.

In the context of overdiagnosis, healthism becomes a key concept for understanding how distinctions drawn between 'responsible' and 'irresponsible' health behaviours drive demands for more and more tests and examinations. The underlying moral logics foster a sense of obligation to actively manage one's health, often motivating individuals to pursue preventive measures such as check-ups and annual blood tests even in the absence of symptoms. Healthism operates on a societal level, shaped by culture, governmentality, and biopower, and on an individual level, influenced by an uncritical trust in biomedicine, a growing alienation from death, and on moral ideas about health behaviour. These dynamics fuel medicalisation, defensive medicine, and increasing demands from patients, all of which contribute to the problem of overdiagnosis.

Health culture and healthism

In all human societies, beliefs and practices surrounding illness are a central aspect of culture. Culture, however, is defined in different ways, and varies and evolves within societal and historical contexts. In this chapter, we focus principally on the contextual and relational aspects of culture, as something that both limits and enriches human expression. As human beings, we are inherently social: even if a person lives in solitude, they exist in a world that is already populated. Growing up, we learn to perceive the world within a particular framework of understanding from our parents and other people, and this web of meanings can be called 'culture' (Hastrup, 2004a, p. 14).

Health culture refers to how people think about and understand the causes of their health problems, as well as how they believe they should behave to prevent illness. Perceptions of what is healthy vary among different cultures, and the way we handle illness and risk of disease depends, among other things, on political discourses, historical developments, media, and individual perceptions. Therefore, it serves no purpose to define health in the context of discussing overdiagnosis. Instead, we use 'health' as an umbrella term that encompasses different understandings and practices that become the subject of political interventions aimed at improving quality of life and well-being for individuals and the population, based on the understanding that it serves a common good (Wahlberg & Rose, 2015).

While health cultures are often deeply embedded in local contexts shaped by specific understandings and responses to illness, there are also many shared patterns deriving from healthism across societies that follow a biomedical model of healthcare. For instance, while alcohol consumption among the adult population varies greatly between cultures, it is generally believed that large amounts of alcohol are harmful. However, within health cultures there are also subcultures: for example, communities who wrongly believe that vaccines cause autism and therefore refrain from having them or their children vaccinated. In this book, we continually refer to a general health culture that applies to populations in The Global North with easy access to biomedical healthcare including technologies and medications because studies show that the greater the access to healthcare, the greater is the risk of overdiagnosis (Welch & Fischer, 2017). This does not mean that all people in the Global North share the same health culture, but rather that a dominant discourse of healthism can be identified—one that shapes how individuals perceive health and risk as being managed, navigated, and contested. Many of these cultural traces are also likely to be found in other places, including in underserved populations where additional challenges may be more prominent: lack of healthcare services, war, poverty, and humanitarian catastrophes.

Health culture can be viewed from a macro perspective, at the societal level, as a phenomenon shaped by specific historical and cultural contexts. For instance, notions of what comprises a balanced healthy diet change over time and exist in various versions in different countries. Another example is bloodletting, once common in the Middle Ages, but no longer practised in healthcare (except in rare cases, such as polycythaemia vera and haematomachrosis, but that's a different story). Health systems, political structures, and the organisation of healthcare services likewise play a role in shaping health culture. For example, there is a difference in the access individuals have to treatment and care in a country with privatised healthcare services compared to one with publicly funded healthcare.

Health cultures can also be examined on a micro level, at the individual level, focusing on people's perceptions of what constitutes health and illness, or, more relevant here, on how people believe they should act to stay or become healthy. Over the past century, psychology, psychiatry, and psychoanalysis have substantially shaped our understanding of the self. Theories and models emerging from these disciplines provide frameworks for explaining human behaviour and continue to influence how individuals are encouraged to optimise their mental health, well-being, and overall quality of life (Brinkmann, 2014; Madsen, 2015, p. 4–8). At the core of this perspective is the belief that individuals must be proactive. Here, we see sedimented beliefs that 'more is better' and in the benefits of screening healthy people to detect potential diseases at an earlier state (Pathirana et al., 2017). Likewise, there appears to be a widespread lack of awareness among the general population about the limitations and potential harms of medical interventions. This often leads to an overreliance on technologies, such as diagnostic tests, as a source of reassurance about their health status. These ideas permeate health cultures—for example, in popular self-help literature—and are now also traceable in the expectations on individuals to optimise their physical and mental health (Brinkmann, 2014).

Understanding health cultures within their broader social and political contexts is crucial to uncovering the forces that shape how health is defined and pursued and how these forces contribute to overdiagnosis. A central driver lies in the cultural emphasis on personal responsibility for health, reinforced by growing expectations for tests and medical examinations as the assumed path to well-being. These dynamics are not incidental but closely aligned with broader shifts toward neoliberal forms of governance, where individuals are expected to self-manage risk, optimise their bodies, and continuously monitor their health.

Neoliberal governmentality and biopower

Two key aspects of modern societal organisation—biopower and neoliberal governmentality—shape how we approach health maintenance and reinforce the belief that more health intervention is always better. Biopower was first introduced by the French epistemologist and intellectual historian Michel Foucault, who is one of the most influential thinkers in the social sciences, and his ideas and theories have been fundamental in critically examining the understanding of healthcare systems. Biopower refers to the way modern states exert control over populations by regulating bodies and managing life processes such as health, reproduction, and longevity through institutions, norms, and medical knowledge. In his lecture series *The birth of biopolitics* from 1978 to 1979, Foucault demonstrates that neoliberalism is more than an ideology; it is also used as a technology of governance and management. One of Foucault's arguments is that social power has shifted from commands to recommendations (Foucault, 2009 [1979]). In feudal society, power was visible. It was the king or emperor who sovereignly dictated what was acceptable and what would result in punishment. If one had committed something forbidden they would receive a penalty. In the late modern state, however, power is 'invisible' because it is impersonal and omnipresent, existing both in written legislation and in discourses about 'right' and 'wrong' actions. Furthermore, late modernity disrupts the binary system of governance: individuals can now be more or less close to breaking the law, so in principle, everything and everyone can be improved. Power in the modern and late modern state has thus become a matter of optimising the state through the disciplining of citizens.

Foucault conceptualises power as an overarching force that shapes and influences individuals, making certain actions more difficult while facilitating others, ultimately guiding people to act within the moral frameworks deemed acceptable in society (Foucault, 1982). Through these power dynamics, various techniques emerge that seek to control populations by encouraging self-discipline of the body. This process, which Foucault refers to as governmentality and self-technology, reveals the dual nature of biopower: on one side, it is the state's control over its citizens, codified through law; on the other, it is the power that individuals exert over themselves and others. Biopower is predicated on the belief that the state's power serves the best interests of its citizens, providing protection for individual lives. Importantly, biopower operates not through coercion or direct mandates, but through subtle influence. It is important to note here that those governed by biopower must have the opportunity to resist, as power only functions when citizens govern themselves to a certain degree of freedom (Vallgårda, 2005). Governmentality, in turn, becomes a tool for governance, with individuals policing and managing their own behaviour, often without full awareness through implicit power, such as disciplinary measures (Foucault, 1982, 1991).

In this context, neoliberal governmentality differs from classical liberalism. Classical liberalism partly has its roots in the economic and philosophical theories of Adam Smith, which describe how classical liberalism ensures that the market is free from external intervention under headings such as laissez-faire, that is, without any form of interference (Wyatt-Walter, 1996, p. 5). Neoliberal governmentality, instead, takes the market model and generalises it to all spheres of society as a management strategy:

> Applied to health policy, this means that any form of behaviour, both that of the patient's demand for specific health services and the doctor's choice of treatment method, can be guided through the manipulation of economic incentives (Larsen, 2015, p. 18, our translation).

Set in a health culture dominated by healthism and neoliberal notions of individual responsibility, a person's health appears independent of economic, social, and institutional structures in society, disregarding the fact that societal structures often contribute to health inequalities (Navarro, 2009). The neoliberal state therefore promotes the idea that the individual alone can create change, and health becomes a matter of taking personal responsibility for oneself (Bauman, 1999).

However, neoliberal governmentality is not without its potential benefits. Some argue that it can empower individuals and encourage greater participation, especially through technologies that allow for self-monitoring, thereby giving people more control over their health (Petrakaki et al., 2018). In this sense, the concept of individual responsibility is framed more positively, focusing on self-determination and shared decision-making. But neoliberalism is also criticised for shifting the burden away from the healthcare system. This shift is problematic because reducing medical problems to individual challenges fails to take account of the larger political picture and societal structures that may be causing the challenges.

Biocitizenship

The subtle and often unseen pressure for individuals to adopt 'healthy' behaviours has been described by several researchers as biocitizenship (Rose & Novas, 2004; Halse, 2009). Biocitizenship refers to the ways in which individuals act within a society governed by biopower and biomedical understandings of illness. The sociologists Nikolas Rose and Carlos Novas, who introduced the concept, explain how the notion of being a citizen, i.e. one who belongs to a community, is intricately linked to our biological existence (Rose & Novas, 2004). They describe how biocitizenship is formed in a reciprocal relationship: medical and legal authorities impose expectations on individuals, while individuals, in turn, create moral expectations for themselves through a desire to live healthy lives. As Foucault would put it, these are 'self-technologies within biopower', yet they appear as if they originate from the individuals themselves, rather than being imposed upon them. Rose and Novas explain that individuals internalise these notions of responsible behaviour, making them feel routine and expected. They also argue that this gives rise to new forms of problematic citizens: those who fail to meet the expectations of a responsible biocitizen (Rose & Novas, 2004, p. 451). Biocitizenship can also manifest in diagnostic identities, where diagnoses serve as the foundation for social mobilisation, including support groups and patient associations that advocate for rights, access to services, and research dedicated to specific conditions (Rose & Novas, 2004). In societies with a strong health culture, biocitizenship becomes a compelling force, where individuals are not only expected to take responsibility for their own health but also to do so as a societal obligation, rather than simply for personal benefit.

Alongside biopower and biocitizenship (Box 2.1), the concept of 'biosociality' is also essential when analysing health culture. Sociality, in this context, refers to ways

Box 2.1 Definitions (simplified for clarity)

Biopower: Foucault's term for the dominance of biomedical systems, which underpins the state's implicit power and control over the human body.

Biocitizen: The concept of health expectations and obligations becoming an integral part of an individual's identity as a citizen in society.

Biosociality: The integration of biomedically defined categories into the social lives of individuals, shaping social interactions and relationships.

of being together and engaging in communities (Simmel & Hughes, 1949). The term 'biosociality' was introduced in 1996 by American anthropologist Paul Rabinow. He used it to describe how biology, uncovered and controlled by science, becomes the basis for social interactions. In the mid-1990s, when the human genome was still being mapped and expectations were high for the potential of genomic knowledge, Rabinow predicted that genetic testing would lead to new classifications of individuals, thereby creating new social groupings. This form of sociality, shaped by biological knowledge, is what Rabinow refers to as 'biosociality' (Rabinow, 1996). However, the biomedical discourses surrounding physical and mental illnesses that underpin health cultures are rarely applied in their original form. Instead, new categories of biosociality are redefined and adapted to align with existing identities. For instance, membership in a patient organisation for endometriosis may provide information about the condition, treatment options, support for diagnosis, patient advocacy, and opportunities to connect with other women who share the experience of endometriosis (a painful condition where the uterine lining grows outside the uterus). These connections help combat the sense of isolation. Nevertheless such membership rarely becomes a defining feature of a woman's identity, as there are competing and multiple identities in most peoples' self-perception: being a relative, a partner, one's professional identity, or membership in a social club and so on. It is the individual's broader life that remains the central concern, not an identity grounded in illness (Ørtenblad et al., 2018; Sand et al., 2021).

As highlighted by American anthropologist Rayna Rapp, biosociality should be understood as an interaction between biomedicine and the individual's life. The concept of 'biosociality' captures how biomedical science, embedded in society, is applied and transformed into various forms of social human life (Rapp, 1998).

Biopower, biocitizenship, and biosociality as concepts illustrate how biomedical ideas shape not only healthcare systems and state governance but also social relations and individual identities (see Box 2.2). Health is not just a personal matter but is deeply embedded in cultural expectations, moral obligations, and political structures. Illness can become both a social identity and a means of accessing resources, revealing how health and disease are negotiated within broader societal frameworks. In this perspective, health behaviour is never neutral but shaped by power, values, and social belonging. In the following section, we turn to how these broader forces are internalised and expressed in the everyday cultural norms that influence individual health behaviour.

Good health as good citizenship: avoiding the stigma of illness

Oscar was an elderly man whom Alexandra had followed for a couple of years during her fieldwork. He had recently lost his wife and was finding it difficult to adjust to life alone. Suddenly, he had to learn how to cook, manage appointments, and keep up a

Box 2.2 Case: Biocitizenship and the risk of overdiagnosis

A form of biocitizenship can be seen in situations where illness becomes a means of negotiating citizenship and claiming rights, thereby exposing deeper power structures and social inequalities. Anthropologist Adriana Petryna illustrates this through the Chernobyl nuclear disaster and Ukraine's post-Soviet transition. She shows how the lack of scientific certainty about the long-term effects of radiation exposure, combined with political instability, gave rise to new forms of biological uncertainty. In the early 2000s, amid Ukraine's economic crisis and widespread poverty, Petryna argues that biological damage from radiation was one of the few recognised pathways to receive state financial assistance. As a result, many sought to be classified as sick due to Chernobyl-related injuries. Illness thus became economically instrumental at the individual level, leading Petryna to coin the term 'biological citizenship' (Petryna, 2004). In this context, it is plausible that many individuals were overdiagnosed with radiation-related conditions precisely because such diagnoses were their only route to financial support.

social life. Newly diagnosed with type 2 diabetes, he offered coffee and cake, a classic Danish gesture when welcoming guests, and quietly admitted that he probably had only himself to blame for getting sick. He didn't eat well enough, he said, and didn't exercise as much as he should have. Whether or not Oscar could have prevented his illness is impossible to know, but what is clear is that he believed he was at fault. His story reflects how deeply ingrained ideas of personal responsibility and healthism can become; acting both as a moral compass and as a hopeful belief that illness can be avoided, if only one tries hard enough.

Conditions such as type 2 diabetes can be experienced as stigmatising, especially because it is associated with obesity, which in turn is considered self-inflicted. The term *stigma* originates from Greek, meaning 'mark' or 'brand'. One of the most influential analyses of stigmatisation comes from Canadian sociologist Erving Goffman, who explored the social mechanisms involved in labelling individuals as deviant. A key insight in Goffman's work is that stigma does not arise solely from a specific condition such as an illness or disability but from how that condition is managed in social interactions (Goffman, 1963). He identifies three primary sources of stigmatisation:

1. **Physical deformities** or bodily differences, such as visible disabilities.
2. **Character blemishes**, including mental illness, addiction, or criminality.
3. **Tribal stigmas**, referring to group identities such as ethnicity, religion, or nationality.

Stigmatisation arises when a person with one or more of these deviations becomes visibly marked in social settings, attracting negative attention that overshadows their other traits. Goffman emphasises that individuals often describe their experience of stigma through the reactions of those around them such as visible discomfort, overly cautious interactions, averted gazes, or forced friendliness, and exaggerated sociability (Goffman, 1963). In this way, stigma undermines the individual's social identity, positioning them as discredited in the eyes of others and rendering them outsiders in a rejecting world.

Not all diseases carry the same connotations of guilt or moral judgment (Lupton, 1994, p. 89). For instance, common infectious illnesses such as colds or norovirus infections are generally not associated with personal blame. In contrast, other conditions are heavily stigmatised and often interpreted as the result of personal failure. So-called 'lifestyle diseases' imply that the patient's choices such as poor diet, lack of exercise, or substance use have directly or indirectly caused their illness. This is particularly evident with diseases such as lung cancer or chronic obstructive pulmonary disease (COPD), which are frequently linked to smoking. Patients with these diagnoses are often subject to moral judgement for having neglected what is perceived as a civic duty to maintain their health and are often met with prejudices of suffering the consequences of self-inflicted harm (Marlow et al., 2010).

Stigmatisation can even occur within the healthcare system itself. For example, studies show that general practitioners may hold both implicit and explicit biases against obese patients (Bøker et al., 2018). Negative reactions such as blame, fear, and disgust have been documented in both healthcare professionals and the public towards individuals living with human immune deficiency virus (HIV), hepatitis C, or COPD (Lupton, 1994). These responses reflect broader societal attitudes in which patients who presumably do not follow medical advice or fail to adhere to treatment guidelines are subject to moral scrutiny, calling into question their management of the body (Kirmayer, 1988).

Health morality may also be evident in prenatal screenings; in one study, pregnant women were asked why they chose to accept a foetal anomaly scan:

> If you're offered it, and it's paid for by the public ... then you think that it's something you should say yes to. Although they try to present it as a choice, the mechanisms are different. When the healthcare system chooses to offer it, it does influence you. (Birgitte in Lou et al., 2007, p. 916, our translation)

Although Birgitte acknowledges that the decision influences her, she does not critically reflect on her own role in making it. Instead, she states that it is simply 'something you should say yes to', revealing an implicit sense of what is considered the right thing to do. Similar logics are visible in healthcare systems driven by insurance markets and out-of-pocket payment, where the *availability* of medical technologies itself produces a sense of obligation. Whether mediated by public provision, insurance coverage, or private payment, the mere existence of diagnostic options carries normative force. In this example, screening uptakes are not simply individual acts of interpretation or consumption, rather they are moral responses to systems that increasingly equate responsible citizenship with anticipatory medical action. As Charles Taylor (1989) argues, morality and identity are deeply connected; our sense of what is right is tightly bound to how we understand ourselves as individuals. Being 'as healthy as possible' becomes a socially observable behaviour, where morally correct choices are met with recognition and respect. This helps explain why many people readily follow public health recommendations especially when authorities use persuasive strategies in their communication, such as encouraging participation in screening programmes (Rahbek et al., 2021). The key point to highlight is that participation in, for example, screening programmes cannot be understood as independent individual choices. On the contrary, strong cultural and social expectations shape and influence people's decisions. As Nikolas Rose puts it: '[M]odern individuals are not merely "free to choose", but are obliged to be free, to understand and enact their lives in terms of choice' (Rose, 2007, p. 87).

Fearing death

However, it is not only moral considerations that influence people's health behaviours. Research suggests that healthism and health culture can also increase uncertainty, worry, and anxiety about not being healthy enough. On a societal level, this contributes to major healthcare spending on unnecessary tests, examinations, and referrals, all driven by the pursuit of health (Greenhalgh & Wessely, 2004) and the illusion of achieving zero risk (Fugelli, 2006). The fear of illness and death is a powerful motivator for seeking medical examinations and participating in screenings, and this fear itself becomes a key driver of overdiagnosis (see Chapter 8 for more on these driving forces). Paradoxically, one can be overdiagnosed precisely because of the fear of not getting sick. In an anthropological study exploring how patients and general practitioners interpret symptoms, Johnny, a man who previously worked with chemicals, explained that he constantly wonders whether he might be developing cancer:

> So, I try to go for regular check-ups. Not long ago, I had my 50,000 km service, where they took some blood tests and an X-ray of my lungs. And everything was as it should be . . . so now I feel much better, you know, I feel healthier because everything was normal, and you know, today is not the day I have to say goodbye to family and friends. There is still time. (Johnny in Kristensen et al., 2022, p. 7)

As Johnny's story illustrates, death is both something we fear and something we try to manage. Before the rise of modern medicine—and especially epidemiology—death was often seen as the result of misfortune, accidents, or other unpredictable forces. But in the late nineteenth century, with the systematic collection of data on mortality, it became possible to calculate life expectancy based on living conditions, age, and gender. Death was translated into numbers, embedded in tables, and analysed through mathematical laws rendering it seemingly rational and predictable. Even today, epidemiology and statistics shape our sense of what counts as a 'normal' or 'average' lifespan (Prior & Bloor, 1993). When death is no longer viewed as entirely random, it becomes something we believe we can control or delay. Ironically, this shift has contributed to a growing fear of death: once accepted as a natural part of life, it is now seen as something to be postponed, fought, or even, in some cases, avoided altogether.

Our everyday lives are shaped by a distance to death while constantly being aware of the threat it poses. Illness often precedes death, and therefore, preventing illness becomes a way of preventing death. In his book *Mortality, immortality, and other life strategies* (1992), the renowned Polish sociologist Zygmunt Bauman argues that, in postmodern society, mortality has been broken down into specific causes of death. Bauman asserts that all cultures are built on the recognition of death's inevitability, though cultures also strive for something permanent and lasting that life itself cannot offer. Death thus becomes a problem that forces humans to create meaning in the face of life's undeniable end. This creates a paradox in postmodern thought: on one hand, humans are constantly in search of meaning, yet on the other, they stubbornly attempt to forget the absolute certainty of mortality (Bauman, 1992, p. 8). According to Bauman, this paradox transforms death into a persistent trauma in late modernity. We are unable to truly imagine non-existence, and so the very thought of our own absence scares us. Bauman draws on philosopher Edmund Husserl's concept of intentionality, which suggests that all thought and action must be directed towards something. But Bauman contends that because death is an unknown form of non-existence, we cannot fully conceptualise it (Lund, 2020). As a result, the ultimate human goal becomes living a life that feels meaningful, purposeful, and free of thoughts about death (Bauman, 1992, p. 7). Yet, despite our attempts to avoid thinking about death, it remains a presence in our lives. Family, friends, and loved ones die, reminding us that death is inevitable. In response, we begin to deconstruct aspects of life to better cope with the awareness of mortality. Death thus becomes something we can conceptualise. We no longer simply die; we die from something: a diagnosis that can be identified and perhaps treated. This shift leads us back to a neoliberal framework of individual responsibility, where death is reframed as a curable condition. In doing so, death is transformed from being a distant, unavoidable deadline to becoming a daily, looming threat that we continuously try to manage (Bauman, 1992, p. 140).

As biomedical treatments have developed, our understanding of death and illness has shifted, with illness increasingly being seen as an individual responsibility. In the nineteenth century, treatment often revolved around the bedridden patient who would present their symptoms, and the provider was chosen based on personal qualities and trust. Over time, however, medical treatment became more institutionalised, and the healthcare provider's role became formalised, with specific qualifications and authority (Jewson, 1976). This shift marked the transformation of the sick person into a 'patient', and, with advancements in medical treatments, diseases that were once fatal or debilitating began to be managed as chronic conditions, their symptoms controlled through ongoing medical intervention, including surgery.

However, being healthy has evolved into something more complex. It is no longer just the absence of illness; rather, health is often replaced by the idea of 'being well' as a more aspirational and dynamic concept. Being well is now seen as something that can be cultivated and optimised through various means, including self-care, exercise, medications, screenings, prevention strategies, and more. Pharmacological treatments, in particular, are often viewed as the ideal way to address medical issues efficiently and with minimal disruption, focusing on symptom relief and a return to function (Steffen, 2005, p. 184). The appeal of pharmacological treatment lies in its individual accessibility. As Dutch anthropologist Sjak van der Geest points out, these treatments allow individuals to act independently, without requiring healthcare professionals or family support, empowering them to manage their own health autonomously (van der Geest et al., 1996, p. 154 ff.). This growing reliance on individual responsibility and medical intervention reflects how deeply the medicalisation of health has shaped our modern understanding of what it means to be healthy. The American anthropologist Joseph Dumit argues that in the past, health was associated with not having to take medication, not having to attend numerous consultations at the hospital or with the general practitioner, and not having to worry about one's body. However, today, according to Dumit, health has become the complete opposite. Health is now conceived based on facts derived from clinical trials designed by the pharmaceutical industry to increase medication intake rather than decrease it. Health is no longer solely a matter of an individual's sense of well-being. Staying healthy now means investing major amounts of time, energy, and money into various preventive treatments, including pharmacological prevention (Dumit, 2012). This not only includes disease prevention but also the prevention of risk factors. Risk can be interpreted as (future) illness and can, therefore, be treated (medically) (Dumit, 2012, p. 114). Classic examples are risk factors for cardiovascular diseases, such as high blood pressure, high cholesterol, obesity, fatty diet, lack of exercise, etc. Knowledge of a risk can create unnecessary worry and anxiety in itself, but the uncertainty lies primarily in the fact that risk cannot always be sensed bodily. Some conditions defined as risk, such as obesity and mild to moderate high blood pressure, can be observed just as what we eat can be observed. However, most of the time, risk cannot be felt as a symptom; it must be measured and assessed. This means that, to optimise health, a series of tests and examinations must be conducted so that not only diseases but also risks of diseases can be exposed, and preventive treatment can be initiated based on that. It is difficult to convince a health-conscious citizen that treatments can be ineffective, unnecessary, or even harmful, despite history showing us that health science can be wrong. In the late 1950s and early 1960s, pregnant women were offered the drug thalidomide for nausea, but it turned out that the drug caused foetal damage and deformities, including short arms and legs. It was one of the biggest and most notorious scandals in the history of pharmaceuticals. Nevertheless, we are interested in being examined and treated, not least to take responsibility for ourselves and do what we can to stay healthy. At the same time, it is not only risk conditions for future illness that individuals are expected to prevent by staying healthy. Prevention is increasingly being defined based on salvatory promises of modifying risk factors that individuals are born with or have been exposed to in their lives so far (ranging from harmful substances to the genes we are all born with). There are preventive treatments, for example, that claim to preserve bone mass (which naturally weakens with age) or administer artificial hormones so that individuals can stay young (Lock & Nguyen, 2018 [2010], p. 50). In other words, health has become a question of preventing what was previously inevitable (for a more detailed discussion, see Bakken, 2020). And with the increasing range of opportunities for prevention and treatment, individuals today live with the belief that with enough effort, they can become healthier and avoid diseases. Although it may be an ideal that few can live up to, it leaves a deep mark on our approach to life and illness. For the healthy individual, being or becoming sick is not a life condition but a curse to be avoided at all costs.

Demanding health

'I will not be silent until this procedure has become standard' invoked a mother in the wake of her 22-year-old son's death from a ruptured aorta the hospital failed to detect. In a heartfelt Facebook post, she pledged to fight for electrocardiograms (ECGs) to be mandatory for all patients presenting with chest pain, as she narrated her son's tragic journey of being sent home and told to rest, having his symptoms dismissed as anxiety. 'An ECG that takes less than one minute—ONE MINUTE—could have saved his life' the grieving mother concluded. This happened in Denmark, usually praised for its free and universal healthcare. Here, patients cannot request procedures directly, rather tests like ECGs require a doctor's recommendation, and so the tragedy became a symbol of inadequate care or professional incompetence. The post struck a chord, drawing widespread sympathy and condolences, but also sparked harmful comments directed at the health services in general for underserving and lacking proactive screening, and one commenter suggested launching a citizens' petition to push for ECGs to become standard procedure.

This story is one of many circulating on social media, covered by the press, or depicted in personal narratives, all sharing a common theme: healthcare services have done too little, and therefore, the call is to demand more. The death of a 22-year-old is always tragic and mostly unexpected. Or at least, it is from an able-bodied and privileged point of view that permeates much of the Global North, free from war and hunger, and with available health services and medications. In this context, death as an inevitable part of life seems acceptable only under certain conditions. We have come to expect life to extend well beyond 22 years, and when it does not, the loss is perceived as unjust, a theft of experiences and opportunities. But this story reveals more than just the expectation of longevity and the privilege it implies. The belief that an ECG could have detected the ruptured aneurysm does not align with medical evidence as other methods are required to diagnose such conditions (Shiga et al., 2006), yet that is not the point. What emerges instead is a broader assumption shared by the grieving mother, the commenters, and likely many of us that when practised 'correctly', medical science can identify and treat all diseases, ensuring that long life is not just possible but expected. It is mirrored in stakeholder campaigns, such as patient organisations pleading for earlier detection, which, as described more fully in Chapter 4, is a notion that does not reflect the evidence, yet prevails because it seems so logical and appealing:

> Without a screening program, and often no symptoms in the early stages, detecting prostate cancer early requires proactive action. Currently, men can request a free PSA blood test from their GP, but GPs are recommended not to raise the issue of PSA testing with men unless they have symptoms. This is a crucial moment for the new government to stick to its commitment to earlier prostate cancer diagnosis and to saving men's lives. (*Prostate Cancer UK, campaign: Faster. Fairer. Better.* (PCUK, 2024)

The various personal narratives, popular beliefs, and campaigns reinforce the notion of healthcare as a fundamental right. As the grieving mother on Facebook embarks on a personal crusade to advocate for what she believes could save future lives, her efforts highlight a growing sense of individual responsibility in the expectation that we must actively demand health and the interventions that promise to protect it. Yet this attitude towards the healthcare system is not without its problems. In fact, the increasing pressure from patients and their relatives for more tests and screening of people without symptoms is part of the reason overdiagnosis occurs (Pathirana et al., 2017). If we were to screen all men for prostate cancer and have ECGs on all people presenting with chest pain, we would, despite the curative aim, be finding enormous amounts of conditions that would never have developed or needed treatment. Advocating for more and earlier detection may not consider this balance between benefits and harms, as most lay people are unaware of the harms such as overdiagnosis, overtreatment, and overuse of healthcare services. It is not a straightforward discussion (see Chapter 4), and deeming where the cut-off should be in the benefit/harm balance is beyond the scope of this book.

Defensive medicine

From the other side of the table, the fear of illness and death can also be observed in the practices and decisions of healthcare professionals. Regarding this, Tina Erikson, a Danish practising physician, writes:

> A very common issue is patients who want to be evaluated for various types of food allergies and intolerances . . . And then we have cases of fatigue in younger, healthy individuals without any other illness. How many blood tests should we perform on

them to conclude that they are not suffering from any vitamin deficiencies? (Tina Eriksson, cited in Jessen, 2021)

In many healthcare systems, healthcare professionals face a growing demand from patients for examinations, alongside an increasing juridification of healthcare where the risk of complaints and legal action over diagnostic or treatment decisions has become more pronounced. One consequence is the rise of what is known as defensive medicine, where healthcare professionals order additional tests or procedures not primarily for the patient's benefit, but to protect themselves from potential complaints or litigation (Hermer & Brody, 2010). Defensive medicine is characterised by a healthcare professional performing actions that go against professional judgement but are carried out due to demands and pressure, for example, from patients (Andersen et al., 2019). One study showed that doctors engage in defensive actions in 10–15% of all consultations. These actions can range from extensive medical records and less comprehensive tests such as the C-reactive protein (CRP) test (a simple blood test used to measure possible infection or inflammation in the body) to more resource-intensive referrals and investigations, such as magnetic resonance imaging and computed tomography (Jessen, 2021).

In some healthcare systems, such as in the United States, where medical malpractice lawsuits are relatively common, defensive medicine may manifest as hedging behaviours; proactive actions taken to pre-empt potential blame or as avoidance behaviours, where clinicians avoid certain patients or clinical areas that are perceived as legally or reputationally high-risk (Ries & Jansen, 2021). Fear of legal liability is widely acknowledged as a key driver of low-value care, where clinicians initiate tests, referrals, or treatments not because they are clinically indicated, but as a means of reducing the perceived risk of litigation or complaints. These actions, often described as part of defensive medical practice, typically offer little clinical benefit. Instead, they are carried out 'just in case' they might serve to protect the clinician in future legal or professional disputes. In this way, defensiveness becomes one of the driving forces behind the overutilisation of healthcare services (Brownlee et al., 2017), which can also lead to overdiagnosis (Berra et al., 2014; Berlin, 2017; Kainberger, 2017).

Medicalisation

A final consequence stemming from the health culture described is the increasing medicalisation of everyday life, in which cultural norms influence definitions of diseases. Medicalisation refers to the process by which human experiences, behaviours, or life circumstances become defined and treated as medical problems, often under the authority of biomedicine (Conrad, 1975, 2007; Conrad et al., 1992). Originally introduced by sociologists such as Irving Zola (1975) and Ivan Illich (1976), the concept emerged as a critique of the growing reach of medicine into areas previously regarded as non-medical. These early critics underscored the paradox that in societies where people are living longer and healthier lives, the influence of the medical profession has nonetheless expanded, often to the detriment of individual autonomy and social responsibility.

Conrad and Schneider (1992) proposed a three-part typology of medicalisation: (1) the medicalisation of non-medical conditions such as childbirth, ageing, or grief; (2) the use of medical technologies and treatments to manage ordinary human states or risk factors; and (3) the creation of institutional frameworks that require medical diagnoses for access to social or legal services. This framework highlights how medicalisation is not limited to clinical practice but is embedded in broader institutional and cultural logics.

In recent decades, medicalisation has been extended to conditions like shyness (Moynihan et al., 2002), natural ageing processes (Estes & Binney, 1989; Jønsson, 2024; Kaufman et al., 2004), and muscle loss in older adults, now redefined as 'sarcopenia' (Haase et al., 2022). Such redefinitions often reflect an underlying shift in values: common human variations are reframed as pathologies, prompting medical interventions that may or may not be beneficial. Anthropologists have emphasised that medicalisation is not merely a neutral or scientific process, but a form of biopower (Lock, 2001; Lock & Nguyen, 2018). Moreover, medicalisation shifts the locus of responsibility for health from structural and political domains to the individual (Crawford, 2006; Jønsson et al., 2020; Jønsson & Spalletta, 2023), reinforcing neoliberal ideals of responsibility and risk mitigation.

Overdiagnosis, while related, is conceptually distinct. Unlike medicalisation, which deals with the expansion of the medical gaze into social and cultural domains, overdiagnosis is a harmful outcome of medical procedures. Despite these distinctions, medicalisation and overdiagnosis, in the form of overdefinition, are increasingly entangled. Both concepts reflect an expansion of the boundaries of disease, but they do so in different ways. Medicalisation operates primarily through sociocultural processes of definition and legitimisation, often in non-biomedical domains. Overdiagnosis, by contrast, is a technical and prognostic phenomenon, arising from efforts to identify disease earlier and more broadly, often before symptoms occur. Medicalisation is concerned with sickness, the social role and experience of being unwell, whereas overdiagnosis is concerned with disease, particularly the silent or latent form detected through screening or imaging.

Yet, medicalisation often serves as a cultural and institutional precondition for overdiagnosis. For example, the diagnosis of sarcopenia based on normative muscle mass thresholds relies on a medicalised framing of ageing that defines natural physiological changes as pathological. Additionally, in the age of P4 medicine (predictive, preventive, personalised, and participatory) medicalisation becomes all-encompassing. As these concepts converge, their critical precision may be lost, risking what could be argued to be a total 'iatrogenisation' of health. What was once a critical vocabulary to assess medical excess now risks becoming diluted, even as the harms associated with overdiagnosis such as anxiety, stigma, and unnecessary interventions persist and proliferate.

Finally, it is not only within the healthcare system that conditions are medicalised. There are also subgroups that share the interpretation of bodily and mental reactions and deviations as diseases, even if the diagnosis is not recognised by the official healthcare system. Often, these subgroups disagree with the healthcare system's diagnoses and treatment options. One of the reasons for the existence of overdiagnosis is precisely the paradox that health culture and its subgroups increasingly make individuals responsible for their own lives and health, while at the same time, in a logic of medicalisation, stripping away their responsibility by translating them to challenges to be solved by the biomedical healthcare services.

Self-diagnosis and the influence of social media

Personal statements of disease and diagnostic trajectories increasingly unfold on social media, in podcasts, through online screening tools, therapeutic encounters outside biomedicine, and intimate conversations with friends, partners, or colleagues. It is within these dispersed sites that *self-diagnosis* takes shape. Self-diagnosis is not merely an individual's private suspicion of illness, but a socially organised practice of identifying oneself as having a specific medical or psychiatric condition prior to, alongside, or even in defiance of formal clinical recognition. Self-diagnosis is thus neither accidental nor purely subjective; it is produced through circulating diagnostic narratives, moral economies of suffering, and shared interpretive frameworks that render particular experiences intelligible as symptoms (Jønsson, 2025). Self-diagnosis, particularly in mental health and psychiatry, intervenes *upstream* of medicine because long before a diagnosis is formally conferred (if ever), the diagnosis may already be lived, rehearsed, defended, and moralised.

Alexandra's ethnographic work with adults who identify as having attention deficit hyperactivity disorder (ADHD) without meeting clinical diagnostic criteria show that self-diagnosis is not a marginal phenomenon, but rather is a central mechanism through which diagnostic categories expand their reach into everyday life. People in this study do not passively await medical judgement; they actively interpret their lives through diagnostic lenses, often with remarkable certainty. 'I know I have ADHD', despite repeated rejections by general practitioners or psychiatrists (Jønsson, 2025). This certainty is not irrational but based on recognition of what is being described often in popular media by influencers and celebrities as symptoms of ADHD. It does not mean that a self-diagnosis is simply 'wrong'; claiming a diagnosis has a force that lies precisely in the fact that it *works*. It provides meaning, recognition, and often a sense of moral legitimacy. Several interlocutors described the diagnosis they sought not as deviance-making but as *norm-making*: ADHD, for them, explained why they were not failing but merely different. This resonates with the argument that psychiatric diagnoses function as semiotic mediators simultaneously explanatory, exculpatory, and identity-affirming (Brinkmann, 2014). In a diagnostic culture where being 'normal' increasingly implies productivity, emotional regulation, and continuous self-improvement, self-diagnosis can appear as a rational strategy for survival.

On the contrary, a diagnosis that one claims without medical confirmation may be grounded in what Ian Hacking famously described as the *looping effects* of human kinds: diagnostic categories create ways of being a person, which in turn reshape the category itself (Hacking, 1995). When people recognise themselves in diagnostic descriptions and especially those framed as late-discovered, underdiagnosed, or historically neglected they do more than apply a label. They reorganise biography, re-interpret past failures, and anticipate future relief. Self-diagnosis thus operates as a narrative technology, offering coherence where life has felt fragmented. Yet it is precisely here that the relationship between self-diagnosis and overdiagnosis becomes analytically productive. In Alexandra's study, self-diagnosis of late-onset ADHD frequently rests on what Gregory Bateson would call an *epistemological error*: a mistaken way of knowing the relationship between person and environment (Bateson, 1972). Many interlocutors treated ADHD as a stable, internal trait—something one *is* rather than as a situated description of behaviour that becomes problematic only in certain social arrangements. Exhaustion, distraction, emotional volatility, or difficulty completing tasks were interpreted as evidence of an underlying disorder rather than as responses to divorce, grief, parenthood, precarious labour, or impossible standards of self-optimisation. In this sense, self-diagnosis exemplifies how diagnostic categories can come to stand in for social critique, translating structural strain into individual pathology.

At the same time, self-diagnosis contributes to what Bateson described as *runaway processes*: self-reinforcing feedback loops in which small shifts in perception generate increasingly expansive consequences (Bateson, 1972). As diagnostic narratives circulate through celebrity disclosures, online communities, and commercial screening tools, thresholds for recognition subtly lower. Mild or situational difficulties become legible as symptoms; symptoms demand diagnostic confirmation; diagnostic confirmation retroactively validates the symptoms. In this loop, the pool of normality contracts, and the risk of overdiagnosis grows not because clinicians are careless, but because the cultural ground on which diagnosis rests has already shifted.

Importantly, self-diagnosis also destabilises the assumed opposition between underdiagnosis and overdiagnosis. In public discourse, these are often framed as opposite errors requiring opposite solutions: more awareness versus more restraint. Empirically, however, they coexist. Individuals who self-diagnose frequently experience themselves as *underdiagnosed*—unseen, dismissed, or misunderstood by professionals while simultaneously being at risk of overdiagnosis should diagnostic criteria expand or a more permissive clinician be found. Self-diagnosis thus occupies a liminal diagnostic space: neither fully inside nor outside medicine, but actively shaping what medicine is asked to recognise.

Self-diagnosis reflects a world in which human problems are increasingly expected to have biomedical names, and in which not having a diagnosis can feel like a failure of explanation rather than a sign of health. Overdiagnosis, then, is not merely the accumulation of unnecessary labels, but the gradual normalisation of diagnostic thinking itself.

How cultural norms lead to overdiagnosis

As demonstrated throughout this chapter, overdiagnosis cannot be understood merely as a medical issue isolated from its broader social and cultural context. Rather, it emerges from and is shaped by the dynamic interplay between individuals and the societies in which they live. At the same time, it is crucial to recognise that overdiagnosis is not an issue confined to the Global North (Brodersen, 2017b). While in high-income countries overdiagnosis is often driven by the widespread availability of general health screenings and preventive examinations (see Chapters 4 and 8), similar patterns are increasingly observed in low- and middle-income countries due to the growing diffusion of medical technologies (Albarqouni et al., 2022). A striking example of this trend is the global surge in thyroid cancer diagnoses, particularly among middle-aged women. Epidemiological data suggest that the majority of these cases are attributable to overdiagnosis. In countries such as South Korea and Thailand, estimates suggest that up to 90% of diagnosed cases may fall into this category (Vaccarella et al., 2016; Li et al., 2020). This underscores the need for multifaceted explanatory frameworks to understand the persistence and expansion of overdiagnosis worldwide.

In some instances, overdiagnosis may even serve the immediate interests of patients. First, a diagnosis can provide access to tangible resources such as financial support, psychological care, or accommodations within healthcare and social systems. But beyond institutional benefits, diagnoses may also open pathways to empathy, understanding, and care from one's social network. Crucially, most patients are unaware that their diagnosis might be unnecessary; instead, they often experience the diagnosis as lifesaving or transformative. As a result, many express profound gratitude for what they perceive as early or timely medical intervention. To be told, retrospectively, that a diagnosis may not have been necessary is not only epistemically destabilising, it can carry major social consequences. Such revelations risk alienating individuals from their sense of biocitizenship, the identity and legitimacy they derive from being a medical subject (Davies, 2024). In contrast, it has been argued that overdiagnosis within somatic and psychiatric conditions may lead to hermeneutic injustice (Nielsen, 2025). In this light, overdiagnosis is not simply a clinical misstep but a deeply social event with consequences that reverberate through individual lives and collective systems of meaning.

While neoliberal health culture is not the sole driver of overdiagnosis, it is equally true that the phenomenon cannot be fully accounted for without reference to broader societal and humanistic dimensions. Objectively speaking, health systems could realise substantial cost savings by scaling back or discontinuing many screening programmes (see also Chapter 4). Yet such proposals are often met with moral resistance: What is the value of money when measured against a human life? Overdiagnosis research invites a reframing of this moral calculus by posing a difficult but necessary counter-question: How many lives must be harmed in order to avoid one patient dying from the condition screened for? It is at this ethical juncture that the human dimension becomes inescapable. Thus, overdiagnosis must also be situated within a cultural context where the pursuit of the healthy body and the fear of mortality are deeply ingrained, yet seldom subjected to critical scrutiny.

3 Diagnostics

Sick, healthy, or in between?

Susan got osteopenia

On a dark winter afternoon, Susan slips on the pavement while carrying her shopping home. She falls awkwardly and feels an immediate, sharp pain in her wrist. A passer-by helps her gather her belongings and urges her to go to the emergency department. Susan cannot lift her arm without pain, and a few hours later she is examined at the hospital. An X-ray reveals a fracture. Susan is 55 and has recently gone through menopause. Because women in this age group may have an increased risk of osteoporosis, the fracture prompts further investigation. Her bone density is measured as a proxy for bone strength. Susan describes herself as a responsible and sensible person and finds it important to know whether she is sick or healthy. But the test result does not give her a clear answer. Her bone density is lower than what is defined as normal, but not low enough to meet the criteria for osteoporosis. Instead, she is diagnosed with osteopenia, a condition often described as a precursor to osteoporosis.

Susan is told that she does not need medical treatment for the osteopenia because her risk of future fractures is considered only slightly elevated compared to people with normal bone density. She is advised to continue her everyday activities, maintain a healthy lifestyle, ensure sufficient intake of calcium and vitamin D, limit tobacco and alcohol use, and stay physically active. If she ever requires long-term corticosteroid treatment, she should return for reassessment.

Now, contrary to the doctor's intention, Susan becomes worried. Because if it really isn't a disease, then why are all these measures so particularly important? Susan cycles regularly and enjoys long walks at her summer house. She also enjoys cake. At home, she begins to doubt whether her diet is sufficiently healthy. She buys calcium supplements with vitamin D. She starts avoiding cycling in the dark or on slippery roads. She hesitates about a planned hiking trip on the Camino de Santiago with a friend. When she reads online that the route is recommended only for people who are healthy, she cancels the trip. She does not feel ill, but she no longer feels well either.

We met 'Susan' during a research project on ageing. A retired nurse, she had signed up to participate in an interview to help raise awareness of osteoporosis and osteopenia. As described in the Chapter 2, taking responsibility for one's health is often understood not only as rational, but also as a moral obligation, and Susan is doing exactly that. Yet living in contemporary health cultures adds an extra layer of complexity when the fine line between sick and healthy is blurred, and, in biomedical terms, one is neither but occupies a position in between. Understanding overdiagnosis therefore requires an introduction to diagnostics as a guiding tool of the medical profession, to the uncertainties inherent in diagnostic practices, and to what being sick, healthy, or somewhere in between means for the individual.

Sick and healthy as a false dichotomy

In a less medicalised world, it may not ring true to speak of sickness and health as binary opposites, because the body is experienced as changeable, interpretive, and embedded in everyday life rather than as a stable biomedical object. As anthropologist Arthur Kleinman suggests, people instead distinguish between disease and illness. Disease, he contends, is what the doctor treats, whereas illness is the personal experience embedded in everyday life with disease. The illness experience is what matters to people (Kleinman, 2006). But in today's world of salvatory visions, the diagnosis of a disease or condition is a powerful classificatory act. As sociologist Annemarie Jutel has shown, diagnoses do not merely describe biological states; they organise uncertainty, legitimise suffering, and determine access to treatment, care, and social recognition (Jutel, 2009). A diagnosis translates lived experience into a medical category that can be acted upon, but in doing so it also fixes boundaries between normality and pathology. In contemporary health cultures, diagnoses therefore function not only as clinical tools, but also as social instruments that shape identities, expectations, and life trajectories.

And so, even though clinical practice, epidemiology, and lived experience consistently challenge the distinction between sick and healthy, diagnostics is what we turn to in the quest to classify whether we are healthy or not—sometimes based on symptoms, at other times as part of systematic or opportunistic testing. Yet whether present or absent, symptoms are rarely experienced as stable or self-evident. Anthropological and sociological research has shown that symptoms are often ambiguous, fluctuating, and interpreted through social context, personal biography, and cultural expectations rather than perceived as clear signs of disease (Zola, 1975). What counts as a symptom, and whether it is taken seriously, develops over time through processes of interpretation, negotiation, and comparison with others. Uncertainty is therefore not an exception in the experience of symptoms, but a defining feature.

What is often overlooked outside medicine is that the detection of disease is marked by a similar uncertainty. No examination can guarantee that a person is completely healthy. One of the main ways somatic diseases are identified is through laboratory testing and imaging. But what does a test result actually tell us? How much trust can we place in it? And how do probabilistic test results interact with people's desire for certainty? It is to this diagnostic logic that we now turn.

The binary logic of diagnoses

When, then, are you sick? And when are you well? These questions appear deceptively simple, yet they resist clear answers. Historically, they have been answered in very different ways, depending on how bodies, disease, and uncertainty have been understood at a given time.

The idea that sickness and health are mutually exclusive states is neither self-evident nor timeless. Rather, it is the product of specific medical, cultural, and historical developments. In much of Western medical history, illness was not understood as a discrete entity located within the body, but as a disturbance of balance between bodily fluids, between the individual and their environment, or between human beings and divine forces. In such frameworks, being sick or well was less a matter of classification than of interpretation.

A well-known illustration of the modern unease with these distinctions appears in Jules Romains' satirical play *Doctor Knock*, or *The Triumph of Medicine* (1923). Here, the fictional Dr Knock declares that 'healthy people are simply sick people who do not yet know it.' The joke resonates with many health professionals because it captures a lingering anxiety at the heart of modern medicine: if one looks closely enough, something abnormal can almost always be found. The body, examined with sufficient scrutiny, rarely appears entirely normal. For lay people, however, the purpose of medical examination is often precisely to confirm health rather than to uncover disease. People seek reassurance, not probabilities. They want to know whether they are sick or well. But modern diagnostics rarely offers such certainty. Instead, it produces gradations, risk categories, borderline states, and findings of unclear significance.

Normality as a diagnostic category

From a sociological perspective, a diagnosis can be understood as a cultural expression of what a given society is prepared to accept as *normal* and what it considers to require treatment (Jutel, 2009). The concept of normality is therefore central to diagnostic practice. Yet *normal* is neither a neutral nor a timeless category. It is often used interchangeably with *healthy*, even though the two are not identical.

Historically, the term *normal* did not originate in medicine at all. Until the nineteenth century, it was used primarily in mathematics and physics to describe regularity and standardisation. It was only with the emergence of modern anatomy that the relationship between normal and abnormal acquired biological meaning (Hacking, 1990). As bodies were dissected and compared, differences between organs and tissues became visible. These variations were interpreted as either distinct diseases or different stages of the same disease and could be linked retrospectively to the symptoms patients had reported while alive. In this way, anatomy contributed to the creation of a standardised body against which illness could be measured (Foucault, 2003 [1963]). This development played a crucial role in establishing a binary diagnostic logic. If the body could be standardised, deviations from this standard could be identified, classified, and named. Diagnosis thus became a means of sorting bodies into categories: normal or abnormal, healthy or sick. Over time, this logic came to underpin modern biomedical practice.

Today, *normal* is widely used as the statistically common and clinically acceptable state. Yet, as philosopher Ian Hacking has argued, normality has also become something to aspire to rather than merely a descriptive category (Hacking, 1990). In a broader sense, normality has come to signify the ordinary and therefore something that can be optimised or improved (Lock & Nguyen, 2010 [2018], p. 41). This shift subtly transforms diagnosis from a tool for identifying disease into a mechanism for regulating variation.

The statistical foundations of this logic are particularly evident in epidemiology and biostatistics. Here, the normal distribution is used to describe variation within a population. Conventionally, the central 95 percent of values are defined as normal, while the 2.5 percent at each end are classified as abnormally low or high. These statistical cut-offs are frequently used to establish diagnostic thresholds. Such thresholds are practical and often necessary. Yet they also illustrate how a binary distinction is imposed on phenomena that are inherently continuous. When continuous variation is translated into categorical diagnoses, individuals are divided into those who fall inside and outside defined boundaries, even when the difference between them may be marginal.

Diagnosis across historical time

This tension reflects a deeper historical shift in how disease has been understood. Before the Enlightenment, bodily suffering was frequently interpreted through religious and moral frameworks, where disease was inseparable from questions of fate, meaning, and divine intervention (Daston & Park, 1998; Lock & Nguyen, 2010). With the Enlightenment, the body increasingly came to be understood as governed by natural laws, open to systematic observation and explanation. This was the beginning of a systematic, scientific approach that formed the basis of biomedical medicine. Later, the ravages of various epidemics gave rise to a numerical approach to disease, such as counting the number of sick people. When the British physician John Snow systematically mapped cholera deaths during the London outbreaks of 1849 and 1854, he demonstrated that disease patterns could be traced, measured, and explained without reference to moral or supernatural causes. Society at the time learned that the cholera infection came from the water supply and not the air, and, with this insight, standardised statistical epidemiology was founded. Disease became a population-level phenomenon, and diagnosis a tool not only for individual care but for public health governance.

Advances in microscopy, bacteriology, and pathology made it possible to link patients' symptoms to identifiable pathological conditions in tissues, organs, and bodily fluids. Disease increasingly came to be understood as something visible, localisable, and classifiable. Diagnosis moved from the autopsy table to the bedside. It is during this period that the diagnostic logic familiar today took shape. A diagnosis was expected to rest on coherence between the patient's medical history (anamnesis), the clinician's findings on examination, and observable pathological changes identified through laboratory tests or imaging. Diagnosis thus became a present-time act, aimed at identifying disease in the living patient who experienced suffering. In this setting, the binary distinction between sick and healthy gained practical and institutional importance: it determined whether treatment could be offered and legitimised.

As diagnostic practices developed, the distinction between sick and well hardened into a binary that was both practically useful and administratively necessary. Diagnoses came to function as gateways: to treatment, to exemption from work, to insurance, and to social recognition. Yet the binary never fully captured lived experience. Many people felt ill without being diagnosable, while others received diagnoses without feeling ill. It is within this tension that contemporary diagnostics operates. While the language of sickness and health suggests clarity, diagnostic practice increasingly reveals uncertainty. People are told they are 'at risk' or have a condition that can be considered a pre-disease. They are neither clearly sick nor unequivocally well. Instead, they occupy intermediate positions that challenge the very categories meant to organise them.

From a timeline perspective, diagnoses in the traditional period (see Chapter 1) were understood retrospectively, by examining deceased patients, whereas diagnoses in the modern period are made in the here-and-now through the examination of living patients (see Chapter 1) who present with symptoms and suffering (Figure 3.1).

Diagnosing the future

The past half-century has seen a further shift in diagnostic temporality. Medicine increasingly turned its attention to the future. Early detection, screening, risk factors, and pre-disease states became central concerns. Disease was no longer only something one had, but something one might develop. Diagnosis expanded to include probabilities and predictions. In this period, diagnostic categories multiplied, thresholds were lowered, and new classifications emerged that blurred the line between sickness and health. Seen through Shorter's (1985) historical lens, the persistence of binary diagnostic thinking is understandable (see Chapter 1). It is rooted in a period when disease was conceptualised as a visible, present condition requiring treatment. Yet contemporary diagnostic practices operate in a very different epistemic landscape characterised by uncertainty, probability, and continuous variation. The result is a growing tension between binary categories and lived bodily experience.

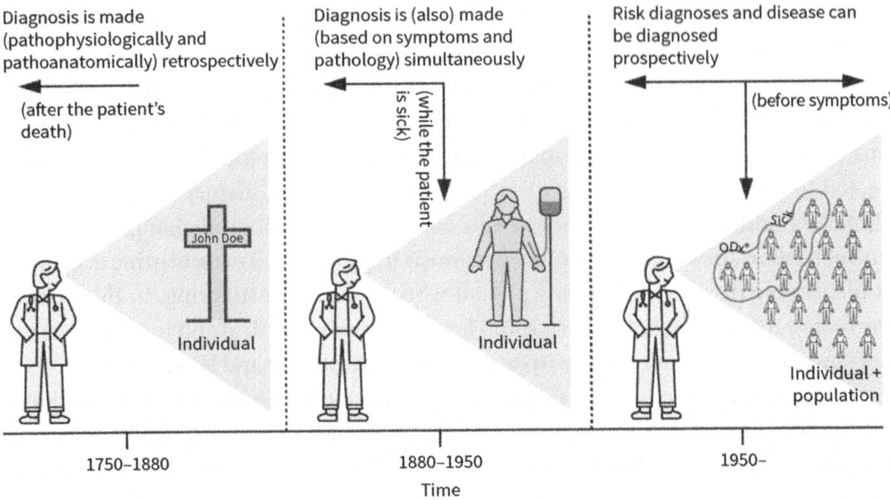

Figure 3.1 Diagnoses understood backwards, here-and-now and into the future in relation to Edward Shorter's three time periods: the *traditional*, *modern* and *postmodern* time periods. Predicting disease in the future will inherently include probabilities, diagnosing some who will be sick in the future but also overdiagnose others.
Reproduced with permission from Samfundslitteratur.

Thus, temporality today becomes a point of attack, where early detection, risk factors, and diagnostics are all about time: the future. Understanding diagnosis is no longer a backwards-looking (as in the traditional period, see Chapter 1) or a here-and-now (as in the modern period, see Chapter 1) picture, but an understanding of possible future illness and disease. This creates space for prevention, which is a core task in healthcare today. The diagnosis, or the possibility of a future diagnosis, becomes a management tool where the individual is expected to take responsibility and change behaviour to avoid a diagnosis or worsening of a diagnosis (see Chapter 2).

Postmodern healthcare has also introduced concepts of *pre-diagnoses* and *at-risk diagnoses* (Reventlow et al., 2006). Pre-diagnosis means that a diagnosis is made that relates to the possibility of another diagnosis in the future (e.g. pre-diabetes possibly turning into type 2 diabetes). At-risk diagnosis is a diagnosis where the 'disease' itself is not noticeable or symptomatic. The at-risk diagnosis expresses an increased risk of another disease or condition, for example, osteoporosis, which increases the risk of fractures due to a lower density of bone tissue. Without taking a position on the justification of issuing pre- and at-risk diagnoses, it is important to note that both diagnoses will necessarily turn more people into patients at an early time in life. For example, if you are diagnosed with pre-diabetes and get type 2 diabetes five years later, you have had five more years as a patient because of the pre-diagnosis.

Consider cardiovascular disease as an example. Measuring risk factors for possible future cardiovascular disease can be done with the variables: blood pressure, body mass index (BMI = [weight in kg]/[height in metres]^2), cholesterol levels, dietary intake, tobacco consumption, alcohol consumption, habits of physical activity (the last four often called modifiable lifestyle risk factors), education level, and income. These are all variables that are measured on a continuum. As time has now turned to the future, this is all about trying to predict what will happen to not-yet-diseased people in perhaps five, 10, or more years. Therefore, the binary understanding of disease and diagnosis is dissolved, because the aforementioned risk factors are all measured as variables along a continuum. The question to be answered then becomes: How well or poorly does a given threshold of risk factors predict future disease? Notably, this threshold is itself defined along a continuous scale.

Based on population studies where randomly selected citizens without cardiovascular disease have been followed over several years, researchers have combined two or more risk factors for cardiovascular disease with the belief that the measure will increase diagnostic test accuracy for future diseases. On the contrary, research shows that the more risk factors that are included in risk calculations, the more citizens are labelled as being at risk, that is people with elevated risk factors, in this specific example with increased risk of cardiovascular disease (Getz et al., 2004; Petursson et al., 2009).

The problem became particularly evident in a study of one of the longest-living populations in Western Europe: Nord-Tröndelag Fylke, an area north of Trondheim in Norway. Here, more than 95% of the population would have at least one elevated risk factor for cardiovascular disease—a kind of inverse normal distribution—defined by the European Society of Cardiology's guideline from 2007, where the thresholds for elevated risk were defined as: blood pressure ≥140/90 mmHg, cholesterol >8 mmol/L, and BMI ≥25 kg/m^2 (Petursson et al., 2009). Despite this, the Norwegians live longer than most other Western Europeans, which can be used to argue that so-called modifiable lifestyle risk factors are poor predictors of future disease and death (see also Chapter 1). This might be the reason why systematic population-level screening programmes do not reduce the burden of cardiovascular diseases (Jørgensen et al., 2024). And even ageing is dangerous: the older you get the higher the risk of death. Even if this was thought of as an ironic remark to make the reader smile, ageing has increasingly become the subject of prevention. Across contemporary healthcare systems, bodily and cognitive changes that once belonged to the ordinary passage of time are now routinely framed as deviations requiring medical attention. From reduced bone density (Box 3.1) and muscle loss to mild cognitive changes or fluctuating blood pressure, ageing bodies are increasingly rendered legible through biomedical categories that promise early detection, prevention, and control. While such interventions are often motivated by care, they also expand the terrain of overdiagnosis by transforming natural, non-pathological aspects of ageing into conditions to be monitored, labelled, and treated. This is when risk of overdiagnosis occur. Within this moral economy, accepting diagnostic interventions appears not merely optional, but ethically correct. If a test is offered, many feel it

Box 3.1 Case: Osteoporosis and the prediction of possible disease

Bone density measurement provides another illustration of future-oriented diagnosis. Bone density peaks around age 25 years and is used as a reference for normality. A deviation of 2.5 standard deviations below this reference defines osteoporosis.

Because bone density decreases with age, and more so in women, many older women will meet this criterion by definition. The logic behind this is that the lower the bone density of any individual, the higher is the risk of a fracture in the future. However, on average, the bone density of an 80-year-old woman has decreased by exactly the standard deviation of minus 2.5 so that her deviation from the 25-year-old woman's normal value results in a diagnosis of osteoporosis. It should be emphasised that not all women aged >80 years will experience a fracture in their remaining lifetime. Women diagnosed with osteoporosis who never fracture are therefore overdiagnosed.

Bone density between 1.0 and 2.5 standard deviations below the reference is labelled osteopenia, often described as a pre-disease of osteoporosis. Osteopenia thus becomes a risk factor for a risk factor.

ought to be accepted. Refusal risks being read as irresponsibility (Jønsson, 2024). To speak of the overdiagnosis of ageing, then, is not to deny illness, suffering, or the need for care in later life. It is to question when medical intervention meaningfully supports ageing well, and when it merely extends biomedical surveillance into domains of life that might otherwise remain untroubled. Ageing is universal, irreversible, and unevenly experienced. Treating it as a condition to be endlessly optimised risks narrowing the space of what counts as a good, liveable, and dignified old age.

Diagnostics of somatic diseases

One of the basic premises of modern medicine is that the human body will always contain pathological abnormalities or biological conditions that *can* be interpreted as disease or as precursors to disease. This does not mean that all such abnormalities will ever cause symptoms, morbidity, or death. Yet their mere presence creates the conditions under which diagnosis becomes possible.

Somatic diagnoses are made by clinicians based on existing medical knowledge and clinical judgement. Depending on the situation, they rest on interpretations of biological findings, bodily signs, and reported symptoms in a particular patient. Central to this process is the patient's *anamnesis*, or medical history. The anamnesis is not simply a collection of facts, but a narrative shaped by the patient's experiences, interpretations, and concerns. It provides the context in which clinical findings acquire meaning.

The diagnostic process typically begins either when a healthcare professional initiates an examination or when a person experiences a bodily change or symptom that prompts them to seek care. Pedersen and colleagues describe the latter as *diagnostic triage*: a process in which patients, or, in the case of children, parents, interpret signs and behaviours in interaction with their surroundings and decide whether medical attention is warranted (Pedersen et al., 2020). This often leads to a back-and-forth process in clinical encounters, where assessments by the clinician and the patient mutually shape the diagnostic trajectory. When diagnosis is uncertain, a range of social, clinical, and organisational factors may influence how the process unfolds and where it ultimately ends.

From the clinician's perspective, diagnosis is a specialised language and a form of practical knowledge that is integral to medical training and professional identity. Diagnosis is part of medicine's craft: a way of thinking, classifying, and acting in the face of uncertainty. Clinicians are well aware that definitive diagnoses are often unattainable and that any diagnosis represents a provisional interpretation rather than an objective truth (Saxtrup & Petersen, 2018). Nevertheless, making diagnoses remains a core competence of biomedicine, and the interpretation of symptoms and findings is central to clinical work.

In most cases, the diagnostic process begins with the patient presenting a complaint or symptom. The clinician conducts a medical interview, followed by a physical and/or mental examination when relevant. This may be supplemented by *paraclinical examinations*; an umbrella term covering blood tests, imaging, and other diagnostic tests. In situations of uncertainty, a tentative diagnosis may be formulated to guide further investigation or follow-up.

Despite the centrality of tests in contemporary medicine, paraclinical examinations are never perfectly accurate. Any diagnostic test may yield *false positive* or *false negative* results. A false positive indicates disease in someone who is not ill, while a false negative fails to detect disease in someone who is. These limitations became widely recognised during the COVID-19 pandemic, when rapid antigen tests were understood to be less reliable than PCR tests. A positive rapid test result often required confirmation, as it could reflect a false positive rather than true infection.

This raises a fundamental question: how do clinicians know how reliable a test result is? The answer lies in the *Bayesian diagnostic paradigm*. Bayesian reasoning provides a set of principles and calculations that allow clinicians to estimate the probability that a test result reflects true disease, given the characteristics of the test and the likelihood that the patient has the condition in question before testing. In other words, test accuracy cannot be assessed in isolation. It depends on both the technical properties of the test and the clinical context in which it is used.

The Bayesian diagnostic paradigm

To understand how diagnostic tests work in practice, it is necessary to distinguish between several related but often confused concepts. The most familiar are *sensitivity* and *specificity*, which describe the technical performance of a test under ideal conditions. Sensitivity refers to the proportion of people with a disease who receive a positive test result. A highly sensitive test correctly identifies most individuals who are ill. Specificity, by contrast, refers to the proportion of people without the disease who receive a negative test result. A highly specific test correctly reassures most individuals who are healthy. These measures are properties of the test itself. They are usually established under controlled conditions and reported in clinical guidelines and scientific publications. Yet sensitivity and specificity alone do not tell clinicians what they most often want to know: *Given this test result, how likely is it that my patient actually has the disease?* To answer that question, two additional concepts are required: *positive predictive value* (PPV) and *negative predictive value* (NPV). The PPV expresses the probability that a person truly has the disease given a positive test result. The NPV expresses the probability that a person is truly disease-free given a negative result. Crucially, both depend not only on the test's sensitivity and specificity, but also on how common the disease is in the population being tested.

The *Bayesian diagnostic paradigm* provides a systematic way of calculating how reliable or unreliable a specific diagnostic test is. In clinical terms, this is referred to as diagnostic test accuracy. At the core of the Bayesian diagnostic paradigm is a simple 2 × 2 table (Figure 3.2).

The table compares the outcome of a diagnostic test with a *reference standard*; a benchmark against which the test result is evaluated. A reference standard represents the best available method for determining whether a person has a given condition. For example, in the case of type 2 diabetes, a long-term blood glucose (HbA1c) value of ≥6.5 percent is commonly used as the reference standard indicating disease, while values below this threshold indicate absence of disease. The term reference standard has replaced the older term *gold standard*, reflecting a growing recognition that certainty is rarely absolute in medicine. Diagnostic accuracy always depends on which reference standard is chosen, and different standards may yield different results.

The sensitivity and specificity of a diagnostic test can be calculated in the Bayesian diagnostic paradigm using simple formulas:

- Sensitivity = $a/(a + c)$, the proportion of people with the disease who are correctly identified by the test.
- Specificity = $d/(b + d)$, the proportion of people without the disease who are correctly identified as disease-free.

In this context, being 'sick' is defined solely by what the test is designed to detect. For example, when measuring HbA1c to diagnose type 2 diabetes, sensitivity refers to the proportion of individuals with type 2 diabetes who receive a true positive test result. Specificity refers to the proportion of individuals without type 2 diabetes who receive a true negative result.

In theory, ruling out all disease with absolute certainty would require a diagnostic test with 100 per cent sensitivity. In practice, such a test would almost inevitably have

		Binary division of a population into stick and healthy compared to a reference standard*		
		Stick	**Non-Stick**	
Diagnostic test	Positive Test	True positive answer (a)	False positive answer (b)	a + b
	Negative Test	False negative answer (c)	True negative answer (d)	c + d
		a + c	b + d	N = a + b + c + d

Figure 3.2 Bayesian diagnostic paradigm.
Outcomes of a diagnostic test compared with a reference standard. Results are divided into sick and non-sick individuals and positive or negative test results, producing four categories: true positive, false positive, false negative, and true negative, with totals calculated for each group.
*A reference standard is the benchmark against which a diagnostic test is evaluated and compared. It serves as the best available method for determining the true disease status of an individual. For example, a reference standard for type 2 diabetes may be an HbA1c blood test result of ≥ 6.5%. If the HbA1c value is 6.5% or higher, the individual is considered to have type 2 diabetes according to the reference standard. Conversely, if the HbA1c value is below 6.5%, the individual is considered not to have type 2 diabetes. Historically, the reference standard was often referred to as the gold standard. However, because the true disease status is rarely known with absolute certainty, the term reference standard is now preferred as a more cautious and scientifically appropriate designation. Estimates of diagnostic accuracy depend on the particular reference standard used, as different reference standards may classify individuals differently.
Reproduced with permission from Samfundslitteratur.

low specificity, resulting in a large number of false positive findings among people who are disease-free. Diagnostic testing thus always involves a trade-off between missing disease and falsely identifying it.

For clinicians, the key question is therefore not only whether a test is sensitive or specific, but how trustworthy a given test result is in practice. When a test result is positive, how likely is it that the person truly has the disease? When a test result is negative, how confident can one be that the person is disease-free? Within the Bayesian diagnostic paradigm, these questions are addressed through the PPV and the NPV. PPV expresses the probability that a positive test result reflects true disease, while NPV expresses the probability that a negative test result reflects true absence of disease.

- PPV = $a/(a + b)$, the percentage of how many of the positive test results that are true positives.
- NPV = $d/(c + d)$, the percentage of how many of the negative test results that are true negatives.

As a hypothetical example, let us say the PPV of a diagnostic test for HbA1c is 80 percent (Figure 3.3). This means that of all the people who have an abnormal result (those we interpret as sick), 80 percent of the results are true, while 20 percent are false positives. Similarly, the NPV of this diagnostic test for HbA1c could conceivably be 90 percent, meaning that of all the people who have normal diagnostic tests for type 2 diabetes (those we interpret as healthy), 90 percent of the results are true, while 10 percent are false negatives.

Bayesian reasoning makes explicit what is otherwise implicit in medical practice: test results must always be interpreted in light of *pre-test probability*; the estimated likelihood that a person has the disease before testing, based on symptoms, medical history, and epidemiological context (Box 3.2). A test does not create certainty; it updates an existing probability.

Within the Bayesian diagnostic paradigm, outcomes other than sensitivity, specificity, PPV and NPV are also used to express diagnostic test accuracy, namely: positive likelihood ratio, negative likelihood ratio, the *ROC curve* (receiver operating characteristic curve) and the area under the ROC curve. It is beyond the scope of this book to explain these diagnostic test accuracy outcomes, but in short, likelihood ratios and ROC curves are also calculated from the information included in Figure 3.3. Likelihood ratios and ROC curves are outcomes that also characterise diagnostic test accuracy, but in a different way than sensitivity, specificity, PPV and NPV.

To understand what happens to the diagnostic paradigm when overdiagnosis occurs, it is sufficient to consider sensitivity, specificity, positive predictive value and negative predictive value (for more information, see Guyatt et al., 2015).

		Type 2 diabetes	Not type 2 diabetes	
Diagnostic test	Positive Test	80 (a)	20 (b)	100
	Negative Test	10 (c)	90 (d)	100
		90	110	200

Sensitivity 80/90 = 89%

Specificity: 90/110 = 82

Positive Predictive Value (PPV): 80/100 = 80%

Negative Predictive Value (NPV): 90/100 = 90%

Figure 3.3 Hypothetical example of what the diagnostic test accuracy might be of a long-term blood glucose (HbA1c) test estimated from sensitivity, specificity, positive and negative predictive values.
Diagnostic test results for type 2 diabetes. Of 200 people, 80 true positives, 20 false positives, 10 false negatives, and 90 true negatives are identified. Calculations are for sensitivity (89%), specificity (82%), positive predictive value (80%), and negative predictive value (90%).
Reproduced with permission from Samfundslitteratur.

Box 3.2 A worked example

Consider a disease that affects 1 percent of a population. Imagine a diagnostic test with a sensitivity of 90 percent and a specificity of 90 percent, These figures would generally be considered good.

If 1000 people are tested, 10 will have the disease. Of these, 9 will correctly test positive, while 1 will receive a false negative result. Among the remaining 990 people who do not have the disease, 981 will correctly test negative, but 99 will receive a false positive result.

In this scenario, a total of 108 people receive a positive test result, but only 9 of them actually have the disease. The positive predictive value of the test is therefore just over 8 percent. In other words, more than nine out of ten positive test results are false positives.

Nothing is wrong with the test. The problem lies in the context in which it is used. When a disease is rare, even a technically good test will generate many false positives. Conversely, when a disease is common, the same test will appear far more reliable.

Diagnostics of mental illnesses

Over the past half century, the diagnostic nomenclature of psychiatry has undergone substantial change. Contemporary psychiatric diagnoses are defined almost exclusively through clinical assessment: the patient's medical history, reported symptoms, and observed presentation. Unlike most somatic diagnoses, psychiatric diagnoses are not anchored in identifiable biological markers or pathological findings. They are, instead, clinical judgements based on interpretation. As a consequence, psychiatric diagnoses do not operate according to a strict binary logic. They are inherently matters of degree, severity, duration, intensity, and functional impairment. Symptoms are assessed along continua rather than as present or absent. Anxiety provides a clear example. At one end of the continuum are individuals who experience little or no anxiety; at the other are those whose anxiety is so severe that it profoundly impairs mental, physical, and social functioning. Epidemiological research consistently shows that populations are distributed along such continua. Most people experience no or only mild anxiety, while progressively fewer experience moderate or severe forms. This distribution resembles the right-hand side of a normal curve, with a long tail extending towards more severe suffering. Drawing a diagnostic boundary along this continuum is therefore inherently difficult. At the extremes, classification is relatively uncontroversial. It is in the broad middle ground where symptoms are present but ambiguous, fluctuating, or only mildly impairing that interpretive dilemmas arise.

Over time, psychiatric diagnostic categories have expanded. New diagnoses have been added, and existing definitions have been revised to include increasingly mild manifestations of mental distress. This is an example of overdefinition, one of the central mechanisms of overdiagnosis discussed in Chapter 1. When diagnostic thresholds are shifted towards the milder end of a continuum, a much larger proportion of the population is captured by the category. Given the underlying distribution of symptoms, even small definitional changes can lead to substantial increases in the number of people diagnosed. From this perspective, overdiagnosis in psychiatry is not an anomaly but a structural consequence of continuum-based classification. Like risk factors and pre-disease states in somatic medicine, psychiatric diagnoses lack clear natural boundaries. It therefore follows that the likelihood of overdiagnosis increases as diagnostic definitions expand toward less severe symptoms and lower levels of impairment (Moynihan et al., 2019).

These dynamics have been critically examined by a number of scholars and clinicians. Allan Frances, former chair of the *Diagnostic and Statistical Manual of Mental Disorders* (DSM-IV), has argued forcefully that diagnostic expansion risks pathologising ordinary distress (2013). Similar concerns are raised by Joel Paris (2015), Svend Brinkmannn (2010), Trond F. Aarre (2018), and Alastair Santhouse (2025), all highlighting how expanding diagnostic categories can transform normal variations in human experience into medical problems requiring intervention. This does not mean that psychiatric diagnoses are meaningless or illegitimate. Rather, it is that their continuum-based nature demands particular caution. Readers with specific interest in overdiagnosis in mental disorders are encouraged to orient themselves in this body of work.

The importance of the diagnosis for the individual patient

While theoretical discussions of diagnosis are essential for understanding medicine and society, they often recede into the background when individuals are confronted with symptoms, test results, or screening outcomes. At that point, the central question becomes deeply personal: *Am I sick or am I healthy?* Diagnosis, risk of diagnosis, or the absence of diagnosis can take on very different meanings in an individual life (see also Chapter 7). For some, a diagnosis provides explanation, reassurance, and a sense of control. It can legitimise suffering and make experiences intelligible. A diagnosis may also open the door to treatment options be it curative, life-prolonging, or palliative, and to social and institutional support. In this sense, diagnosis can be experienced as relief.

These experiences must be understood within the broader context of contemporary health cultures. As discussed in Chapter 2, neoliberal health governance increasingly frames health as an individual responsibility, and risk as something that should be managed proactively. The French sociologist Robert Castel described this development as *hyperrationalism*: a mode of reasoning in which individuals are encouraged to continuously monitor, calculate, and manage health risks (Castel, 1991).

Paradoxically, such rationalisation may have iatrogenic consequences, including the proliferation of chronic anxiety generated by the healthcare system itself.

To understand what diagnosis means for individuals, social science has developed several theoretical frameworks. In the following, we introduce two such perspectives: the *labelling effect* and the *looping effect* (Box 3.3).

From an overdiagnosis perspective, the looping effect is particularly instructive. A diagnosis not only names a condition but also creates interpretative frameworks and opportunities for action. As anthropologist Susan Reynolds Whyte has argued, uncertainty is not something individuals can simply choose to accept or reject. Uncertainty is an inherent feature of life; what matters is how uncertainty can be acted upon (Whyte, 2005). A diagnosis may offer a way of managing uncertainty, especially when treatment options exist. At the same time, diagnosis can also generate new forms of uncertainty, because what ultimately matters to individuals is often not the diagnosis itself but the prognosis, namely what the diagnosis means for the future. A cancer

Box 3.3 Possible psychosocial consequences of a diagnosis

A diagnosis can produce what sociologist Thomas Scheff termed a *labelling effect*. According to labelling theory, assigning a diagnostic label does not merely describe a condition; it can shape identity, behaviour, and social interaction (Scheff, 1966). While originally developed in relation to mental illness, the labelling effect applies more broadly to medical diagnoses. Later work has identified several dimensions that influence how labelling operates, including whether individuals anticipate discrimination, the timing of the diagnosis, how they relate to the label, the practical consequences of being labelled, and whether the label leads to further forms of categorisation (Link et al., 1989; Link & Phelan, 1999). Empirical research shows that such effects are not limited to psychiatric diagnoses but also occur in somatic conditions and risk factors, such as hypertension (Gyuricza, 2020).

Another theory about the effect of diagnoses, which is less commonly associated with mental illness, is Canadian philosopher Ian Hacking's *looping effect* theory. Hacking argues that classifications of people such as diagnostic categories do not merely describe individuals but interact with them. Once classified, people may come to understand themselves and behave in ways that align with expectations associated with the category (Hacking, 1995). This feedback mechanism means that classifications can change the very phenomena they are meant to describe. A diagnosis such as schizophrenia, for example, carries implicit assumptions about behaviour, limitations, and life course. These assumptions may shape how patients interpret their own experiences and how others respond to them, potentially reinforcing the category itself. Importantly, Hacking's theory concerns classification systems rather than individual psychology, and his claim that classifications themselves change because of looping has been debated (Tsou, 2007).

diagnosis, for example, says little on its own about how life will unfold. Prostate cancer may represent an indolent condition that will never cause symptoms, or it may develop into a life-threatening disease. From the patient's perspective, the diagnosis is only meaningful insofar as it informs expectations about future health, functioning, and life possibilities. In other cases, diagnosis may bring long-awaited recognition and support. A diagnosis of ADHD in a child, for instance, can help explain long-standing difficulties at school and in social life, while also alleviating parental guilt or shame. It may grant access to educational support, respite care, or medical treatment, and provide a framework for understanding everyday challenges (see Ryborg, 2011; Jønsson, 2014). In such contexts, diagnosis becomes a way of controlling uncertainty and legitimising the need for assistance. Here, the problem arises when diagnostic categories are diluted. As criteria become less stringent, increasing numbers of individuals with mild or transient symptoms come to fit diagnostic definitions which may reflect genuine need, but they also raise concerns about overdiagnosis. Part of the rise may be driven by institutional structures in which access to public support depends on diagnosis. Part may reflect the medicalisation of behaviour previously considered within the range of normal variation. And part may result from the progressive expansion of diagnostic definitions. Longitudinal studies suggest that some children diagnosed with ADHD no longer meet diagnostic criteria for extended periods, placing them at risk of unnecessary long-term treatment (Rabiner et al., 2010).

In places with insurance-based healthcare systems, yet another challenge occurs. A chronic diagnosis can have long-term consequences that extend far beyond access to care. Diagnoses may shape eligibility for health insurance, life insurance, disability insurance, and even educational or occupational opportunities. Rather than merely enabling support, a diagnosis can become a marker of risk that follows individuals across institutional contexts. Adding to that, diagnoses are central to risk stratification in insurance-based systems. Insurance logic is built on the differentiation between low-risk and high-risk individuals, and diagnostic labels are routinely used to justify higher premiums, exclusions, or denial of coverage. Prior to the introduction of the Affordable Care Act in the United States, for example, mental health diagnoses, including ADHD, were commonly treated as *pre-existing conditions*, allowing private insurers to exclude coverage or impose substantial financial penalties (Rowan et al., 2013). Although some protections have since been introduced in certain jurisdictions, diagnostic information continues to circulate across insurance, employment, and welfare systems in ways that can disadvantage individuals with chronic or psychiatric diagnoses.

For children diagnosed with ADHD, autism spectrum disorders, or other neurodevelopmental conditions, these consequences may only become apparent later in life. Diagnoses acquired in childhood are often difficult, in some settings even impossible, to remove from medical records, and may affect access to life insurance, mortgage insurance, fertility treatment, or certain professions in adulthood, including military service, aviation, and policing (Paris, 2015; Owens, 2020). In this sense, diagnosis may close off future possibilities at the very moment it appears to offer help.

From a sociological perspective, this reflects a shift in the function of diagnosis. Rather than serving solely as a clinical tool for care, diagnosis increasingly operates as an administrative device that sorts populations according to actuarial risk (Rose, 2007). In insurance-based systems, the diagnostic label becomes less about present suffering and more about predicted future costs. The problem is compounded in cases of overdiagnosis. When diagnostic thresholds are lowered and more individuals with mild or transient symptoms are classified as chronically ill, increasing numbers of people may be exposed to the long-term social and financial consequences of patienthood without proportional benefit. As Allan Frances has argued, individuals who are overdiagnosed are uniquely vulnerable: they receive the burdens of diagnosis without the compensatory advantages of effective treatment or improved prognosis (Frances, 2013). It may also produce enduring structural harms, binding individuals to identities and risk categories that shape life chances in ways that are difficult to reverse. What appears, in the short term, as access to care may, in the longer term, function as a constraint.

The importance of diagnosis for the individual, then, lies precisely in its ambivalence. Diagnosis can offer explanation, predict prognosis, access to care, and relief. But it can also constrain lives, generate uncertainty, and produce harms that extend far beyond the clinic. Understanding this ambivalence is essential for grasping why overdiagnosis matters, not only statistically or clinically, but ethically and socially.

Diagnostics and overdiagnosis

Research over the past three decades has demonstrated that far from all early identified pathological changes in otherwise healthy individuals develop into disease later in life (Welch et al., 2011). Many such findings remain harmless throughout a person's lifetime. For example, a tissue alteration or lesion in an asymptomatic individual that can be visualised microscopically and classified as malignant according to established medical criteria will not necessarily progress into a symptomatic or life-threatening disease. The core problem, and the source of much of the complexity surrounding overdiagnosis, lies at the individual level. Among asymptomatic people, it is impossible at the time of diagnosis to determine who is correctly diagnosed and who is overdiagnosed. When a pathological condition meets diagnostic criteria but causes no future morbidity or mortality, this distinction can only be made retrospectively, often not until the person dies of other causes (Brodersen et al., 2014). By that point, any unnecessary treatment, psychosocial consequences, and use of healthcare resources can no longer be undone.

To illustrate how overdiagnosis affects diagnostic reasoning, we return to the Bayesian diagnostic paradigm. In the standard 2 × 2 table (Figure 3.2), individuals with true disease who test positive are placed in box (a). However, when overdiagnosis occurs, this box inevitably contains two distinct groups: those who are correctly diagnosed (including symptomatic patients and asymptomatic individuals who will later develop symptoms or die from the disease) and those who are overdiagnosed. At the time of diagnosis, the asymptomatic people in these two groups are indistinguishable (see also Chapter 4, Figure 4.1).

As a result, standard calculations of diagnostic test accuracy, particularly sensitivity and positive predictive value, are flawed if overdiagnosis is not explicitly accounted for. To address this, the diagnostic paradigm must be expanded from a 2×2 table to a 2×3 table (Figure 3.4), which distinguishes between true disease, overdiagnosed conditions, and absence of disease.

In this expanded model, the category of false negatives among the overdiagnosed (box c^*) is always empty. By definition, overdiagnosed individuals never develop symptoms or die from the condition in question. They therefore cannot later be identified as false negatives. Apparent false negatives arise only because either the diagnostic technology is not yet sensitive enough to detect very small changes, or because findings that are biologically present are interpreted as normal according to prevailing pathological criteria despite being irrelevant from a prognostic perspective.

Once overdiagnosis is introduced into the diagnostic paradigm, the calculation of test accuracy changes (Box 3.4). Sensitivity and PPV are particularly affected. Sensitivity is now calculated as the proportion of all sick *and overdiagnosed* individuals who test positive, while PPV reflects the proportion of all positive test results that include both correctly diagnosed disease and overdiagnosis.

As the formulas demonstrate, sensitivity and PPV are systematically inflated when overdiagnosis occurs. Mathematically, the fraction $(a + a^*)/(a + a^* + c)$ will always be larger than $a/(a + c)$ as long as at least one overdiagnosed individual is present

		Dividing a population into sick, overdiagnosed and healthy in relation to a reference standard and prognosis/cause of death			
		Stick	**Overdiagnosed**	**Non-Stick**	
Diagnostic test	Positive Test	True positive answer (a)	"True" positive answer (a*)	False positive answer (b)	a + b
	Negative Test	False negative answer (c)	"False" negative answer (c*)	True negative answer (d)	c + d
		a + c	a* + c*	b + d	N = a + a* + b + c + c* + d

Figure 3.4 The diagnostic paradigm including overdiagnosis.
Extension of the diagnostic test framework to include overdiagnosis. The population is divided into sick, overdiagnosed, and not sick groups. Test results include true positives, false positives, false negatives, and true negatives, showing how overdiagnosed cases complicate interpretation of diagnostic accuracy.
Reproduced with permission from Samfundslitteratur.

Box 3.4 Calculating diagnostic test accuracy when overdiagnosis occurs

- Sensitivity = $(a + a^*)/(a + a^* + c)$: percentage of how many sick + overdiagnosed out of all sick and overdiagnosed people the test finds.
- Specificity = $d/(b + d)$: percentage of how many non-sick people out of all non-sick people the test finds.
- Positive predictive value (PPV) = $(a + a^*)/(a + a^* + b)$: percentage of how many positive results are true positives, including the overdiagnosed.
- Negative predictive value (NPV) = $d/(c + d)$: percentage of how many negative results are true negatives.

($a^* \geq 1$). The greater the extent of overdiagnosis, the greater this inflation. The same applies to PPV.

This has an important implication: diagnostic tests may appear to perform better precisely because they detect conditions that will never cause harm. In other words, overdiagnosis artificially improves apparent diagnostic accuracy. Specificity and NPV remain unchanged only if the absolute numbers of true negatives and false positives are unaffected; if these distributions shift, they too may change.

For this reason, Brodersen and colleagues (2014) have suggested that terms such as *artificial sensitivity* and *artificial positive predictive value* more accurately describe test performance in contexts where overdiagnosis is present. Strictly speaking, it is not possible to calculate the true sensitivity or PPV of a diagnostic test unless the extent of overdiagnosis is known, a condition that is rarely, if ever, met in empirical settings.

4
Screening

Did screening save Lisa?

Lisa is aged 61 years and has had regular mammograms since her early fifties, usually scheduled through her primary care physician and carried out at a large imaging centre affiliated with her local hospital. Each time, the results have appeared in her online patient portal a few days later, accompanied by a brief message stating that no abnormalities were found. This time, the notification is different. Lisa receives an automated message informing her that an abnormality has been detected and that she will be contacted for further imaging. Before she speaks to a clinician, she opens the report herself. It contains unfamiliar terms such as 'suspicious findings' and 'BI-RADS category' and recommends additional tests. Lisa feels a jolt of fear. Like many families, hers has been touched by breast cancer. She calls her daughter. Within days, Lisa undergoes further imaging and a biopsy. The diagnosis is breast cancer. Her clinician explains that the cancer was caught early and that treatment options are available. Lisa and her family feel relieved and grateful that the screening found the malignant cells.

What Lisa and her family is unaware of is the uncertainty that underlies diagnosis based on screening results in asymptomatic healthy people. Was it cancer that was found, or was it perhaps an indolent cluster of neoplastic cells that would never have developed into something dangerous for Lisa? The language of early detection suggests clarity and success, but the reality is more complex. From a medical perspective, Lisa's diagnosis could reflect several different scenarios. She may be among the minority of women who benefit from screening because early detection genuinely improves prognosis. She may also be among the larger group of women whose cancer would have become symptomatic and been treated effectively even without screening, through a timely visit to a physician. A third possibility is that the cancer is aggressive, and that the timing of detection makes little difference to outcome. And then the fourth possibility rarely discussed in clinical encounters or media narratives: Lisa may have been overdiagnosed. The cancer detected on screening may never have caused symptoms or threatened her life. It might have remained indolent or regressed. In many countries, where screening is widely promoted and often framed as a personal responsibility, such distinctions are difficult to articulate. Screening results are delivered directly to screening participants, most often before they have spoken with a clinician, and abnormal findings are experienced as urgent and actionable. Within this system, early detection becomes a moral good, while the possibility of overdiagnosis remains largely invisible.

As authors, we are neither for nor against screening, and the benefits and harms of screening are also likely to depend on culture, local epidemiology and healthcare organisation. In this chapter, we assess screening in contexts where patients have easy and regular access to healthcare services.

There is a growing body of literature on the iatrogenic effects of screening, including overdiagnosis, overtreatment, anxiety following false positive results, false reassurance after false negative results, and downstream harms from unnecessary interventions (Welch et al., 2011; Brodersen & Siersma, 2013; S.M. Carter et al., 2015a; Raffle et al., 2019). Readers seeking a detailed account of screening practices are referred to the specialist literature. However, because screening is one of the major drivers of overdiagnosis, we provide an introduction to *why* screening produces overdiagnosis, followed by a critical and up-to-date assessment of the evidence underpinning the most widely implemented screening programmes.

What is medical screening?

> Medical screening is defined as the presumptive identification of unrecognized disease or defect by the application of tests, examinations, or other procedures which can be applied rapidly. Screening tests sort out apparently well persons who probably have a disease from those who probably do not. A screening test is not intended to be diagnostic. Persons with positive or suspicious findings must be referred to their physicians for diagnosis and necessary treatment.
>
> **(Commission on Chronic Illness, 1956)**

This now ageing definition of medical screening, which has also been adopted in the longstanding World Health Organization (WHO) report by Wilson and Jungner from 1968, is still largely valid. What has changed is not the underlying logic of screening, but the context in which it is applied. In particular, the criterion that screening procedures should be 'applied rapidly' has lost much of its relevance. In the mid-twentieth century, screening primarily targeted infectious diseases such as syphilis and tuberculosis, as well as conditions such as schizophrenia, where speed was central to large-scale population testing. Today, screening examinations can be time-consuming and technically complex. A general health check may last half an hour or more, and prenatal screening by ultrasound, which is otherwise considered a typically brief procedure, can take substantially longer depending on foetal position and the feasibility of obtaining specific measurements.

The term *screening* itself offers a useful metaphor. Linguistically, it derives from practices such as 'screening the coal', where coal and slag were separated and coal pieces sorted by size using metal grids or rollers. This was a coarse sorting process rather than a precise one. Similarly, airport security screening functions as a rough form of sorting: passengers are classified as posing either a higher or lower risk and are channelled accordingly. As many travellers have experienced, this process is imperfect. False positives are common, individuals are searched or scanned further despite carrying no prohibited items. False negatives are also possible, allowing restricted items to pass through undetected, as demonstrated by quality control studies of airport security systems (Linos et al., 2007). These examples illustrate a central characteristic of screening: it is inherently imprecise.

Medical screening operates according to the same principle. As the definition makes clear, screening does not diagnose disease. Instead, it divides a population of apparently healthy individuals into two groups. One group receives a positive or abnormal screening result and, on average, has a higher probability of disease than the screening population as a whole. The other group receives a negative or normal result and, again on average, has a lower probability of disease than the population mean. This coarse sorting produces four possible outcomes: true positives, false positives, true negatives, and false negatives (see also Chapter 3).

The stated purpose of medical screening is to identify pathological conditions at an earlier point in time before individuals develop symptoms or die as a consequence of those conditions. However, the scope of screening is not only to detect manifest disease, but also to identify precursors to disease and markers of increased risk. In cervical cancer screening, for example, the primary target is not invasive cancer itself, but abnormal cells of the cervix, some of which may develop into cancer over time. Similarly, bowel cancer screening seeks to detect both colorectal cancer and bowel polyps, acknowledging that certain polyps can act as precursors to malignancy. In the case of cardiovascular disease, screening does not target acute myocardial infarction or stroke directly. Instead, it focuses on identifying individuals at increased risk of developing these conditions later in life. This is achieved through the detection of risk factors such as elevated blood pressure, high cholesterol levels, evidence of atherosclerosis, increased body mass index, and other measurable indicators associated with future cardiovascular events.

Opportunistic screening refers to unorganised and unsystematic testing that takes place outside formal, population-based screening programmes. It typically occurs in clinical encounters for other reasons, for example, when a test is ordered 'just to be sure', added to a routine consultation, or performed because diagnostic technology is readily available rather than because the individual meets predefined screening criteria. Unlike organised screening programmes, opportunistic screening is not governed by explicit eligibility rules, quality assurance, or systematic evaluation of benefits and harms. As several of the examples discussed later in this chapter illustrate, opportunistic screening plays a substantial role in driving overdiagnosis, precisely because it targets individuals with a low pre-test probability of disease and operates without the safeguards that structured screening programmes are intended to provide.

Screening for precursors and risk factors rests on a different hypothesis from that underpinning early disease detection. Here, the aim is not only to improve outcomes for individuals who will develop disease, but to prevent disease from occurring at all.

In public health terms, this approach is referred to as primary prevention, as it seeks to reduce or eliminate causal pathways leading to disease incidence (see Chapter 5) (Brodersen et al., 2014). Thus, some screening programmes are designed to operate at multiple preventive levels. They may function as secondary prevention by detecting disease earlier, and simultaneously as primary prevention by identifying precursors or risk factors whose modification may reduce disease incidence at the population level. Later in this chapter, we return to this distinction when we examine empirical evidence for screening programmes that claim to reduce the incidence of disease.

Difference between screening and diagnosis

A positive (abnormal) screening result does not constitute a diagnosis. This distinction is fundamental, yet often blurred in public discourse. A diagnosis is based on a synthesis of information that extends well beyond the result of a single test, whether the diagnostic process unfolds in response to symptoms or follows a screening invitation. In clinical practice, diagnosis emerges through consistency across several domains: the patient's medical history, findings from the clinical examination, and results from relevant paraclinical investigations such as blood tests, biopsies, or imaging. These elements are interpreted together, and diagnostic reasoning is shaped by the patient's presentation, complaints, and context. Screening differs in several crucial respects. Screening programmes target *apparently healthy individuals*, not patients seeking care. Participants have not presented symptoms, and the examination is not prompted by a clinical concern. Screening therefore begins in the absence of a medical history oriented towards a specific problem, and it rarely includes a full clinical examination except in cases where screening takes the form of a general health check or where the screening test itself involves a focused examination. This structural difference has important consequences. In clinical settings, paraclinical tests are selected and interpreted in light of a patient's history and clinical findings. This targeted approach increases the likelihood that abnormal results are clinically meaningful. Therefore, the positive predictive value of diagnostic tests is generally higher in clinical contexts than in screening, and the risk of false positives is correspondingly lower. Moreover, incidental findings, so-called *incidentalomas*, are less likely when investigations are guided by a specific clinical question.

It is therefore also emphasised in national screening guidelines globally, and in the WHO principles for screening, that screening participants with a positive (abnormal) screening result should be referred for further diagnostic investigations to find out if the positive screening result is true or false. In contrast, screening applies the same test to large numbers of people regardless of individual risk profiles or symptoms. Abnormal findings are therefore more likely to include deviations that are unrelated to future disease, including indolent or non-progressive conditions. For this reason, the imaging modalities and thresholds used in screening often differ from those used in diagnostic work-ups. These differences underpin a key principle in screening guidelines worldwide, including those articulated by WHO: individuals with a positive screening result should be referred for further diagnostic evaluation. The purpose of this step is to determine whether the screening finding represents a true disease state or a false alarm.

However, even when screening findings are confirmed diagnostically, an additional layer of uncertainty remains. As discussed in Chapter 1, not all screen-detected pathological conditions will progress to symptomatic disease. Screening therefore does not merely involve distinguishing between true and false positives, but also between conditions that will cause harm and those that will not. This distinction cannot be resolved at the time of detection.

Screening should thus be understood not as a single test with four possible outcomes, but as described by Harris and colleagues as the starting point of a cascade of investigations, surveillance, and prognostic judgements. The possible trajectories are illustrated in Figure 4.1. This cascade may lead to benefit for some individuals, but it

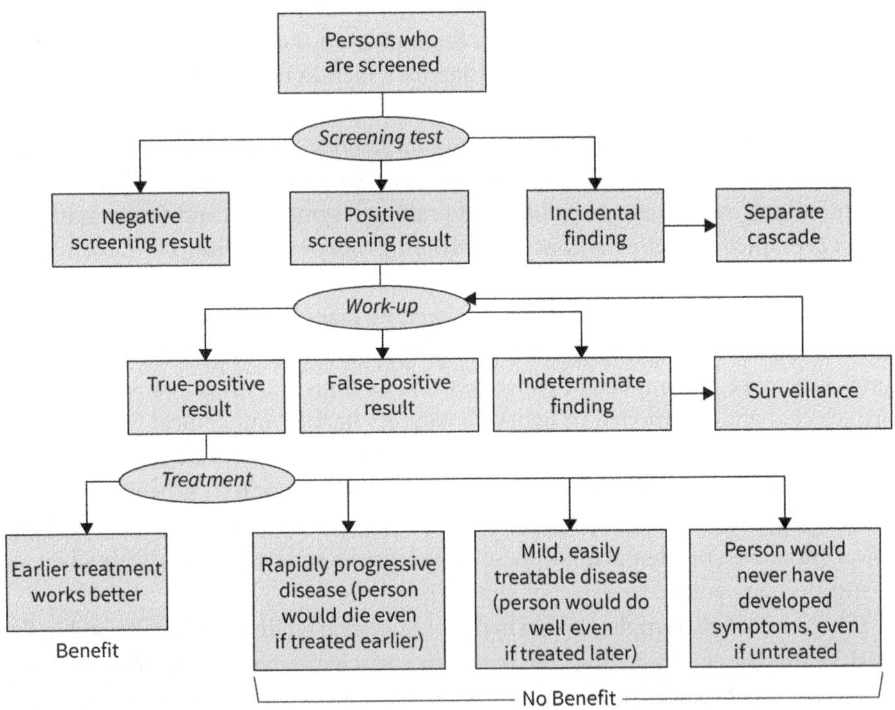

Figure 4.1 The screening cascade. Source: modified from Harris et al. (2015). Screened individuals may receive negative or positive results or incidental findings. Further work-up may identify true positives, false positives, or indeterminate findings. Treatment may benefit some patients but often leads to no benefit, including cases of mild disease or overdiagnosis.

Reproduced with permission from Samfundslitteratur.

can also expose healthy people to harm through overdiagnosis, overtreatment, and prolonged patienthood.

Benefits and harms of medical screening

In the foreword to their book *Screening. Evidence and practice*, Raffle, Mackie, and Gray write:

> All screening programmes do harm. Some do good as well and, of these, some do more good than harm at reasonable cost. (Raffle et al., 2019)

They go on to elaborate:

> It is the responsibility of policy-makers, public health practitioners, managers, and the clinicians involved in screening to ensure that only programmes that do more good than harm at reasonable cost are implemented and, when they are implemented, that they are managed in such a way as to achieve a level of quality which will ensure that the balance of good and harm demonstrated in research is reproduced in the ordinary service setting. Unfortunately, many screening services either have been introduced on the basis of inadequate evidence that they do more good than harm at reasonable cost or, even if introduced on good evidence, are managed so badly that the efficacy demonstrated in research is not translated into effectiveness in practice. This results in waste of resources and in harm to those individuals who accept the offer of screening (Raffle et al., 2019)

This formulation captures a central tension running through this chapter. Screening is not a neutral intervention. It is an organised medical practice that inevitably produces harm, even under optimal conditions. The ethical and political justification for screening therefore rests not on the absence of harm, but on whether the anticipated benefits outweigh those harms and whether this balance can be realised outside controlled research settings, in everyday clinical practice.

Therefore, both benefits and harms are central to the evaluation of any screening programme. Yet the scientific literature on screening is markedly asymmetric. Studies are far more likely to report intended beneficial effects than unintended harms. This pattern has been documented in a comprehensive review of randomised trials of cancer screening (Heleno et al., 2013) and more recently in systematic reviews of the physical harms associated with colorectal cancer screening (Kindt et al., 2023; Martiny et al., 2024; Bie et al., 2025). This phenomenon is known as *reporting bias* and poses a serious ethical, democratic, and political challenge. When benefits are investigated and reported more consistently than harms, it becomes difficult, and sometimes impossible, to weigh the two against each other in an evidence-based manner (Heleno et al., 2013; Kindt et al., 2023; Martiny et al., 2024; Bie et al., 2025).

As a consequence, evidence of benefit is often readily available, whereas evidence of harm is limited, incomplete, or absent. The potential *intended* benefits of screening include (Brodersen et al., 2010a; Østerø et al., 2014; Rasmussen et al., 2015):

- reduced mortality
- more conservative or less invasive treatment
- reduced incidence of disease
- reduced morbidity

At the same time, screening may give rise to a range of *unintended* harms, including:

- false negative screening results
- false positive screening results
- overdiagnosis (through overdetection and overdefinition)
- overtreatment
- overexamination and surveillance
- prolonged patienthood (more years lived as a patient)
- increased morbidity
- increased mortality
- increased insecurity and anxiety

At the societal level, these benefits and harms must be weighed when deciding whether a screening programme should be introduced, continued, modified, or discontinued. In many countries, this task is assigned to advisory committees responsible for monitoring existing screening programmes and assessing applications for new ones. When new screening programmes are proposed, they are typically assessed against the WHO screening principles, alongside national screening criteria where these exist. The available evidence on benefits and harms is usually synthesised through systematic reviews, often using the GRADE approach. Yet, even when evidence is carefully appraised, balancing benefits and harms remains a value-based judgement rather than a purely technical exercise (Jensen et al., 2021, 2025).

Ongoing monitoring is particularly important because the balance between benefit and harm may shift over time. Changes in primary prevention, diagnostic technologies, and treatment effectiveness can alter the justification for screening programmes long after their implementation (Ropers et al., 2021). The introduction of human papillomavirus vaccination into childhood immunisation programmes and the global decline in tobacco use are two prominent examples of primary prevention that may justify de-intensifying, de-implementing, or never implementing certain screening programmes, such as cervical cancer screening, abdominal aortic aneurysm screening, or low-dose computed tomography (CT) screening for lung cancer (Johansson et al., 2018; Duffy & Wald, 2022; Winsløw et al., 2026).

At the individual level, international democratic norms require that invited citizens are provided with understandable and balanced information about both benefits and harms, enabling them to make an informed decision about participation. In practice, this ideal is difficult to realise. Several studies suggest that deeply rooted cultural assumptions complicate informed choice. Screening is widely perceived as inherently beneficial and only minimally harmful, a perception shared by experts, authorities, and citizens alike (Gram et al., 2023a). One study shows that US primary care physicians struggle to distinguish between beneficial and harmful hypothetical screening programmes (Wegwarth et al., 2012). Other studies demonstrate that both doctors and the general population systematically overestimate the benefits of screening and underestimate its harms (Hoffmann & Del Mar, 2015, 2017).

This mismatch between evidence and beliefs can produce what has been described as a *perception gap*, in which individuals experience cognitive dissonance when confronted with information that challenges deeply held assumptions about screening (Damhus et al., 2018; Petersen et al., 2020). One hypothesis is that when the discrepancy between factual information and existing beliefs becomes too great, individuals are unable to internalise the information, making informed choice difficult or even impossible (Petersen et al., 2020). Another is that key concepts and especially overdiagnosis are poorly understood even by health professionals in a context of screening (Piessens et al., 2025). An Australian study found that overdiagnosis is largely incomprehensible to the general population, further complicating efforts to balance benefits and harms (Moynihan et al., 2015).

Deliberative approaches such as citizen juries and deliberative polls have been proposed as ways of addressing these challenges. However, they yield mixed results. Citizen juries typically involve small, non-representative groups, raising democratic concerns if their conclusions are used to guide population-level policy (Rychetnik et al., 2013; Degeling et al., 2015; Pickles et al., 2018; Degeling et al., 2019). A large representative deliberative poll showed substantial gains in knowledge about mammography screening: from 1 to 56 percent demonstrating high knowledge and greater opinion stability (Jensen et al., 2021). After deliberation, participants were generally less supportive of the screening programme. Yet, a majority still made recommendations inconsistent with the levels of mortality reduction and overdiagnosis they themselves considered acceptable (Jensen et al., 2025).

Intended beneficial effects of screening

The overarching goal of screening is to reduce the burden of disease in a population by identifying disease, precursors to disease, or risk factors for disease at an earlier point in time. Screening is therefore justified by a set of anticipated benefits, both for individuals and at the population level. These benefits are typically framed as reductions in mortality, the possibility of more gentle treatment, reduced incidence of disease, and reduced morbidity. In the following, we examine each of these claims and explain how they are measured.

Reduced mortality

The primary justification for screening is the expectation that it will reduce mortality—either disease-specific mortality (death from the condition targeted by screening) or all-cause mortality (death from any cause). But as discussed in Chapter 1, cancers and diseases more broadly do not behave uniformly. Screening can only reduce mortality in the diseases that are progressive and potentially lethal. Assessing whether screening reduces mortality therefore requires careful choice of outcome measures. Although increased survival is often reported, survival statistics are misleading in the context of screening and say little about whether screening improves outcomes (Welch et al., 2007). Overdiagnosis and earlier detection alone will inflate survival figures without affecting the number of deaths. A worked example:

- Before screening: 10 people die from 'xyz cancer', 90 survive.
- With screening: 10 people die from 'xyz cancer', 900 survive.

It looks like the screening is working because survival appears dramatically improved, yet mortality is unchanged. The apparent benefit arises because screening has identified more people, of which the majority have an indolent disease that would never have caused harm. Mortality is therefore the most appropriate outcome, but it is also the most difficult to demonstrate. It requires substantially greater statistical power to detect a reduction in all-cause mortality than in disease-specific mortality, because deaths from any one cancer typically account for a small proportion of total deaths. For example, colorectal cancer accounts for approximately 3–6 percent of deaths among individuals aged 55–75 years in Nordic countries (Sigurdsson et al., 2013). While screening may reduce colorectal cancer mortality by 15–30 percent (Jodal et al., 2019), this corresponds to only a 0.45–1.8 percent reduction in overall mortality, which is extremely challenging to detect statistically. In addition, survival often yields results that look much more convincing and thereby get a lot of media attention, creating potential conflicts of interest among researchers in showing such convincing biased results (Welch et al., 2007; Abraham, 2008). However, testing all-cause mortality for multicancer screening is feasible, as cancer-related deaths constitute a major proportion of overall mortality (Welch & Dey, 2023).

Meaningful reductions in all-cause mortality through screening are therefore only plausible when two conditions are met:

1. the screening targets diseases that cause substantial and premature mortality in the screened population, and
2. that mortality is not primarily driven by lack of symptoms or suboptimal treatment, care, or rehabilitation.

If these conditions are not met, trials must include very large populations; hundreds of thousands, perhaps millions, of ordinary people must be included in a scientific trial, and the trial participants must be followed for 10, 20, or even 30 years before a difference in total mortality can be expected. Otherwise, only individuals with a very high risk of dying prematurely should be included in the trial.

Against this background, it is notable that a large meta-analysis including randomised trials with more than nine years of follow-up found no substantial reduction in all-cause mortality for six common cancer screening programmes (Bretthauer et al., 2023). Only sigmoidoscopy screening for colorectal cancer showed a marginal reduction; however, this meta-analysis result might be biased by unknown confounding (Juul et al., 2022; Olsen et al., 2023).

Only two screening trials have demonstrated reductions in all-cause mortality: the US National Lung Cancer Screening Trial (NLST) and the Danish VIVA trial.

The NLST showed a 6% reduction in all-cause mortality and a 15% reduction in lung cancer-specific mortality among current and former heavy smokers (Aberle et al., 2011). Participants were randomised to either low-dose CT scanning or chest X-ray. By contrast, seven European randomised trials of CT lung cancer screening, most comparing CT with no screening, did not demonstrate reductions in all-cause mortality, though several showed reductions in lung cancer-specific mortality (Bonney et al., 2022).

These discrepancies may reflect differences in healthcare systems. One hypothesis is that participation in the NLST led to improved detection and treatment of cardiovascular risk factors among high-risk smokers, thereby reducing deaths from non-cancer causes which could be argued to be a form of performance bias. A similar explanation has been proposed for the Danish VIVA trial, which screened men for cardiovascular risk factors and abdominal aortic aneurysm (Lindholt & Søgaard, 2017). The study reported a small absolute reduction (0.006 percent, with a statistical uncertainty of 0.001–0.011 percentage points in a 95% confidence interval[1]) in all-cause mortality, corresponding to an estimated 169 men needing to be invited to prevent one death, but this number is rather uncertain.[2] This effect was attributed primarily to improved pharmacological management of hypertension, hypercholesterolaemia, and peripheral arterial disease rather than reduced mortality from aneurysm rupture. However, the absence of reductions in cause-specific cardiovascular mortality and a paradoxical trend towards reduced cancer mortality, which could be a

[1] The confidence interval is an expression of the statistical uncertainty. In statistical analysis, a parameter is estimated by a number (e.g. the mean value of a number of measurements) but that is affected by statistical uncertainty. This uncertainty can be conveyed in a simple way in the form of a confidence interval, which is defined so that the interval with a certain probability (often 95% is chosen) contains the true value of the parameter.

[2] The 169 men are calculated with a statistical uncertainty of 89–1811 in a 95% confidence interval. In other words, the exact number of men who need to be invited for screening in order to hit the target with 95% certainty is somewhere between 89 and 1811.

statistical coincidence, have raised concerns about bias and randomisation problems (Jørgensen & Johansson, 2018).

More broadly, evidence from general health checks is convincing. A high-quality Cochrane review found no reduction in all-cause, cardiovascular, or cancer mortality from invitations to general health checks among seemingly healthy adults aged 40–65 years (Krogsbøll et al., 2019). Similar conclusions were reached in a WHO-commissioned review of screening for cardiovascular risk factors (Jørgensen et al., 2024).

The large US PLCO trial, which offered screening for prostate, lung, colorectal, and ovarian cancer to more than 150,000 participants, likewise showed no reduction in all-cause mortality (Prorok et al., 2018). Only colorectal cancer mortality was reduced, consistent with findings from colorectal-specific screening trials (Jodal et al., 2019). This is similar to what has been found in the screening trials targeting only one type of cancer: prostate cancer (Ilic et al., 2018), lung cancer (Manser et al., 2013) and ovarian cancer (Henderson et al., 2018). Notably, ovarian cancer screening in PLCO was associated with a possible excess mortality, suspected to result from overdiagnosis and overtreatment (Buys et al., 2011; Temkin et al., 2017; Henderson et al., 2018).

Increased survival

In evaluations of screening programmes, increased survival is often presented as evidence that screening is effective. Yet survival is a deeply misleading measure. As Welch and colleagues have shown, survival can increase even when screening does not reduce the number of people who die from the disease in question (Welch et al., 2007). This is because survival time is measured from the moment of diagnosis rather than from the onset of symptoms. Two mechanisms in particular inflate survival statistics without improving outcomes. First, screening leads to earlier diagnosis and therefore more years lived with a diagnosis, what we described as patienthood. Second, screening detects pathological conditions that would never have caused symptoms or death, that is, overdiagnosis. In both cases, survival increases simply because the clock starts earlier, not because lives are saved.

Prostate cancer provides a paradigmatic example. Across Europe, the incidence of prostate cancer has more than doubled since the mid-1990s, coinciding with the widespread introduction of the prostate-specific antigen (PSA) blood test in primary care (Vaccarella et al., 2024) (Figure 4.2). Over the same period, prostate cancer mortality has remained largely unchanged (Figure 4.2), although modest declines have been observed in some countries e.g. Denmark (Figure 4.3), most likely due to improvements in treatment and palliative care rather than earlier detection. In contrast, 10-year survival has increased dramatically. In Denmark, for example, relative survival has increased approximately fourfold, closely tracking the rise in incidence rather than a fall in mortality (Figure 4.4).

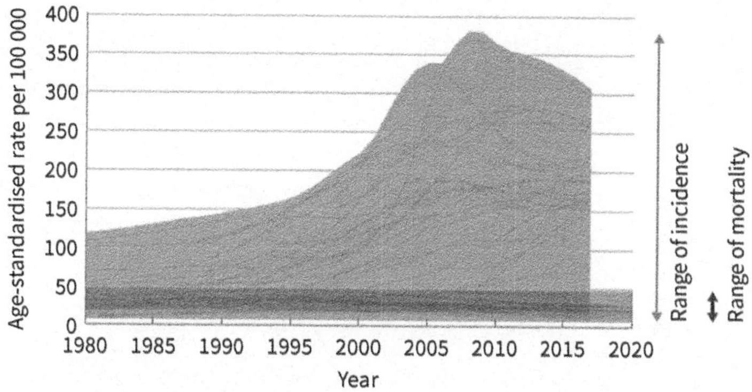

Figure 4.2 Age-standardised incidence and mortality of prostate cancer in Europe from 1980 to 2017. The lighter grey area shows incidence rising sharply over time; the darker grey area represents mortality remaining relatively stable. This demonstrates how increasing diagnosis rates can occur without a corresponding increase in deaths.
Source: Vaccarella et al. (2024).

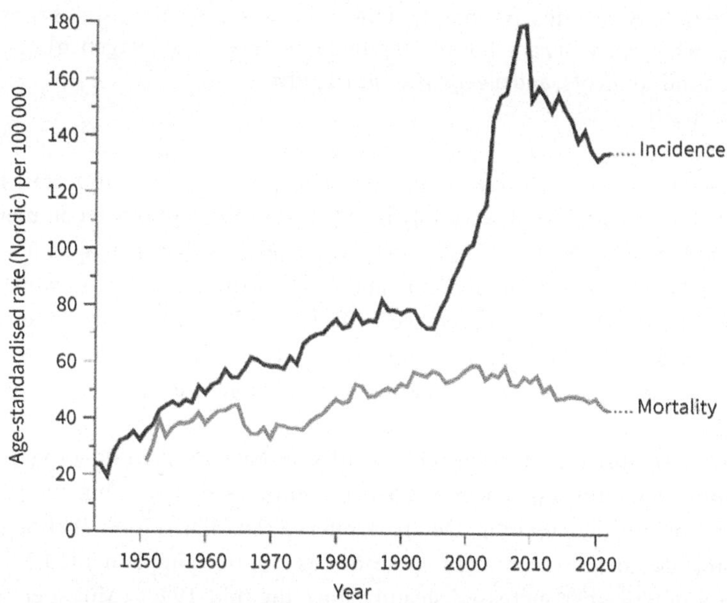

Figure 4.3 Age-standardised incidence and mortality of prostate cancer in Denmark from 1943 to 2025. Incidence rates (dark grey line) rise sharply, especially after the late 1990s, while mortality rates (lighter grey line) increase only slightly and later decline. There is a divergence between diagnoses and deaths.
Source: NORDCAN.

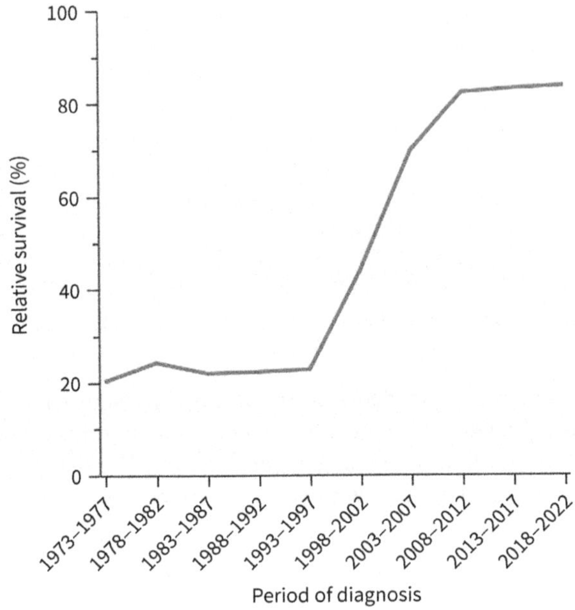

Figure 4.4 Age-standardised 10-year survival rate of prostate cancer in Denmark from 1973 to 2022. Survival rates rise sharply at the same time as incidence rates rises in Figure 4.3, while mortality are more of less the same. There is convergence between diagnoses and survivors, and divergence with deaths.
Source: NORDCAN.

The effectiveness of PSA screening in reducing prostate cancer mortality is uncertain (Ilic et al., 2018). This uncertainty is reflected in the cautious recommendations of the US Preventive Services Task Force, which advises that men aged 55–69 years should make an individual decision about PSA-based screening, while recommending against screening in men aged ≥70 years (USPSTF, 2018). In an evidence synthesis and drafted recommendation from November 2025, the UK National Screening Committee does not recommend population screening for prostate cancer (UKNSC, 2025).

Despite the absence of organised population-based screening programmes in many countries, prostate cancer incidence continues to rise. This suggests widespread opportunistic screening. Denmark offers a clear illustration. Although no national prostate cancer screening programme has ever been implemented, PSA testing in general practice has increased steadily since the mid-1990s (Mukai et al., 2010). Part of this increase has been driven by clinical guidelines that, until recently, recommended PSA testing in men presenting with lower urinary tract symptoms (LUTS), such as difficulty initiating urination, weak stream, nocturia, or a sense of incomplete bladder emptying—symptoms that are extremely common and largely age-related.

Crucially, there is no association between LUTS and clinically consequential prostate cancer leading to morbidity or death (Østerø í Jákupsstovu & Brodersen, 2018).

Given that most older men experience some degree of LUTS, PSA testing in this context effectively functions as screening (Ilic et al., 2013). Thus, there is a higher risk for men with LUTS being overdiagnosed with prostate cancer compared to men who do have LUTS (Østerø í Jákupsstovu & Brodersen, 2018; Widding et al., 2025).

More gentle treatment

Screening may allow disease to be detected at an earlier stage, when treatment can be less invasive. Localised cancers may require less extensive surgery or shorter courses of chemotherapy than advanced disease. Similarly, abdominal aortic aneurysms detected through screening are typically smaller and may be managed more conservatively than those detected after rupture or symptoms. However, as illustrated in the screening cascade (Figure 4.1), only some screen-detected cases benefit from gentler treatment. Any treatment offered to overdiagnosed individuals, regardless of how conservative, is by definition overtreatment and constitutes harm.

Reduced incidence of disease

When screening targets precursors or risk factors, it may theoretically reduce disease incidence. Evidence for such effects varies substantially between screening programmes. There is low-quality evidence that cervical cancer, where the goal is to identify abnormal cells on the cervix that may be precursors to cervical cancer, incidence is reduced through screening (Peirson et al., 2013). The same outcome is found in high-quality evidence showing that sigmoidoscopy screening reduces the incidence of colorectal cancer by removing pre-cancer polyps (Jodal et al., 2019). By contrast, screening for cardiovascular risk factors has not been shown to reduce disease incidence, morbidity, or mortality (Krogsbøll et al., 2019; Jørgensen et al., 2024).

Reduced morbidity

Screening may reduce morbidity either indirectly through gentler treatment or reduced incidence, or directly, by preventing irreversible harm. Newborn screening for phenylketonuria is a classic example: varying between countries, the newborn is screened for approximately 18 different congenital diseases, one of these being phenylketonuria (congenital disease where a specific enzyme is missing). If phenylketonuria is diagnosed in the first days of life, it allows for dietary treatment that prevents severe intellectual disability and severe brain damage.

Another example is screening for diabetic retinopathy, which aims not to reduce mortality but to prevent vision loss and blindness among patients with diabetes. This programme is widely regarded as effective, with benefits outweighing harms, and is cost-saving for both individuals and society.

Unintended harmful effects of screening

We refer to the harmful effects of screening as *unintended* because none of the actors involved in screening be it clinicians, researchers, policymakers, or screening participants intends to cause harm. On the contrary, screening thresholds are typically set with the explicit aim of minimising false positive and false negative results. Nevertheless, harm is an inherent feature of screening, not an accident, and cannot be eliminated without also eliminating potential benefits. In the following, we outline the major unintended harms of screening and explain how they arise, so that the benefits and harms of screening programmes can be meaningfully weighed.

False negative screening results

Screening is a coarse sorting process, and one of its inevitable outcomes is the false negative screening result. A false negative occurs when a screening participant receives a normal (negative) screening result but is later diagnosed with the disease for which they were screened before the next screening round. False negatives can occur for several reasons:

- The disease is present at an early stage, but biological variation means that the screening marker remains below the threshold.
- The disease exists, but the test result is mismeasured or misinterpreted.
- The disease develops rapidly between screening rounds and was not present or detectable at the time of screening.

Individuals who receive a false negative screening result are given a false sense of security. Empirical studies show that when such individuals later receive a diagnosis, they often experience disappointment and anger directed at the screening programme (Danish Health Authority, 2004).

More seriously, false negatives may worsen prognosis. Individuals may delay seeking care when symptoms arise (*patient delay*), and clinicians may be less likely to investigate symptoms aggressively if a recent screening result was normal (*doctor delay*) (Weller et al., 2012; Woloshin et al., 2020). Although difficult to study empirically, both delays are plausible mechanisms through which false negatives may increase harm and healthcare costs. Screening is structurally poor at detecting diseases with rapid progression and poor prognosis, a phenomenon we have described as *bird cancers* in Chapter 1. By contrast, screening preferentially detects slow-growing conditions with good prognosis (*turtle cancers*). This phenomenon, often referred to as *length-time bias*, can create the illusion of benefit when localised-stage disease is detected in large numbers, particularly during the first screening round. For this reason, early and incomplete screening results are unreliable indicators of benefit. Drawing conclusions from prematurely terminated screening trials or from localised-stage detection alone constitutes poor scientific practice and risks overstating benefit while underestimating harm.

False positive screening results

The second false outcome of screening is the false positive result, sometimes described as a *false alarm*. A false positive occurs when a screening participant receives an abnormal screening result but subsequent diagnostic investigations reveal no disease. All participants with abnormal screening results must undergo further diagnostic testing. When these tests rule out disease, the individual is retrospectively identified as having received a false positive screening result. The psychosocial consequences of this process are substantial. A large body of qualitative and quantitative research demonstrates that false positive results in screening for serious diseases such as breast, cervical, lung, and colorectal cancer, as well as abdominal aortic aneurysm cause short-term psychological distress (Brodersen & Thorsen, 2008; Brodersen et al., 2010a, 2010b, 2018b, 2018c; Bond et al., 2012; Damhus et al., 2021b; Malmqvist et al., 2021). Long-term effects have been less studied, but existing evidence suggests that harms may persist for years. In mammography screening, a Danish cohort study showed that women with false positive results experienced worse psychosocial outcomes across multiple domains up to 36 months after screening (Brodersen & Siersma, 2013). A long-term follow-up of the same cohort found persistent negative psychosocial consequences 12–14 years later (Gram et al., 2023c). These women also had increased general practitioner visits for up to seven years after the false positive result (Gram et al., 2024).

Qualitative studies suggest that false positives may alter individuals' sense of bodily vulnerability, producing a chronic perception of being 'at risk'. Some individuals respond by seeking repeated medical reassurance, including more frequent testing and screening (Lindberg et al., 2013). Contrary to common assumptions, false positives do not appear to lead to disengagement from healthcare; instead, they are associated with increased healthcare utilisation (Barton et al., 2001; Lafata et al., 2004; Rasmussen et al., 2014; Jensen et al., 2020; Gram et al., 2024).

Overdiagnosis

As outlined in Chapter 1, overdiagnosis occurs through two mechanisms: *overdetection* and *overdefinition*.

Overdetection

Overdetection occurs when screening identifies pathological conditions that would never become clinically relevant. These findings meet diagnostic criteria but are biologically indolent (see Chapter 1). When individuals with harmless pathological conditions fall above the screening threshold, they receive a 'true' positive test result in a technical sense but are nevertheless overdiagnosed.

Figure 4.5 illustrates the normal distributions of a 'healthy population' and a 'sick population' on an arbitrary scale, assuming that the concepts of healthy and sick are defined by certain criteria. The dotted vertical line is a set threshold for when a screening test is set to be positive (abnormal) or negative (normal). This creates the four possible outcomes for a screening test: true positive, false positive, true negative, and false negative.

Figure 4.5 illustrates the considerable biological variation that exists within what we label as 'healthy' and 'sick' populations. On the arbitrary scale shown, individuals classified as healthy fall between 1 and 8, while those classified as sick fall between 4 and 11. This overlap is not a flaw in the figure; it reflects the biological reality that health and disease are not neatly separated states. If the threshold for a screening test is set at 4, all individuals defined as sick will be detected. However, this comes at a cost: more than half of those classified as healthy will also receive a false positive result. If, on the other hand, the threshold is set at 8, false positives are avoided entirely, but more than half of the sick population will now receive a false negative result.

Figure 4.5 therefore demonstrates a fundamental feature of screening: false positives and false negatives are inseparable. Any choice of threshold inevitably creates both. This helps explain why some screening participants who later develop disease may nevertheless receive a normal (negative) screening result. When the threshold is

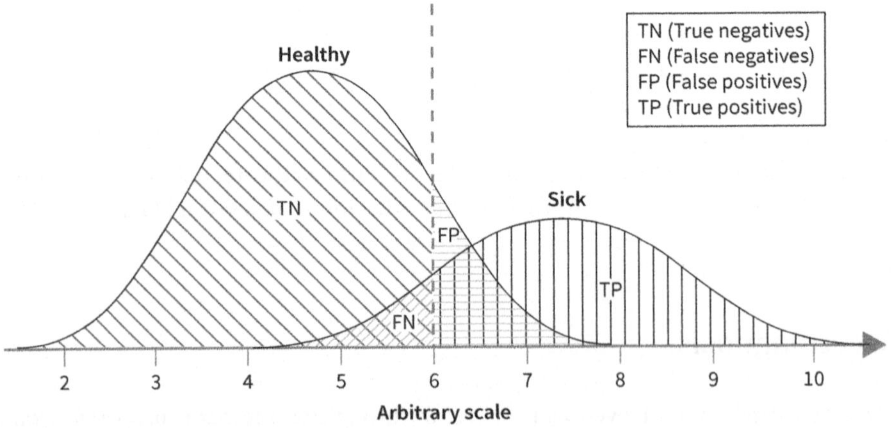

Figure 4.5 The distribution of a 'healthy' and 'sick' population.
Reproduced with permission from Samfundslitteratur.

placed somewhere between 4 and 8, both types of erroneous results occur, and their relative frequency depends entirely on where that threshold is drawn.

Note that Figure 4.5 depicts only two populations: those labelled healthy and those labelled sick. If we also include individuals who carry pathological conditions that will never lead to symptoms or harm, one of the key mechanisms leading to overdetection, the picture becomes more complex. This expanded situation is illustrated in Figure 4.6.

In Figure 4.6 individuals located between 3 and 9 on the horizontal axis all have pathological conditions in their bodies. If we imagine a screening test where the threshold for being classified as sick is set at approximately 6, some of those tested will have pathological conditions who will not be categorised as sick. As a consequence, screening produces not four but six distinct outcomes:

- **True negatives (TN)**: Individuals without pathological conditions who receive a negative test result.
- **False negatives (FN)**: Individuals with pathological conditions that will later develop into disease but who receive a negative test result.
- **'False' negatives (FN*)**: Individuals with pathological conditions that are too small to be detected at the time of screening and that will never progress into disease, and who therefore receive a negative test result.
- **False positives (FP)**: Individuals in whom pathological conditions are detected, but where subsequent diagnostic investigations show that these findings do not represent disease.
- **'True' positives (TP*)**: Individuals in whom pathological conditions are detected and classified as disease, but where these conditions will never lead to symptoms, morbidity, or death.
- **True positives (TP)**: Individuals with pathological conditions that will later develop into disease and who receive a positive test result.

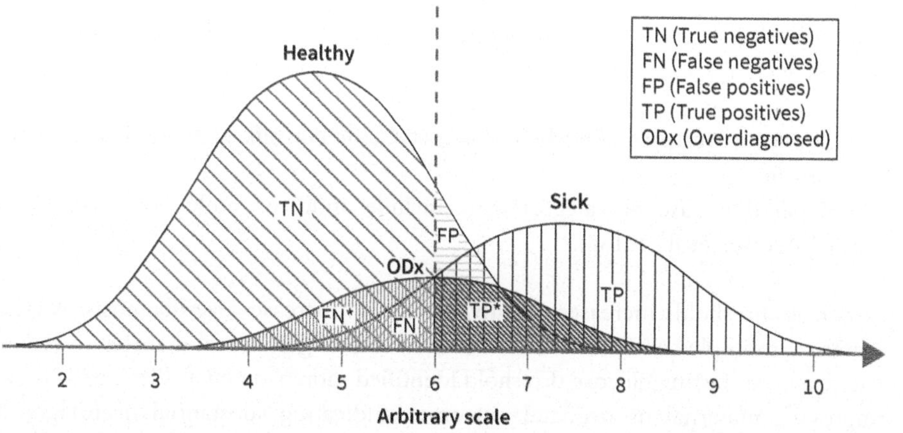

Figure 4.6 Distributions of a 'healthy' population, a population that has harmless pathological conditions in their bodies that can be overdiagnosed ('ODx') and a 'Sick' population.
Reproduced with permission from Samfundslitteratur.

Which individuals fall into each category depends entirely on where the screening threshold is set, illustrated by the dotted vertical line in Figure 4.6.

These six outcomes correspond directly to the expanded 2 × 3 diagnostic table introduced in Chapter 3. In that framework, two of the outcomes, the 'true' positive screening result (TP*) and the 'false' negative screening result (FN*), occur among individuals with harmless pathological conditions. Those in the TP* category are overdiagnosed, while those in the FN* category represent individuals who could have been overdiagnosed had the screening threshold been set lower.

Although the following empirical example is somewhat technical, it provides a clear illustration of overdetection in contemporary screening practice. In a study of women aged 50–69 years undergoing biennial mammography screening, outcomes from a period before the implementation of artificial intelligence (AI) were compared with outcomes after AI was introduced into the screening process. Before AI implementation, all mammograms were double-read by radiologists. After implementation, examinations assessed by AI as likely normal were single-read, while the remaining examinations were read by two radiologists with AI-assisted decision support.

The study found a reduction in false positive results. At the same time, however, there was a marked increase in diagnoses of both carcinoma in situ and invasive breast cancer, without any change in the proportion of node-positive cancers. This pattern suggests an increase in overdiagnosis rather than earlier detection of clinically relevant disease (Lauritzen et al., 2024). We return to this study in Chapter 6, where we discuss in more detail how AI may contribute to overdiagnosis in screening programmes.

Overdefinition

Overdefinition occurs when diagnostic thresholds or disease definitions are expanded without evidence that doing so improves outcomes. This may involve:

- Lowering treatment thresholds or risk-factor cut-offs without demonstrable benefit.
- Expanding disease categories to include mild or ambiguous symptoms (Brodersen et al., 2018a).

Lowering thresholds increases sensitivity but also increases overdiagnosis. A clear empirical example comes from a randomised trial of gestational diabetes screening where a lower fasting glucose threshold identified more women as diseased without improving maternal or neonatal outcomes, indicating substantial overdiagnosis (Hillier et al., 2021).

As discussed in Chapter 3, when overdiagnosis occurs, sensitivity and positive predictive value become misleading metrics. Without knowing how many individuals are overdiagnosed, diagnostic accuracy cannot be meaningfully calculated.

Overtreatment

Most overtreatment arises from poor clinical practice rather than screening. However, all treatment of overdiagnosed individuals is, by definition, overtreatment. These treatments expose individuals to physical harm, psychological distress, and long-term side-effects without the possibility of benefit. We return to overtreatment in detail when discussing specific screening programmes later in this chapter.

Overexamination

Finally, screening inevitably leads to overexamination. All individuals with false positives undergo unnecessary diagnostic procedures, and all overdiagnosed individuals have undergone examinations that would never have been initiated outside a screening context.

At an individual level, false positives can be identified and studied; overdiagnosis cannot. It is impossible to determine, in any given case, whether a diagnosed individual would ever have developed disease. This epistemic asymmetry lies at the heart of screening-related harm.

Patienthood from screening

Screening intends to change the timing of diagnosis. Individuals are identified as patients earlier than they would otherwise have been, or they are diagnosed with conditions that would never have caused symptoms at all. In both cases, screening extends the period of life lived as a patient.

All screening participants who receive a true positive screening result therefore enter patienthood. They become subject to follow-up examinations, surveillance, treatment protocols, and behavioural expectations associated with their diagnosis. This applies regardless of whether the diagnosis is timely, clinically beneficial, or the result of overdiagnosis. From the individual's perspective, the distinction is often unknowable at the time of diagnosis and remains unknowable in many cases throughout life. Those who are overdiagnosed are the most profoundly affected. They may live for decades with a diagnosis of a potentially serious disease that would never have caused them harm. Depending on the screening programme and the age at which screening begins, this may mean living 10, 20, 30, or even 50 years as a patient without any corresponding gain in health or longevity. These years are not neutral. They are often marked by repeated medical appointments, monitoring, anxiety about progression or recurrence, side-effects of treatment, insurance implications, and subtle but persistent changes in self-understanding and life planning.

From a population perspective, the expansion of patienthood through screening is largely invisible in traditional outcome measures. Mortality statistics do not capture years lived under medical surveillance. Survival statistics actively obscure them. Yet from an individual and societal perspective, extended patienthood represents a substantial cost: psychosocial, institutional, and economic, even when screening is well intentioned and technically well executed.

Increased morbidity

In some screening programmes, the screening test itself may cause harm. For example, imaging-based screening exposes participants to ionising radiation. In such cases, screening may directly contribute to increased morbidity. More commonly, however, increased morbidity arises indirectly through the processes set in motion by screening, namely what we have referred to as the screening cascade. This includes overexamination and overtreatment following positive screening findings.

In their original conceptualisation of the screening cascade (Figure 4.1), Harris and colleagues focus primarily on morbidity arising during diagnostic follow-up and treatment (Harris et al., 2015). Less attention is paid to morbidity that may occur after the cascade has formally ended. Yet screening findings whether true or false can have lasting effects on people's behaviour, symptom perception, and healthcare utilisation. A positive screening result may alter how individuals interpret bodily sensations, how readily they seek medical care, and how healthcare professionals subsequently assess and manage their complaints. These effects may be particularly pronounced among individuals who have been overdiagnosed. Several cost and utilisation studies support this concern. Analyses from lung cancer screening with low-dose CT and mammography screening for breast cancer show major increased healthcare utilisation among individuals who received false positive results and among those who were diagnosed through screening, including those likely to have been overdiagnosed (Rasmussen et al., 2014; Jensen et al., 2020; Gram et al., 2024). This increased use of healthcare services can be interpreted as a surrogate measure of increased morbidity. At the same time, it may itself generate additional morbidity through unintended iatrogenic effects, as increased contact with healthcare inevitably entails exposure to further examinations, interventions, and treatments, each carrying its own risks.

As described earlier, false positive screening results are associated with short- and long-term negative psychosocial consequences, which should also be understood as forms of morbidity. In addition, individuals with false positives are, by definition, overexamined. Because no medical examination is entirely risk-free, these individuals may experience complications or late effects from follow-up tests, leading to both short- and long-term harm.

People who are overdiagnosed are exposed to similar risks, but with two important differences. First, overdiagnosed individuals are often treated. Since no medical treatment is without potential adverse effects, overtreatment may lead to additional morbidity, sometimes severe and irreversible. Second, while individuals with false positives can be identified retrospectively, overdiagnosed individuals cannot be distinguished at the individual level from those who have been correctly and beneficially diagnosed.

This distinction has important implications for the evaluation of screening programmes. When screening leads both to more gentle treatment for some and to overdiagnosis with overtreatment for others, scientific trials can usually only capture the net effect on morbidity. It is not possible to disentangle the harms experienced by those who benefit from early treatment from those experienced by individuals who were unnecessarily diagnosed and treated. Moreover, many of the complications and adverse effects associated with treatment occur along a continuum, differing in degree rather than in kind between gentle treatment and overtreatment.

As a result, increased morbidity attributable to screening may be underestimated or obscured in aggregate outcome measures, even when it represents a substantial burden for individuals and healthcare systems alike.

Increased mortality

The most serious unintended harm of medical screening occurs when participation in a screening programme leads to the death of individuals who would otherwise have remained healthy. Some screening tests involve invasive procedures with known, albeit rare, risks. Colonoscopy, for example, is used both as a primary screening test and as a follow-up investigation after positive results from stool-based tests or sigmoidoscopy. Colonoscopy is not without danger. One of its most serious complications is bowel perforation, where the colonoscope or an associated intervention causes a rupture of the bowel wall. Though uncommon, bowel perforation can lead to severe morbidity and, in rare cases, death (Reumkens et al., 2016; Martiny et al., 2024).

Deaths among screening participants who initially received false positive screening results have been documented across several screening programmes. Such cases have been reported in ovarian cancer screening (Tabor et al., 1997), colorectal cancer screening (Reumkens et al., 2016; Martiny et al., 2024), and lung cancer screening (Saghir et al., 2012; Manser et al., 2013; Bonney et al., 2022). In these instances, individuals underwent further diagnostic investigations or treatment based on a suspected disease that was ultimately not present, with fatal consequences.

Psychological pathways may also contribute to mortality, although they are far more difficult to document systematically. A widely cited case report describes a woman who died by suicide after receiving a letter informing her of an abnormal mammography screening result and urging further diagnostic evaluation (Weil & Hawker, 1997). While such reports remain anecdotal and cannot be used to estimate frequency, they nonetheless underscore the profound distress that screening-related uncertainty and fear can provoke.

In prenatal screening, deaths of otherwise healthy foetuses have occurred as a direct consequence of invasive diagnostic procedures such as amniocentesis or chorionic villus sampling, performed following false positive screening results (Tabor et al., 2009). These procedures carry a small but real risk of miscarriage, meaning that screening can lead to the loss of foetal life in cases where no serious abnormality was present.

Finally, mortality related to overtreatment has been documented in screening for abdominal aortic aneurysm. Men who are overdiagnosed with small aneurysms may undergo preventive surgery that carries a risk of perioperative death or fatal postoperative complications (Johansson et al., 2015). In such cases, the harm arises not from the aneurysm itself, but from the intervention prompted by its detection.

Increased insecurity

Several qualitative studies suggest that one of the most important motivations for participating in screening programmes is the desire for reassurance, that is, the wish to be told that one is healthy (Brodersen et al., 2011). Screening is thus often perceived as a way to reduce uncertainty and alleviate latent worries about disease. Yet empirical evidence complicates this assumption. A systematic review shows that among people who are apparently healthy or, more precisely, who have a low pre-test probability of serious disease, screening does not reduce anxiety or worry about being ill (Rolfe & Burton, 2013).

At the population level, perceptions appear more ambiguous. A Danish questionnaire survey conducted in 2007 and repeated in 2012 found that women reported feeling safer when they lived in areas where mammography screening was offered compared to areas without screening (Brodersen et al., 2011; Østerø et al., 2014). However, this finding must be interpreted with caution. A critical limitation of the study is the absence of baseline measurements prior to the introduction of screening, making it impossible to determine whether screening increased feelings of safety or whether women in screened areas already felt more secure to begin with.

Baseline measurements were incorporated into a later Danish questionnaire study embedded within a randomised trial of low-dose CT screening for lung cancer (Rasmussen et al., 2015). This study revealed a different pattern. Across the trial, all participants experienced increased worry and insecurity over time. Notably, this increase was greatest among participants in the control group who were not offered screening. The authors interpreted these findings as indicating that participation in the screening trial itself heightened concern about disease. Screening did not eliminate this concern, but rather redistributed it, with those receiving negative screening results experiencing partial, but not complete, reassurance.

Alas, screening programmes may contribute to the creation or amplification of disease-related concern in the general population. At the same time, screening offers a conditional form of reassurance to those who receive a normal result. This reassurance is neither absolute nor lasting, but it may nonetheless be experienced as meaningful by individuals navigating uncertainty about their health.

Benefits and harms of existing screening programmes

This section reviews the benefits and harms of selected screening programmes based on the best available evidence. It is intended to function as a reference section, allowing readers to consult individual screening programmes selectively rather than sequentially.

As noted earlier, bowel cancer screening reduces disease-specific mortality by approximately 15–30% among adults invited for screening. This proportion represents a *relative risk reduction*. Relative risk reductions, however, are difficult to interpret in isolation, because they do not convey how common death from the disease is in the population being screened. To understand what such a reduction means in practice, it must be accompanied by absolute measures of risk, which denote the number of percentage points by which the risk of a participant dying is reduced.

The effects of screening can be expressed in several ways. It can be reported as relative risk reduction, as absolute risk reduction, and as the number needed to invite to screening (NNIS). NNIS is the number of people who must be invited to prevent one death.

The examples in Box 4.1 illustrate why this distinction matters.

Some studies also report the number needed to screen (NNS). NNIS will always be higher than NNS because not everyone who is invited for screening participates. However, NNIS cannot be converted into NNS by adjusting for participation rates alone. Screening participants differ systematically from non-participants: on average, they have higher educational attainment and income, better baseline health, and are more often non-immigrants; factors that independently influence morbidity and mortality (Brodersen & Lunde, 2002; Hestbech et al., 2011).

Research on the communication of screening outcomes consistently shows that absolute risk reductions either expressed in percentage points or absolute numbers are the least misleading way to present benefits and harms (Woloshin & Schwartz, 2011; Edwards et al., 2013). To allow meaningful comparison, benefits and harms should be presented using the same denominator and follow-up period, for example, outcomes per 1000 people invited for screening over a period of 10 years (Gøtzsche et al., 2009). In the sections that follow, we therefore present the intended benefits and unintended harms of different screening programmes using absolute numbers wherever possible, applying consistent denominators and, when feasible, comparable follow-up periods.

Box 4.1 Three cases: the same relative risk reduction, but very different absolute effects

Case 1

A disease kills two out of every 1000 people aged 50–69 over a 10-year period. Screening reduces mortality from two deaths to one death, with around 80% of those invited for screening participating.

- Relative risk reduction: 50%
- Absolute risk reduction: 1 per 1000 (1‰)
- NNIS: 1000

Case 2

A second disease kills two out of every 100 people over a 10-year period. Screening again reduces mortality from two deaths to one death.

- Relative risk reduction: 50%
- Absolute risk reduction: 1%
- NNIS: 100

Case 3

A third, highly aggressive, disease kills two out of every ten people over a 10-year period. Screening reduces mortality from two deaths to one death.

- Relative risk reduction: 50%
- Absolute risk reduction: 10%
- NNIS: 10

These cases show that relative risk reduction alone tells us very little about how effective a screening programme actually is. Although the relative reduction is identical in all three scenarios, the absolute benefit differs by a factor of 100 between case 1 and case 3.

Our assessment is based on the best available evidence, and is updated on January 2026. For outcomes such as mortality reduction and overdiagnosis, this primarily means systematic reviews that include formal quality assessments of the underlying studies. Where available, Cochrane reviews are prioritised, as they usually apply the most stringent methodological standards. In their absence, we rely on reviews from independent bodies such as the US Preventive Services Task Force, provided that comparable principles for evaluating evidence quality are used.

Estimating overdiagnosis poses particular challenges, as it can be calculated in multiple ways, limiting comparability across studies and screening programmes (Biesheuvel et al., 2007; Bae, 2015; Gulati et al., 2016). Where data permit, we follow Welch and Black's proposal to estimate overdiagnosis as the proportion of screen-detected diagnoses that would never have become clinically relevant (Welch &

Black, 2010). This approach facilitates comparison across screening programmes and offers a meaningful estimate of an individual screening participant's risk of being overdiagnosed.

Bowel cancer: stool sample and endoscopic examination

Broadly speaking, colorectal cancer screening is conducted using either a stool sample or an endoscopic examination. As described above, screening has been shown to reduce bowel cancer mortality by approximately 15–30%, with the lowest effect observed for stool sample-based screening and the highest for colonoscopy-based screening (Hewitson et al., 2007; Holme et al., 2013; Jodal et al., 2019). A relative risk reduction of 15–30% corresponds, in absolute terms, to inviting 10,000 citizens aged 50–69 years to biennial bowel cancer screening over a 10-year period. Assuming a participation rate of approximately 60%, this would prevent between seven and 15 deaths from bowel cancer (Hewitson et al., 2007). Expressed differently, this corresponds to an NNIS of between 667 and 1429 over 10 years to prevent one death of colorectal cancer (Hewitson et al., 2007).

However, there is evidence suggesting that the beneficial effects of stool sample-based screening may be overestimated. In a methodological review of four randomised trials comparing stool sample screening with no screening, several sources of bias were identified (Riboe et al., 2012). Five of the six types of bias detected were found to inflate estimates of mortality reduction, indicating that the evidence base for stool sample screening is less robust than that for colonoscopy-based screening (Riboe et al., 2012).

In contrast, endoscopy screening, particularly once-only sigmoidoscopy, has been shown not only to reduce mortality but also to reduce the incidence of colorectal cancer itself. Approximately one in five cases of bowel cancer can be prevented if individuals aged 60–65 years are invited to undergo a single sigmoidoscopy during their lifetime (Juul et al., 2022).

Regardless of the screening modality used, colorectal cancer screening is associated with substantial overdiagnosis of colon polyps (Kalager et al., 2018). Between 30% and 50% of the general population have colonic or rectal polyps, the vast majority of which are not pre-cancer. Some polyps may even regress spontaneously (Øines et al., 2017; Vleugels et al., 2017). This creates a major potential for overexamination, overtreatment, and overdiagnosis. A concrete illustration can be drawn from the Danish national colorectal cancer screening programme, which uses an immunochemical stool test. In the first screening round, nearly two million citizens were invited, of whom 62.6% participated (Njor et al., 2018). Among participants, 6.9% (approximately 84,000 individuals) received a positive screening result. Almost 90% of these underwent colonoscopy, which revealed the following outcomes: false positive results in 33.7%, low-risk polyps in 18.6%, medium- or high-risk polyps in 32.0%, colorectal cancer in 5.9%, while results were unclassified in 9.8% of cases (Bowel Cancer Screening Database Steering Group, 2020).

A systematic review scrutinised the physical harms of colorectal cancer screening using the PRISMA harms checklist, published in two articles (Kindt et al., 2023; Martiny et al., 2024). The overall conclusion was sobering. The evidence was highly heterogeneous and characterised by substantial limitations in the measurement and reporting of harms. Therefore, the estimates about physical harms are conservative, not only because of the heterogeneity and low quality of the evidence, but also due to underreporting of harms in national quality databases in France and Denmark (Denis et al., 2013; Mikkelsen et al., 2018). Moreover, these underestimated physical harms are poorly reported in systematic reviews, raising concerns about how to evaluate the safety of colorectal cancer screening (Bie et al., 2025).

Meta-analyses suggest that between three and 23 deaths occur per 100,000 individuals screened for colorectal cancer. Cardiopulmonary events could not be reliably quantified due to inadequate reporting, although studies with a critical risk of bias tended to report lower estimates of both deaths and cardiopulmonary complications (Martiny et al., 2024). Across the 89 studies included on bleeding and perforation following sigmoidoscopy or colonoscopy, reporting was generally poor. More than 95% of studies were judged to have a serious or critical risk of bias, and all GRADE assessments were rated as very low (Martiny et al., 2024). Estimated risks of bleeding per 100,000 screened individuals were:

- 8 [2; 24] for sigmoidoscopy
- 229 [129; 408] for colonoscopy following a positive faecal immunochemical test
- 68 [39; 118] for once-only colonoscopy
- 698 [443; 1045] for colonoscopy following any screening test

Corresponding risks of bowel perforation were estimated at 88 [56; 138] per 100,000 for colonoscopy following a faecal immunochemical test, and 53 [25; 112] per 100,000 for once-only colonoscopy (Martiny et al., 2024).[3]

Breast cancer: mammography

Mammography screening has been shown to reduce breast cancer-specific mortality by approximately 15%. In absolute terms, this corresponds to inviting around 2000 women to biennial mammography screening over a 10-year period to prevent one death from breast cancer (Gøtzsche and Jørgensen, 2013). Participation rates are difficult to estimate and vary by country but are typically around 80% (Gøtzsche and Jørgensen, 2013). These estimates are based on evidence from nine randomised trials

[3] Values in brackets indicate 95% confidence intervals.

included in a Cochrane review. However, the estimated benefit depends strongly on the methodological quality of the underlying trials. Of the nine trials, four were assessed as being of high quality, while five were judged to have substantial methodological limitations and a high risk of bias (Gøtzsche and Jørgensen, 2013). When the analysis is restricted to the four high-quality trials, the relative risk reduction falls to approximately 10% and is no longer statistically significant. In plain terms, this means that the highest-quality evidence does not demonstrate a statistically significant reduction in breast cancer mortality from mammography screening. In contrast, analyses based solely on the five lower-quality trials suggest a relative risk reduction of 25% (Gøtzsche and Jørgensen, 2013). There is thus a clear inverse relationship between trial quality and the estimated magnitude of benefit: the lower the methodological quality, the greater the apparent mortality reduction.

Alongside these modest and uncertain benefits, mammography screening is associated with substantial harms. When 2000 women are invited to participate in biennial screening over 10 years, approximately 10 women will be overdiagnosed with breast cancer (Gøtzsche & Jørgensen, 2013). In addition, more than 200 women will receive a false positive screening result. As discussed earlier in the chapter, false positives can lead to substantial psychosocial harms, some of which may persist for many years.

Recent estimates suggest that approximately 25% of breast cancers detected through mammography screening represent overdiagnosis (95% CI: 0.12–0.38) (Voss et al., 2023). In other words, around one in four women diagnosed with breast cancer via screening are diagnosed with a cancer that would never have caused symptoms or death. It is important to emphasise that this figure applies only to screen-detected cancers among apparently healthy women invited on the basis of age alone; it does not include women who undergo mammography because they present with symptoms.

For individual women whose cancers are detected through screening and who are not overdiagnosed, mammography may lead to more conservative treatment. Compared with symptomatic presentation, a higher proportion of screen-detected cancers can be treated with breast-conserving surgery (lumpectomy) rather than mastectomy. However, at the population level, overdiagnosis leads to overtreatment. Overall, mammography screening results in approximately 30% more lumpectomies and 20% more mastectomies than would occur in the absence of screening (Gøtzsche and Jørgensen, 2013). Thus, although treatment may be gentler for some individuals, the net effect of screening is an increase in surgical interventions among women who do not stand to benefit.

Cervical cancer: smear

Evidence on the mortality effects of cervical cancer screening is largely based on non-randomised studies (Peirson et al., 2013). Only one randomised trial exists, and this trial has been subject to substantial criticism due to multiple sources of bias. With these limitations in mind, and based on the best available evidence, cervical cancer screening is estimated to reduce cervical cancer-specific mortality by approximately 35%. The quality of the evidence underlying this estimate is judged to be moderate (Peirson et al., 2013).

Unfortunately, this relative risk reduction has not been converted into absolute numbers by the authors of this systematic review. An assessment of the cervical cancer screening programme from Bristol in England from 1976 to 1996 shows that 1000 women need to be screened for 35 years to avoid one death from cervical cancer (Raffle et al., 2003).

As with colorectal cancer screening based on endoscopic examination, cervical cancer screening also has a primary preventive effect, as it aims to identify and treat a pre-cancer cellular condition. The best available evidence suggests that screening may reduce the incidence of cervical cancer by approximately 65%. However, the quality of this evidence is very low (Peirson et al., 2013), and the estimate should therefore be interpreted with caution.

Cervical cancer screening based on smear testing is associated with substantial overdiagnosis of cellular abnormalities. Again, the evidence base is limited, but the Bristol screening programme provides a concrete example of the scale of this issue. When 1000 women are screened over a 35-year period, approximately 150 will receive a positive (abnormal) screening result (Raffle et al., 2003). Of these women, around 80 will be referred for further gynaecological assessment, and approximately 50 will undergo treatment for presumed cervical cancer or its precursors, most commonly in the form of conisation. A substantial proportion of these treatments are likely to represent overtreatment (Raffle et al., 2003).

Conisation is not a benign procedure. Short-term complications are relatively common: within 30 days of the procedure, bleeding occurs in 2.81% of cases, infections in 0.48%, and additional gynaecological surgery in 3.95% (Aagaard et al., 2025). In the longer term, women who undergo conisation have an almost 15-fold increased risk of cervical stenosis and a two- to threefold increased risk of requiring cervical dilatation. Cervical suturing to control bleeding is rare, but when performed it is associated with a markedly increased risk of both stenosis and subsequent cervical dilatation (Aagaard et al., 2025).

Ovarian cancer: transvaginal ultrasound and blood test

Screening for ovarian cancer using transvaginal ultrasound and/or the CA-125 blood test does not reduce mortality, neither ovarian cancer-specific mortality nor all-cause mortality (Henderson et al., 2018). At the same time, ovarian cancer screening is associated with substantial harm, particularly in the form of overexamination and overtreatment among women who receive false positive screening results (Buys et al., 2011).

When screening raises suspicion of ovarian cancer, women are referred for further diagnostic procedures, most often surgical exploration of the abdominal cavity by laparoscopy. In the PLCO trial, 28,745 women were screened for ovarian cancer. Of these, 3285 women (11.4%) received a false positive screening result. Approximately one-third of these women (1080) subsequently underwent surgery, and many had one ovary removed despite not having ovarian cancer. Among those who underwent surgery, 163 women (15%) experienced at least one serious complication. Thus, ovarian cancer screening exposes large numbers of otherwise healthy women to invasive procedures with a non-trivial risk of harm. In rare cases, iatrogenic deaths following diagnostic surgery have also been reported (Tabor et al., 1997).

Beyond these immediate harms, ovarian cancer screening may also increase mortality. The PLCO ovarian cancer screening substudy found a possible excess ovarian cancer mortality of 18% in the screened group compared to the control group (Buys et al., 2011). Subsequent analyses have suggested that this excess mortality may be explained by overdiagnosis followed by overtreatment, particularly surgical interventions and their complications (Temkin et al., 2017; Henderson et al., 2018).

Supporting this interpretation, the PLCO trial found that 21% more women were diagnosed with ovarian cancer in the screened group than in the control group, despite no reduction in mortality (Buys et al., 2011). This excess incidence is consistent with overdiagnosis. An overview of systematic reviews estimates that approximately 18% of screen-detected ovarian cancers represent overdiagnosis, whereas the proportion is much lower, around 1%, when screening is based on transvaginal ultrasound alone (Voss et al., 2022). However, even this lower estimate does not translate into demonstrable benefit at the population level.

Finally, routine gynaecological examination of apparently healthy, asymptomatic, non-pregnant adult women has also been evaluated as a screening strategy for pelvic malignancies. The best available evidence shows that such examinations do not confer benefit and are instead associated with harm, leading to recommendations against their use for screening purposes (Qaseem et al., 2014).

Lung cancer in heavy smokers: CT scan

A Cochrane review including a meta-analysis of eight randomised trials of low-dose CT screening for lung cancer shows a relative reduction in lung cancer-specific mortality of 21% (Bonney et al., 2022). In absolute terms, this corresponds to approximately seven lung cancer deaths avoided per 1000 heavy smokers screened (Brodersen et al., 2020). Screening intervals varied across the trials: annual, biennial, and other schedules. Screening duration ranged from one to ten years, with mortality follow-up periods of approximately 5–12 years (Bonney et al., 2022). Importantly, none of the eight trials was assessed as having a low risk of bias across all methodological domains (Bonney et al., 2022).

At the same time, screening leads to a substantial degree of overdiagnosis. Approximately 20 out of every 1000 screened individuals will be overdiagnosed with lung cancer (Brodersen et al., 2020). This corresponds to an estimated overdiagnosis proportion of 49%, meaning that for every two individuals diagnosed with lung cancer through CT screening, one is overdiagnosed while the other is correctly diagnosed (Brodersen et al., 2020).

This finding does not suggest that smoking or tobacco use is less dangerous than commonly assumed. Rather, it reflects the fact that heavy smokers are not only at increased risk of lung cancer and chronic obstructive pulmonary disease but also have a markedly elevated risk of dying from cardiovascular diseases, including myocardial infarction and stroke. Consequently, many individuals diagnosed with lung cancer through screening will die from competing causes before the lung cancer becomes symptomatic or life-threatening (see also Chapter 1).

False positives are another prominent harm of CT screening for lung cancer. Reported false positive rates vary widely, ranging from 3% to 23% per screening round in randomised trials (Rasmussen et al., 2020), and reaching nearly 60% per round in an ongoing large-scale screening programme (Kinsinger et al., 2017). In practical terms, this means that at least 150 out of 1000 screened individuals will experience a false positive result after five screening rounds, while as many as 600 may do so after just a single screening round.

Getting a false positive result in CT screening for lung cancer has severe negative psychosocial consequences (Brodersen et al., 2010b; Rasmussen et al., 2020; Damhus et al., 2021a), which can also be seen in the fact that these screening participants subsequently use more healthcare services, presumably as an expression of an increased degree of concern and morbidity (Rasmussen et al., 2014; Jensen et al., 2020).

Taken together, the balance of outcomes in CT screening for lung cancer among heavy smokers can be summarised approximately as follows: for every one lung cancer death avoided, there are around three individuals overdiagnosed and between 21 and 86 individuals who experience a false positive screening result.

Prostate cancer: the prostate-specific antigen blood test

A meta-analysis of five randomised trials shows no reduction in prostate cancer mortality. However, none of these five trials are of high quality. The least-poor-quality randomised trial shows a limited reduction in mortality, with the NNS in 10 years being 1000 to avoid one death (Ilic et al., 2018).

The evidence base for estimating the extent of overdiagnosis associated with PSA screening is likewise of low to moderate quality. A major methodological challenge is that opportunistic PSA testing occurred in the control groups of the randomised trials (Ilic et al., 2018). Generally, the more opportunistic screening that takes place among the control groups in randomised studies, the more the degree of overdiagnosis attributable to screening is underestimated. This problem is explicitly demonstrated in a meta-analysis of three of the five trials, which nonetheless shows a substantial degree of overdiagnosis despite contamination of the control groups (Ilic et al., 2018).

Across trials, PSA screening increases the incidence of prostate cancer by an average of 39%, with estimates ranging from 13% to 75% (Ilic et al., 2018). Importantly, this variation closely reflects the extent of opportunistic PSA testing in the control groups. In the trial reporting a 75% increase in incidence, only 20% of men in the control group had been PSA-tested at least once (Schröder et al., 2009). By contrast, in the trial reporting only a 13% increase, PSA testing in the control group was substantial with 40% in the first year, rising to 52% by the sixth year (Andriole et al., 2009). This inverse relationship between the observed increase in incidence and the level of opportunistic screening in control groups suggests that the average estimate of 39% overdiagnosis is likely conservative. Under conditions of widespread PSA screening, it is therefore plausible that the incidence of prostate cancer could approach a doubling as a consequence of screening.

There is limited evidence of overtreatment as a result of prostate cancer screening with the blood test PSA (Heleno et al., 2013; Ilic et al., 2018). Using the best available evidence and modelling studies, it is estimated that when 1000 men are PSA screened and followed for 10 years, one man will be hospitalised due to bacteria in the blood (sepsis), three will experience urinary incontinence requiring treatment, and 25 experience erectile dysfunction (impotence) (Ilic et al., 2018).

Evidence from settings without organised PSA screening further illustrates the harms of widespread testing. In Denmark, where no national PSA screening programme exists, substantial variation has been documented in PSA testing practices across general practices (Hjertholm et al., 2015) (see also Chapter 1). Comparing men registered with general practices in the highest quartile of PSA testing with those in the lowest quartile, Hjertholm and colleagues found no differences in prostate cancer-specific mortality or all-cause mortality and a small statistically non-significant reduction in prostate cancer-specific mortality. However, they observed markedly higher rates of prostate biopsies, prostatectomies, and radiotherapy in the high-testing practices. These practices also had a higher incidence of localised prostate cancer, increased survival rates, and no reduction in advanced-stage disease (Hjertholm et al., 2015). Another Danish cohort study concludes that data from the death registry is prone to misclassification, potentially overestimating the proportion of deaths from prostate cancer (Nguyen-Nielsen et al., 2019). If this also applies to Hjertholm et al.'s data, then the above-mentioned non-statistically significant reduction in prostate-specific mortality may also disappear.

Thyroid cancer: ultrasound

Screening for thyroid cancer can be performed in at least three ways: by ultrasound examination of the neck, by clinical examination (palpation) of the thyroid gland, or through blood tests assessing thyroid function. A systematic review conducted by the US Preventive Services Task Force (USPSTF) found no evidence that any of these screening approaches confers a beneficial effect on mortality or morbidity

(Bibbins-Domingo et al., 2017). At the same time, the review identified low-quality evidence suggesting that thyroid cancer screening is associated with a substantial risk of overdiagnosis.

Observational 'ecological' data from several countries provide compelling evidence that opportunistic screening for thyroid cancer leads to marked overdiagnosis (Park et al., 2016). South Korea offers the clearest illustration of this phenomenon. From 1999 to 2008, the incidence of thyroid cancer increased 6.4-fold, a development widely described as an epidemic (Ahn et al., 2014; Park et al., 2016). This dramatic rise was not driven by changes in disease biology, but rather by the widespread introduction of ultrasound technology into routine clinical practice. As physicians increasingly examined the thyroid glands of apparently healthy individuals using ultrasound, large numbers of small, indolent thyroid cancers were detected. Importantly, thyroid cancer mortality in South Korea remained essentially unchanged throughout this period (Ahn et al., 2014; Park et al., 2016). Subsequent registry data show that the elevated incidence has persisted beyond 2008, with no corresponding decline in mortality (Ahn et al., 2014; Park et al., 2016; Li et al., 2020).

International comparisons further underscore the role of screening practices in shaping thyroid cancer epidemiology. The estimated proportion of thyroid cancer diagnoses attributable to overdiagnosis varies widely between countries, reflecting differences in opportunistic screening and diagnostic management of thyroid-related symptoms (Vaccarella et al., 2016; Li et al., 2020; Hueber et al., 2023). In countries such as South Korea, Belarus, China, Italy, Croatia, Slovakia, and France, listed here in order of highest estimated overdiagnosis, between 83% and 93% of thyroid cancer diagnoses are estimated to represent overdiagnosis (Li et al., 2020). In contrast, lower but still substantial proportions, ranging from 44% to 66%, have been estimated in Thailand, Japan, the UK, Ireland, Norway, and Denmark (Li et al., 2020).

Notably, none of the population-based registry studies examining thyroid cancer trends show evidence that the extent of overdiagnosis is declining (Ahn et al., 2014; Park et al., 2016; Vaccarella et al., 2016; Li et al., 2020). The most recent data included in these analyses extend to 2012. It remains possible that overdiagnosis rates have decreased more recently, as awareness of the problem has grown and international organisations, including WHO, have begun to advise against opportunistic screening for thyroid cancer. However, robust empirical evidence to support such a shift is currently lacking.

Abdominal aortic aneurysm: ultrasound

Screening for abdominal aortic aneurysm (AAA) has been shown in a systematic review to reduce mortality related to ruptured aneurysms by 35%, based on a meta-analysis of four randomised trials (Guirguis-Blake et al., 2019). In absolute terms, this corresponds to an absolute risk reduction of 0.3%, meaning that approximately 30 men avoid death from AAA when 10,000 men are invited for screening and followed for 13–15 years (Johansson et al., 2018; Guirguis-Blake et al., 2019).

However, the underlying trials show substantial heterogeneity, with reported mortality reductions ranging from 8% to 63%. This variation weakens confidence in the pooled estimate. In addition, these trials are now 20–30 years old. Over the same period, the incidence of AAA has declined by more than 70%, largely attributed to reduced smoking prevalence (Svensjö et al., 2011; Darwood et al., 2012). For this reason, it was no surprise that a large Swedish study conducted after the introduction of national AAA screening was unable to replicate the earlier mortality reductions. In this study, the estimated mortality reduction was reduced by 93% and was no longer statistically significant (Johansson et al., 2018). In absolute terms, two AAA-related deaths were avoided per 10,000 men invited for screening over a 6-year follow-up period. One of the four original randomised trials (the UK MASS study) reported sufficient data to estimate overdiagnosis (Thompson et al., 2012). In this trial, 44% of screen-detected AAAs were estimated to be overdiagnosed, corresponding to 176 men per 10,000 invited over 13 years (Johansson et al., 2015, 2018). In the Swedish programme, the sharp decline in AAA incidence was accompanied by a 79% reduction in overdiagnosis. Nevertheless, this still equated to 37 men being overdiagnosed per 10,000 invited (Johansson et al., 2018).

As discussed in Chapter 1, overdiagnosis is highly sensitive to diagnostic and treatment thresholds. In AAA screening, vascular surgeons have debated lowering the diagnostic threshold from the current ≥30 mm to 25 mm, prompted by concerns that some men with diameters between 25 and 29 mm may receive false negative screening results and later experience rupture (Johansson et al., 2015). However, lowering the threshold inevitably increases overdiagnosis nearly exponentially. In the MASS study, overdiagnosis varied markedly by aneurysm size (diameter found in screening; Johansson et al., 2015):

- 25–29 mm: 87% overdiagnosis
- 30–39 mm: 56% overdiagnosis
- 40–54 mm: 34% overdiagnosis
- ≥55 mm: 17% overdiagnosis

The overall degree of overdiagnosis with a lower threshold would therefore exceed 44%, although the precise figure is difficult to estimate given the declining incidence of AAA.

Screening also increases the number of surgical interventions. A meta-analysis of five randomised trials shows a 44% increase in aneurysm surgeries following screening[4] (Johansson et al., 2015; Johansson et al., 2018). In absolute terms, this

[4] Scheduled aneurysm surgeries performed preventively increase by 75% and emergency aneurysm surgeries performed when the aneurysm has ruptured are reduced by 33% (Guirguis-Blake et al., 2019), resulting in 44% more aneurysm surgeries overall.

corresponds to 37 of the 176 overdiagnosed men undergoing unnecessary preventive surgery per 10,000 invited. Preventive AAA surgery carries a mortality risk of 4–5%, implying that one to two men die as a direct consequence of unnecessary treatment (Johansson et al., 2015).

Data from ongoing screening programmes further show that 59% of men treated with endovascular vascular prostheses (surgery) had aneurysms smaller than 55 mm, the threshold below which surgery is known to do more harm than good (Johansson et al., 2015). Some of these men are therefore both overdiagnosed and overtreated.

Beyond surgical risks, being diagnosed, whether correctly or not, with AAA has substantial psychosocial consequences. Qualitative and quantitative studies show that receiving an AAA diagnosis through screening often produces ambivalent and negative psychosocial effects, consistent with the labelling effect described in Chapter 3 (Hansson et al., 2012; Brodersen et al., 2018c; Damhus et al., 2021b).

The ratio between deaths avoided and cases of overdiagnosis has worsened markedly over time. In the original randomised trials, the ratio was approximately 30 deaths avoided to 176 overdiagnoses (1:6). In the Swedish screening programme, the ratio was 2 deaths avoided to 37 overdiagnoses (1:19). This threefold deterioration illustrates a broader principle: when the incidence of a screened disease declines, both benefits and harms decrease in absolute terms, but benefits tend to decline more rapidly than harms. As a result, the balance between benefits and harms becomes increasingly unfavourable.

Summary

As this chapter has demonstrated, the beneficial effects of screening are not always commensurable with its unintended harms. Some outcomes such as mortality, disease incidence, and treatment rates can, in principle, be compared using quantitative methods grounded in utilitarian reasoning. From this perspective, benefits and harms may be weighed against one another using population-level calculations. However, from other ethical standpoints, such comparisons become deeply problematic. It is not self-evident that a death avoided through screening can be ethically equated with a death caused iatrogenically in an apparently healthy individual who has been overdiagnosed or harmed following a false positive result. Ethical frameworks such as deontology, and principles such as *primum non nocere* (first, do no harm), resist such trade-offs.

Moreover, many of the consequences of screening are not directly comparable at all. Outcomes such as patienthood, false negatives and false positives, overdiagnosis, overexamination, and increased anxiety do not lend themselves to simple mathematical balancing. They differ not only in magnitude, but in kind. Weighing the benefits and harms of screening therefore requires more than numerical comparison; it demands an understanding of what each outcome entails and how probabilities translate into lived experience.

In practice, this balancing must occur on two levels. At the societal level, decisions about implementing, continuing, or withdrawing screening programmes involve collective judgements about acceptable harm, resource use, and public values. At the individual level, invited citizens are asked to make sense of probabilistic information and to decide whether the potential benefits of participation outweigh the possible harms in their own lives. Recognising this dual responsibility is essential to any ethically defensible approach to medical screening.

5
Risk and prevention

Should Matthew be worried?

Matthew is attending a wedding reception. By his table, one of the guests produces a small device, straps it around his wrist, and notes down a number in a pocket notebook. When asked, he explains that it is a blood pressure monitor that allows him to keep track of his blood pressure throughout the day. The device quickly becomes a topic of curiosity around the table, and later several guests, including Matthew, take turns trying it. Matthew, who is 37 years old, works as a primary school teacher. Like many of his colleagues, he has felt under considerable pressure in recent years, not least because pupils are expected to 'catch up' academically after the COVID-19 pandemic. When the device flashes red on his wrist, signalling elevated blood pressure, he laughs it off. Stress comes with the job, he says, and everyone nods in agreement. Later that evening, however, the moment lingers. At home, Matthew and his wife talk about the reading, and they agree that he should contact his GP. He expects reassurance, perhaps even dismissal. Instead, the GP takes his concerns seriously. She asks about family history: have any close relatives had heart disease or blood clots? And she asks about headaches, stress, sleep. Matthew explains that two of his uncles died from heart-related blood clots, that he sometimes experiences severe headaches requiring painkillers and rest, and that work has felt relentless. Before drawing conclusions, the GP sends him home with a National Health Service (NHS)-issued blood pressure monitor and asks him to measure his blood pressure three times a day for three days. Matthew feels uneasy. When he tells his wife about the monitor, she becomes anxious too. The first reading is high. With that, thoughts of his uncles' illnesses and deaths intrude. By the second reading, his blood pressure is higher still. Now he is frightened. Will his children grow up without a father? His wife tries to calm him. 'Prevention is better than cure', she says. 'Let's wait and see what the doctor says.'

At the follow-up appointment, Matthew admits that he has taken far more measurements than agreed. His readings, he says, seemed to rise the more he measured. He also tells the GP that he has been worried, sleeping badly, and feeling increasingly on edge since the initial consultation. The GP explains that home measurements can be misleading, particularly when anxiety is high. Instead, she refers him for 24-hour ambulatory blood pressure monitoring at the local NHS hospital. Matthew is fitted with a cuff around his upper arm connected to a small portable device that records his blood pressure every 15 minutes over a full day and night. He can feel the cuff inflate, but he cannot see the readings. When he returns the device, the results show that his blood pressure is entirely within the normal range, following a typical circadian pattern: slightly lower at night, higher during the day. 'So, I won't have a blood clot tomorrow?' Matthew asks, relieved. 'Well, no one can know for sure, but it's highly unlikely' the GP replies. Matthew is confused again. The GP explains that risk is never absolute. Everyone is at risk of different conditions at different times, and the task is not to eliminate risk entirely, because that is impossible, but to manage it sensibly. She advises him to reduce stress where he can and reassures him that, at present, no treatment is needed. Matthew leaves with a lingering sense of uncertainty. Is he at risk after all? He and his wife decide to buy a blood pressure monitor of their own. That way, they reason, they can keep an eye on things themselves and perhaps prevent something serious from happening. What Matthew and his wife do not realise is that many blood pressure monitors available for private purchase are poorly validated and can produce inaccurate readings. Nor do they fully appreciate that uncertainty and risk are inescapable features of human life, and that no amount of monitoring can guarantee freedom from disease or a long life. What this form of self-monitoring does offer, however, is a heightened risk of overdiagnosis, particularly when technologies designed for clinical contexts are used repeatedly by healthy individuals. Such devices are sensitive to fluctuations that have little or no clinical significance, yet can nevertheless trigger anxiety, medical consultations, and further testing.

In this chapter, we place overdiagnosis within the broader landscape of risk management, prevention, and self-monitoring among people who are, by clinical standards, healthy.

Managing risk

Uncertainty is an inherent part of human life, yet man has always sought explanations and solutions. Visiting a classic example from the Azande people in English anthropologist E.E. Evans-Pritchard's book *Witchcraft, oracles and magic among the Azande* can illustrate how uncertainty is both accepted and constantly navigated. The 1937 book describes how misfortune is explained through witchcraft and magic. If a group of Azande sit beneath a wooden shade structure and it collapses, killing those underneath, the event is understood through magic and fate. Still, the Azande recognise the rationality of these common occurrences: that termites have gnawed on the tree, causing it to crack, and that people often seek shade beneath the structure. What calls for explanation, however, is why *this* particular structure collapsed at *this* particular moment, with *these* particular people beneath it (Evans-Pritchard, 1976 [1937], p. 22f.). Much of Azande social life has been transformed through colonisation and civil war since the book was first published, but the example illustrates a persistent human concern: that explanation is not only about understanding misfortune, but also about locating points of intervention and possibilities for action. What is historically specific, however, is the modern concept of *risk* itself. As Lock and Nguyen note, the notion of 'being at risk' is epistemologically a product of late modernity, profoundly shaping how we think about, and try to control, risk today (Lock and Nguyen, 2018 [2010], p. 267).

In healthcare, managing risk in an individual is about monitoring or even treating risks for diseases, but at the population level, categorisation of individuals into 'risk groups' has become a central feature. Such groups are typically defined either by the risk individuals are thought to pose to themselves, for instance through behaviours associated with future illness such as smoking, by specific traits such as 'old age' or having particular genes, or by the risk they may pose to others, for example through transmitting infectious disease (Lupton, 1995; Petersen & Lupton, 1996). Once identified, these groups often become the target of public health interventions. These interventions increasingly rely on emotionally resonant messaging to encourage such change (Lupton, 2013). Rather than moralising or blaming, such campaigns often appeal to care, relationships, and everyday aspirations. An international example can be found in the US Centers for Disease Control and Prevention's long-running *Tips from former smokers* campaign. Rather than relying on abstract risk statistics, the campaign features former smokers describing how smoking has altered their everyday lives and relationships. One participant states: 'I wish I had quit sooner', while others focus on the loss of ordinary pleasures such as breathing easily, eating, or playing with their children (CDC, 2012; McAfee et al., 2013). The campaign deliberately mobilises emotional identification and embodied experience, framing smoking cessation as a way to regain everyday life rather than merely avoid future disease. Risk, in this sense, is communicated not only as a biomedical probability, but as a moral and relational concern.

When individuals worry about risk of disease, it not only creates uncertainty about how we should behave but also uncertainty about our very existence (Steffen et al., 2005). Political philosopher François Ewald has argued that modern risk thinking reflects a radical shift in how responsibility, time, and fate are understood. In increasingly secular societies, risk replaces providence: 'in a world without God, all control is left to man himself' (Ewald, 1991, p. 208, our translation). Risk thus becomes something to be managed, anticipated, and governed. In that sense, risk management has moved into the everyday life sphere, 'embedded in routine decisions about how to live' as German sociologist, known for his theories on risk, Ulrich Bech has described (Beck, 1997, p. 135). American anthropologist Mary Douglas similarly observed that risk has been transformed from a condition of unavoidable danger into a supposedly neutral, technical concept amenable to scientific calculation and prevention (Douglas, 1992). In this framing, being *at risk* becomes a state in its own right, neither sick nor healthy, but suspended between the two, and this translates into health through everyday mundane practices: 'Health promotion encourages people to view their everyday habits—eating, exercise, sleep—as sites of constant self-surveillance and moral responsibility' (Lupton, 1995, p. 63).

This lived experience of risk is seldom at the tip of the tongue in everyday conversations; however, when asked directly, most people can access whether they see themselves at risk and to what degree, and how they potentially try to manage the perceived risk. Here, diagnosis plays an important but dark role in blurring—even when unharmful or not severe disease is detected—the way that one understands one's state of risk. In an interview study of Norwegians diagnosed with high cholesterol, one man described his situation as follows: 'I am not sick, but one day it may become a disease. I have a threat of illness hanging over me' (Anderssen, 2000, p. 88, our translation). Others described how they attempted to manage risk through small, routine actions. As one participant put it, 'I take the stairs instead of the lift and go for a walk every evening, just small things, but it feels like I'm doing something' (Steffen et al., 2005, p. 21). Such practices do not eliminate uncertainty, but they create a sense of agency in the face of it. Being 'at risk' thus came to be understood as a position between health and illness. In Anderssen's study, older participants emphasised that this state was unstable: if they failed to 'follow the doctor's orders', they believed they would eventually become ill. In this way, the doctor, or more broadly, the medical profession is endowed with the capacity to intervene in what might otherwise be experienced as silent dangers. As anthropologist Susan Whyte has argued, people act not to remove uncertainty, but to render it tolerable and morally manageable (Whyte, 1997). Within this framework, biomedicine presents itself as capable of controlling both body and mind. Yet, as with all efforts to manage uncertainty, such attempts often generate new forms of uncertainty in the process (Steffen et al., 2005, p. 17). In this context, risks are no longer primarily associated with external dangers or accidents, but are increasingly produced through technological and scientific advances themselves. This includes the proliferation of self-monitoring technologies that allow individuals to measure bodily indicators and calculate their own risk profiles. As we will see later in this chapter, such technologies promise control and reassurance, yet often generate new forms of uncertainty, anxiety, and overdiagnosis in the process.

Risk perceptions

Ulrich Beck famously characterised late modern societies as *risk societies*, in which risk becomes a dominant organising principle of social life. In this formulation, the risk society begins where nature ends: risks are no longer understood primarily as accidents or external dangers, but as phenomena produced through human activity and technological development (Beck, 1997). In health contexts, this includes an expanding array of biomedical technologies, among them self-monitoring devices that allow individuals to measure bodily indicators and translate them into assessments of personal risk. We return to these technologies later in the chapter. With health, understandings of risk are socially embedded. They are shaped by health cultures, institutional practices, and broader societal preoccupations with anticipation and prevention, much as Beck describes. For this reason, risk perceptions are analytically important. How a phenomenon is perceived largely determines how the associated risk is assessed, interpreted, and acted upon. Risk only becomes meaningful in everyday life when it is linked to a concrete 'what' and a particular 'who' (Tulloch &

Lupton, 2005). Abstract statements about risk are difficult to grasp, whereas the idea that a father, partner, or close friend might be at risk of a blood clot makes the threat tangible and actionable.

Not all risks, however, can be modified. Genetically determined risks, for example, are largely beyond individual control, raising distinct ethical and existential questions that we return to in Chapter 7. Risk perceptions are therefore closely entangled with social relations and lived contexts, and, as pointed out, risk is not detached from everyday life (as it sometimes appears in Beck's macro-level analyses), but embedded in social networks, biographies, and moral expectations (Jensen et al., 2008).

Risk perceptions are central to overdiagnosis, because they foreground some of the cultural and social drivers that lead to practices of overdetection and overdefinition. And the focus on perception places emphasis on how actors, relationships, and practices give risk its meaning (Tulloch & Lupton, 2005), including medically defined risks and risk groups. But what counts as a medical risk is not fixed, but continuously redefined as scientific knowledge, technologies, and treatment paradigms change, requiring individuals to constantly reassess what they know and how they should act. One example is oestrogen therapy, which was once considered the treatment of choice for osteoporosis. This changed when epidemiological studies demonstrated that the risks of treatment, including an increased likelihood of breast cancer, outweighed its benefits. Individuals, therefore, must repeatedly integrate new and sometimes contradictory knowledge about osteoporosis risk, alongside information about other health risks. The intensified focus on risk also plays a role in self-understanding and identity formation (Reventlow et al., 2006).

Practices and behaviours now widely regarded as risky were not always understood in this way. Once upon a time, smoking tobacco, having high blood cholesterol levels, or driving a car without a seatbelt were not considered to pose a risk to human health, but today these three examples are all categorised and treated as health risks. Smoking, especially, clearly has severe negative health consequences, as demonstrated by epidemiological research, yet it has been practised in various cultures for centuries before being perceived as dangerous (Lupton, 2013, p. 42). This historical shift illustrates how risk is not simply discovered but socially constructed and reinterpreted over time.

Although most of us are socialised from an early age to recognise and manage health-related risks, which Australian sociologist Deborah Lupton refers to as 'risk scenarios' (Lupton, 2013), the uncertainty and shifting definitions of what constitutes risk can make navigation difficult. Psychological research helps explain why. American psychologist Paul Slovic argues that humans rely heavily on emotions when evaluating risk.

Risk perception is shaped by the experimental system, which is an unconscious system of intuition and associations linked to emotions (that something is good or bad). This rapid automatic response has helped humans survive, and here risk is an emotion that tells us whether it is safe to drink smelly water, for example. This system should be seen in conjunction with a rational approach to risk, where we consciously analyse the situation, but studies have shown that an analytical approach does not work without emotional guidance (Slovic et al., 2004). At the same time, emotional responses can harden into preconceptions that are difficult to revise. In the context of medical screening, studies show that pre-existing beliefs strongly shape how individuals interpret information about benefits and harms. Petersen and colleagues describe this as a *perception gap*, which emerges when evidence-based information conflicts with deeply held assumptions (Petersen et al., 2020). When individuals strongly believe that screening can only do good, information about potential harms may be discounted, reinterpreted, or resisted. The individual uses strategies and defence mechanisms to maintain their preconceptions, even if these are contradicted by the evidence presented (Petersen et al., 2020). In a study of women's understanding of information material about cervical cancer screening, the women were asked to reproduce in their own words the material's points about the benefits and harms of screening. In this instance, several of them refrained from mentioning the side-effects of conisation, which had just been described to them but instead added emotional counterarguments. Thus the participants created a greater degree of consistency between what they had read and their perception (Petersen et al., 2020).

Risk perceptions are also influenced by broader health cultures. Within neoliberal health cultures, individuals are expected to act responsibly by monitoring their health, modifying risky behaviours, and participating in preventive interventions such as screening. In this context, it is often biomedicine itself that generates uncertainty through risk estimates, test results, and probabilistic knowledge rather than bodily symptoms or existential concerns. Risk calculations become tools for rendering potential dangers visible and governable (Skolbekken, 1996). This can lead to overdiagnosis, as discussed in Chapters 1, 4, and 6.

Health examinations and interventions that focus on risk states rest on the assumption that knowledge enables control: by knowing one's risk profile, the individual is expected to navigate recommendations, adjust behaviour, and reduce future illness. Yet risk calculations are not truths; they are estimates derived from population-level data, often based on large datasets and statistical modelling (see Chapter 6). What constitutes a risk factor at the population level cannot be straightforwardly translated to the individual level. At the population level, the risk is calculated epidemiologically, where sociodemographic factors such as education level, income, and place of residence, together with lifestyle and what is defined as risk behaviour (e.g. smoking), become key parameters (Risør, 2005). This slippage between population risk and individual meaning is one of the mechanisms through which overdiagnosis can arise.

But risk definitions based on epidemiological research and population-level estimates can also be used as a management tool (Lupton, 2013). Here, risk is dependent on individuals voluntarily acknowledging, accepting and working with their health in the interest of the state. This logic fits well with neoliberal health policies, where responsibility for health is individualised and framed as a moral obligation to avoid becoming a burden on society (see also Chapter 2). Those who do not modify their risk and continue to smoke, not exercise, or perform other preventive actions can be subject to harsh judgement. The prevailing assumption is linear and moralised: risk factors will eventually lead to preventable disease, and some may be met with the implicit or explicit assumption that they are personally responsible for having become ill (Jønsson, 2018).

Prevention plays a central role in this moral economy of risk. Mundane practices such as handwashing have become powerful symbols of infection control, taught from early childhood as acts of responsibility and care. The same applies to brushing teeth and other everyday routines aimed at maintaining health and avoiding unnecessary exposure to danger (Lupton, 2013).

Yet prevention is not merely a private concern; it is also a longstanding state project. Preventive efforts have expanded from targeting specific groups to encompassing entire populations. While the effects of prevention as such fall outside the scope of this book, the preventive practices, especially those centred on risk, can lead to overdiagnosis.

Prevention

Prevention can be understood as a medical strategy that situates itself precisely at the boundary between health and illness. It not only addresses conditions already defined as disease but reaches into people's everyday lives and ordinary ways of being (Risør, 2005). As such, prevention is never merely clinical but operates simultaneously through medical encounters, public health campaigns, media narratives, and political debate.

Although it is often claimed that authoritarian and paternalistic forms of prevention belong to the past, this is easily contested. Contemporary prevention continues to rely heavily on prescriptive language and imperatives (Vallgårda, 2005, p. 24) as health authorities still issue guidance in forms that closely resemble commands. The Australian health authorities write on their website: 'To stay healthy, you should drink plenty of water and eat a wide variety of nutritious foods from the 5 food groups every day' (GOV.AU, 2025). In this sense, the authoritarian dimension of prevention has not disappeared; it has been reformulated. Rather than overt coercion, contemporary prevention often works through implicit influence and self-regulation, aligning closely with neoliberal forms of governmentality in which individuals are encouraged to manage themselves through internalised norms and self-technologies. Vallgårda identifies three particularly striking tendencies in modern prevention. First, there has been a steady expansion in the number of professionals tasked with guiding citizens toward healthier lifestyles. New occupational groups have emerged, and the volume of guidance materials, interventions, and campaigns has increased markedly. Second, prevention has become embedded in a broader health culture characterised by a neoliberal emphasis on individual responsibility. Citizens are increasingly addressed as autonomous decision-makers who are expected to choose correctly. That is, to choose health. Third, preventive messages are often delivered in the form of prescriptions and appeals to fear, particularly fear of illness, disability, and premature death (Vallgårda, 2005). Prevention thus conveys the impression that one should constantly strive for improvement: more health, less risk, fewer signs of bodily imperfection.

Within public health and medicine, prevention is conventionally divided into three types: primary, secondary, and tertiary prevention (see Box 5.1). In addition, general practice and family medicine have proposed a fourth category: quaternary prevention. All four forms of prevention can operate at the level of the individual or at a structural and societal level, or through a combination of both (see Figure 5.1).

Relating to overdiagnosis, primary and secondary prevention are particularly important, as both can involve the identification and management of conditions or risks in people who are otherwise asymptomatic. American paediatrician Barbara Starfield and colleagues have argued that these types of prevention, while intuitively appealing, have increasingly drifted away from its original ethical and clinical grounding (Starfield et al., 2008). Starfield shows how preventive interventions are often implemented without sufficient evidence that benefits outweigh harms, particularly when applied to asymptomatic populations. In such cases, prevention risks expanding medical activity into everyday life in ways that generate overdiagnosis, overtreatment, and unnecessary anxiety rather than improved health outcomes. From this perspective, prevention becomes not inherently benign, but a domain that requires the same critical scrutiny as diagnosis and treatment.

Tertiary prevention, by contrast, is directed at patients with established disease and aims to prevent deterioration, relapse, or complications. Here, a paradox arises in relation to overdiagnosis. For individuals who have been overdiagnosed, tertiary prevention is largely meaningless, since these 'patients' will, by definition, never

Box 5.1 Definitions: types of prevention and their target groups

- **Primary prevention** targets healthy individuals and seeks to reduce or eliminate causes and/or causal factors of disease in order to prevent this disease from occurring.
- **Secondary prevention** targets primarily healthy individuals, but may also include patients screened for diseases other than those they are currently experiencing. It is defined as early disease detection and the main goal is to reduce morbidity and mortality.
- **Tertiary prevention** targets patients and aims to prevent disease progression, exacerbation, or recurrence.
- **Quaternary prevention** targets both healthy individuals and patients, aiming to protect them from medical interventions that do more harm than good, including overmedicalisation, overdiagnosis, overtreatment, and other unintended iatrogenic harms (Brodersen et al., 2014).

	Individual-oriented	Structural
Primary prevention	Talk to a healthy person about their diet, tobacco, alcohol and exercise habits.	Limit car traffic with narrower lanes and promote cycling with wider bike lanes.
Secondary prevention	Advertising a self-pay screening examination, e.g. a general health check.	A population study where a specific target group is invited for screening, e.g. lower colonoscopy (sigmoidoscopy) for all 60-64-year-olds once in a lifetime.
Tertiary prevention	Conversation with a patient diagnosed with a blood clot in the heart about their diet, tobacco, alcohol and exercise habits.	Offer a 12-week exercise program to all patients who have recently been hospitalized with a heart attack.
Quaternary prevention	Conversation with a healthy person about the harm outweighing the benefit of taking low-dose aspirin.	Abolish the system whereby low-dose aspirin can be bought over the counter at the pharmacy, but instead make this medicine prescription-only, so that only patients are prescribed the medicine.

Figure 5.1 Examples of individual-oriented and structural prevention in the four types of prevention.

experience progression or relapse of the condition with which they have been diagnosed. The disease trajectory that tertiary prevention seeks to alter simply does not exist. Nevertheless, many overdiagnosed individuals live with long-term consequences of overtreatment, including physical side-effects and psychosocial burdens. In such cases, evidence-based rehabilitation may be entirely appropriate, even though the original diagnosis was unnecessary. Quaternary prevention explicitly addresses these issues by seeking to protect individuals from excessive or harmful medical intervention. One of its central aims is precisely to prevent overdiagnosis and its downstream consequences.

With prevention, the state, through technologies, seeks to influence the future through interventions in the present (Rose, 2007, p. 18). Preventive strategies are framed as investments in population health, with anticipated benefits that may only become visible over time. As epidemiologist Geoffrey Rose famously observed, the most effective preventive measures often have little perceptible impact at the individual level, even though they may substantially shift risk distributions at the population level (Rose, 1985). Seatbelt legislation provides a classic example: hundreds of thousands of people must wear seatbelts to prevent a single fatality, even though most individuals will never directly experience that benefit.

Yet prevention is never a purely technical exercise. Decisions about which risks to target, which behaviours to modify, and which interventions to promote are shaped by cultural values, political priorities, and assumptions about responsibility. It is within this space where prevention intersects with risk, responsibility, and everyday life that the potential for overdiagnosis becomes particularly salient.

Primary prevention

In primary prevention, strong emphasis on individual responsibility for health shape the priorities of decision-makers who seek to deliver measurable and politically viable preventive initiatives. As a result, societal structures that influence a person's opportunities and choices are rarely taken into account. This seems logical: if the problem of smoking is seen as a consequence of people *choosing* to smoke, and obesity is seen as a result of overeating, then the solution is to educate people about the harmful effects and suggest that they stop. Yet this represents a highly simplified understanding of complex practices such as smoking or eating, reducing them to matters of individual, freely made choice. Unsurprisingly, even large, randomised trials have shown that it is difficult to change individual behaviour in a sustained way at the population level (Speyer et al., 2016; Krogsbøll et al., 2019; Jørgensen et al., 2024). This does not mean that individuals cannot stop smoking or change their diet if they wish to do so. Rather, it highlights that from a population perspective, structural and societal interventions are often more effective.

Smoking prevalence in the Nordic countries provides a clear example of how population-level preventive policies can accompany behavioural change at the societal level. In Sweden, adult smoking rates have fallen from approximately 15% to around 5% over the past 15 years, bringing the country close to the 'smoke-free' threshold much earlier than European targets anticipated (Smokefree Sweden, 2026). Similarly, data from across the Nordic Region show a significant decline in daily smoking overall, from about 15.6% to 9.9% between 2014 and 2024. In Norway, daily smoking has decreased steadily since the late 1990s, reaching roughly 7–8% of adults by 2022 (Fagt et al., 2025). These trends have unfolded alongside smoking bans in public places, advertising restrictions, taxation increases, and other measures designed to de-normalise tobacco use such as graphic depictions of smoking-related diseases on the front of nicotine product packaging.

By contrast, even when individual-level preventive efforts are framed as success stories such as campaigns encouraging people to stop smoking, the responsibility for both action and failure remains firmly located with the individual. This emphasis on personal responsibility is central to understanding why early detection of risk factors and disease has become such a highly valued intervention model in contemporary health systems.

Secondary prevention

In secondary prevention, overdiagnosis arises primarily through the screening of apparently healthy individuals. Despite well-documented harms, including overdiagnosis and overtreatment, new screening programmes continue to be introduced. Some of these programmes are effective, but many do more harm than good. Why, then, are they launched and sustained?

One explanation lies in what has been termed the *popularity paradox*. When the number of diagnosed cancer cases increases while mortality remains unchanged, this does not indicate that more people are suffering from cancer. Rather, it reflects the detection and treatment of small, indolent tumours that would never have caused symptoms or death. The popularity paradox operates by producing visible 'survivors'. These 'survivors' are individuals who appear to have been saved by early detection and treatment. In this way, the healthcare system is publicly affirmed as effective, even when mortality remains unaffected.

This paradox is difficult to grasp, not least because many people are alienated from death and have an understandable fear of severe disease. At the same time, individuals are continuously exposed to secondary prevention campaigns that reiterate the mantra of *early diagnosis*. In such contexts, emotional responses often override epidemiological reasoning. We want to believe that detecting disease earlier prevents progression and death (Damhus et al., 2025) even when the best available evidence shows no, or only minimal, reductions in mortality, as is the case for breast cancer screening (Gøtzsche & Jørgensen, 2013).

The media helps to produce the popularity paradox. When the screening debate rages, stories and interviews with people who have been diagnosed with cancer through screening are presented as 'cancer survivors' and stories proving the salvatory visions of biomedicine, even though this may well be a cancer that would never have caused symptoms or death anyway. By contrast, stories of individuals who die from cancer despite screening attract far less attention and are seldom reported. What circulates publicly, therefore, is not a balanced representation of outcomes, but a selective moral economy of hope.

Government prevention services are, in principle, framed as offers rather than obligations. Not everyone chooses to participate in screening programmes. In Denmark, both the least educated and the most highly educated groups are less likely to attend mammography screening than those in the middle educational strata (von Euler-Chelpin et al., 2008). Whether such non-participation reflects free choice is, however, debatable. Information materials distributed to citizens are not neutral but value-laden and, at times, subtly manipulative (Rahbek et al., 2021). For many lay people, it is difficult to engage meaningfully with information about harms such as overdiagnosis when their prior understanding frames screening as inherently beneficial (Petersen et al., 2020). In some cases, campaigns explicitly target groups underrepresented among screening participants. These initiatives move beyond neutral information, instead functioning as persuasive invitations. Still, not everyone follows recommendations associated with primary prevention, and in some cases this reflects deliberate and considered decisions (Merrild et al., 2016). If prevention strategies are to be meaningful across populations, they must take seriously the diversity of life circumstances and social contexts that shape people's capacity and wish to comply.

Self-monitoring

It can be argued that there is another form of secondary prevention coming from self-monitoring technologies that promise monitoring, prediction, and early detection. We refer to self-monitoring as all digital or other measurement or recording of bodily or mental states, undertaken by individuals themselves and outside formal healthcare settings. Here, individuals consciously and intentionally collect data about themselves in order to interpret that data and say something about, or potentially change, how they live (Lupton, 2016, p. 2).

Self-monitoring is not a new phenomenon. History is filled with collections, numbers, and measurements, all to define what is normal and what is deviant (Beer, 2014). What is new is the scale, speed, and accessibility of such practices. Cheap, portable electronic sensors have made self-monitoring available to large segments of the population. These technologies include wearable devices such as watches worn continuously on the body that measure physiological parameters as well as smartphone-based health applications, often referred to simply as 'health apps'.

For some users, self-monitoring has become a quasi-scientific practice in its own right. The global Quantified Self movement, founded by Gary Wolf and Kevin Kelly under the slogan 'Know yourself by numbers', invites participants to experiment systematically with self-tracking (Quantified Self, 2020). When discussing overdiagnosis, health-oriented self-monitoring oriented towards seemingly healthy people is relevant, where everything from food intake to physical activity is logged in a health app, for example. Here the stated aim is to encourage healthier lifestyles or detect potential health problems through continuous measurement. This may involve sensors that automatically collect bodily data or self-reporting practices in which individuals log food intake, physical activity, sleep, or symptoms in an app. By October 2020, more than 100,000 health apps were available globally, with new ones added daily (European Commission, 2020). The use of such technologies initiated by individuals rather than healthcare professionals has increased markedly, including among young and otherwise healthy people (Mosa et al., 2012; Lupton and Jutel, 2015).

Analytically, health-related self-monitoring can be divided into three broad types, each oriented towards a different purpose (Box 5.2). Other classifications are also possible, for example by distinguishing between monitoring, diagnostic, informational, and therapeutic wearables. For our purposes, however, this tripartite distinction is sufficient.

For many, the performance-related metric can be a welcome motivator. In our research, we have come across men and women of all ages and from all walks of life who use self-monitoring to record, for example, the number of daily steps as a way of reminding themselves to get moving, take the stairs, or walk to the station. Athletes report that they use self-monitoring to engage in a form of competition with themselves to boost performance. Whether the data collected is valid or not is a discussion we will

Box 5.2 Fact: three types of self-monitoring

- **Performance-related self-monitoring**, used to measure parameters such as heart rate, distance, or speed during sports or exercise.
- **Treatment-related self-monitoring**, used in the management of chronic conditions such as diabetes, or to support weight loss through monitoring diet and physical activity.
- **Symptom-related self-monitoring**, used to record bodily functions or sensations such as blood pressure, heart rate, sleep patterns, headaches, or weight among seemingly healthy users in order to detect deviations that may signal disease.

leave for another time, and since performance-related self-monitoring is not related to overdiagnosis, we will not go further into this type of measurement.

Treatment-related self-monitoring may be initiated by healthcare professionals or undertaken independently. Sofie, a young woman who participated in a study of everyday life with mental disorders, described how her psychologist encouraged her to monitor her heart rate and practice breathing exercises during anxiety attacks. This helped her regain control when symptoms escalated. Sofie also used the same device to monitor physical activity and sedentary time, hoping to support weight loss. Daniel, a man in his mid-forties diagnosed with diabetes and stress, invested in a Garmin watch to track physical activity. Combined with dietary changes, he described himself as 'diabetes-free', although stress remained an issue. 'The stress is also monitored,' he explained, 'but that's less useful, because I can feel the stress myself' (unpublished interview data, 2021).

Since the treatment-related branch of self-monitoring focuses on the treatment of already known conditions and diseases, it is less relevant to discuss concerning overdiagnosis.

Detecting risk with self-monitoring

Symptom-related apps and wearables are more problematic from an overdiagnosis perspective. These technologies range from tools that claim to detect depressive symptoms to applications that offer image-based diagnoses of skin lesions. Emily, a woman in her mid-thirties, described how she primarily used her smartwatch to track sleep: 'There are times when I sleep poorly. Sometimes the watch confirms that I've slept badly; other times I'm surprised to see that I've actually slept better than I felt. Then I feel relieved that things are not so bad' (unpublished interview data, 2021)

In Emily's case, self-monitoring provided reassurance. In other cases, however, symptom-related apps promise rapid diagnostics. Some applications ask users to input symptoms, apply algorithmic pattern recognition, and then produce a diagnosis alongside treatment suggestions. Unlike Emily's experience, such apps can easily mis- or overdiagnose, provoke anxiety, prompt unnecessary healthcare consultations, and contribute to overuse and overtreatment.

Unfortunately, many people perceived measures from self-monitoring as credible alternatives to medical diagnostic processes, a perception that is both questionable and risky. Scientifically, many apps are opaque: their algorithms are proprietary, their measurements vary across devices, and their validity is rarely independently assessed (Patel et al., 2015). Consider sleep tracking. For such an app to be meaningful, it must reliably distinguish between light and deep sleep and accurately identify when a person falls asleep and wakes up. Yet even humans themselves cannot always pinpoint these transitions. If an app claims to do so, it is reasonable to ask: according to which definitions, and based on what evidence?

More broadly, self-monitoring technologies rest on implicit assumptions of bodily homogeneity that rarely hold in practice. Bodies age differently, move differently, and respond differently depending on context, life course, and circumstance. Thus, the 'normal variation' is very large in humans. Many algorithms also assume linear improvement, for example, that once exercise begins, it will continue steadily ignoring everyday disruptions such as illness, work pressures, weather, or family obligations. Through these assumptions, symptom-related self-monitoring technologies contribute to a narrower understanding of normality, in which deviation increasingly appears pathological. Yet 'normal values' are statistical constructs, not truths that can be straightforwardly applied to individuals. Several of our current and former interlocutors regularly monitor their blood pressure at home. The question that then arises is simple, but consequential: what happens when a measurement suddenly exceeds what is defined as 'normal'?

Keeping track or installing worry?

While many self-monitoring technologies can be beneficial, they also contribute to a substantial level of anxiety and, in some cases, to overdiagnosis.

In the field of mental health, for example, numerous apps claim to measure symptoms and diagnose conditions such as stress, anxiety, or depression. Although these apps often draw on recognised diagnostic criteria, they risk medicalising ordinary human experiences such as grief, sadness, or periods of emotional strain. Crucially, diagnostic thresholds are operationalised algorithmically, without access to social, relational, or biographical context. Perhaps that is why several apps state, often in small print, that results should be reviewed by a doctor. Yet, as we discuss further in Chapter 7, once knowledge of possible illness or risk has been introduced, it is difficult to neutralise or undo.

When an app raises suspicion of melanoma, depression, or another condition, clinicians may find it difficult to argue against further investigation. A suspicious mole could potentially be more likely to be sent for histopathological analysis; a low mood flagged in a self-monitored app may lead to further assessment of possible depression (Hasse et al., 2023). In this way, algorithmic suspicion may perhaps set clinical processes in motion, even when the initial signal is weak or misleading.

A central problem with self-monitoring technologies is the use of normal values as implicit boundaries between health and disease. These values are often derived from population-level data and do not necessarily correspond to clinically meaningful thresholds at the individual level. When combined with Big Data and artificial intelligence, this problem is amplified. Measurement error is particularly likely when data are generated by apparently healthy individuals, using consumer-grade devices under uncontrolled conditions (Chapter 6). At the population level, such errors may inflate estimates of disease prevalence. At the individual level, they can lead to unnecessary follow-up, treatment, and the long-term consequences of living with an overdiagnosed condition (Chapter 7).

Data generated through self-monitoring rarely remain private. When a measurement deviates from what an individual expects, it can become the reason for contacting a healthcare professional. Such data may also be shared on digital platforms where lay people exchange experiences and collectively interpret numbers. Especially concerning risk perceptions, as described earlier in the chapter, sharing data can help to support not only a sense of being at risk but also that it is good that this risk has been detected through self-monitoring (Lupton, 2012).

Individuals who seek healthcare on the basis of self-generated data such as an anomalous heart rate reading are often described as part of the group known as *the worried well*. These are people who are healthy and socioeconomically privileged, but experience anxiety about their health and struggle to accept reassurance that nothing is wrong. Instead, they may request additional tests or referrals to specialists. The 'worried well' not only consume healthcare resources that might otherwise be allocated to those in greater need (see Chapter 8); they also expose themselves to unnecessary investigations, treatments, and the risks associated with overdiagnosis and overtreatment (Spence, 2016). This does not mean that the worried well should be dismissed or denied care. Rather, it highlights some of the unintended consequences of widespread self-monitoring of bodily functions.

A Danish study provides a striking example. Svendsen et al. (2021) screened people aged 70–90 years for asymptomatic atrial fibrillation defined as a rapid, irregular heart rhythm without symptoms among individuals with hypertension, diabetes, heart failure, or prior stroke. Participants in the intervention group had their heart rhythm continuously monitored for four weeks. If more than six minutes of atrial fibrillation were detected, they were contacted and encouraged to begin blood-thinning medication (anticoagulant treatment). The study detected three times as many cases of atrial fibrillation in the intervention group compared to the control group, leading to a corresponding increase in treatment with anticoagulant treatment. Crucially, however, there was no difference between the groups in terms of clinical outcomes, neither benefits nor harms. The findings indicate a substantial degree of overdiagnosis and, consequently, overtreatment of atrial fibrillation. It clearly demonstrates that seemingly banal forms of heart rhythm monitoring are not neutral or harmless. They can generate overdiagnosis, initiate unnecessary treatment, and ultimately cause harm to individuals, healthcare systems, society, and environment (see also Chapter 1).

The value of numbers

Numbers acquire intrinsic value partly because they are associated with objectivity. A classic example is provided by philosopher Ian Hacking, who describes how the birth weight of a newborn is imbued with meaning that the number itself does not inherently possess. The number, the birth weight, appears on official documents and is shared with family, friends and the workplace. As the weight increases, the difference between the two numbers is a symbol of the child's development. In this way, numbers situate the child within a framework of normality (Hacking, 2002, p. 20).

For patients, numerical values—measurements expressed in numbers—can become a symbolic form of language (Nielsen and Grøn, 2013), or even what has been described as a 'tyranny of numbers' (Kristensen et al., 2022). In people living with asymptomatic conditions, such as high blood pressure, numbers may generate what Danish anthropologist Bjarke Oxlund has termed a numerical ontology. Within such an ontology, numbers become tangible and concrete, shaping how disease is understood, narrated, and lived. Numerical values thus cease to function merely as biomedical parameters and instead become integrated into everyday life (Oxlund, 2012). We suggest that similar mechanisms apply to people who are not (yet) patients but who engage in self-monitoring. When bodily states are translated into numbers, those numbers come to symbolise health and illness. At the same time, they appear modifiable and therefore controllable. This association between numbers and control is central to the appeal of health apps and wearables. Technology becomes a strategy through which individuals seek to prevent illness and suffering by collecting data about themselves (Lupton, 2016, p. 76ff.). Phenomena that are otherwise experienced as diffuse, unstable, or overwhelming: chronic illness, body weight, stress, sleep, mood, medication use, physical activity, hormonal fluctuations, can be rendered legible and manageable through self-monitoring. In this way, numbers promise order where there was previously uncertainty. This sense of control operates not only at the individual level. Self-monitoring is frequently framed through concepts such as patient involvement, empowerment, and self-care. Within this discourse, individuals who self-monitor are seen as acting responsibly and appropriately, becoming what Deborah Lupton has described as 'digitally engaged patients' (Lupton, 2013).

Moreover, self-monitoring is no longer limited to disease or bodily symptoms. As discussed in Chapter 2, biopower has shifted from a primary focus on the body toward human subjectivity (Wahlberg, 2007). New forms of measurement now include self-reported indicators such as quality of life and well-being. As Wahlberg and Rose have argued, when social and personal experiences of illness can be measured and calculated, they become amenable to intervention within neoliberal governance frameworks

(Wahlberg & Rose, 2015). However, numbers are not neutral. They are vulnerable to measurement error, interpretation, and contextual distortion. Psychometric research has repeatedly shown that self-reported data often fails to measure what it claims to measure (Lund et al., 2018; Krogsgaard et al., 2020). Technological self-monitoring is similarly flawed. For example, when a weight-loss app reduces complex physiological and social processes of calorie intake, fat composition, and cholesterol levels into a single numerical output, weight loss is treated as the product of a simple algorithm, despite the fact that the biological mechanisms underlying weight regulation remain poorly understood (Sørensen et al., 2013). At the same time, reference values derived from large epidemiological datasets are not necessarily meaningful at the individual level. Numbers may therefore appear authoritative while failing to correspond to lived bodily experience. This raises a fundamental question for self-monitoring practices: when numbers promise certainty and control, but are themselves uncertain, what and whom should be trusted?

When numerical values become central to how health is understood and experienced, they also begin to structure moral responsibility. In a numerical ontology, numbers do not merely describe bodily states; they demand interpretation and action. A raised value calls for response, monitoring, adjustment, or further investigation. In this way, numbers generate obligations. To ignore a number that signals deviation from what is defined as normal can appear irresponsible, even negligent. This is particularly the case in a neoliberal health culture, where individuals are expected to actively manage risks and optimise their future health. It is here that numerical ontology becomes closely entangled with overdiagnosis. When bodily variation is continuously translated into numerical deviations, the threshold for what counts as a medical problem is lowered. Minor, transient, or clinically inconsequential fluctuations are more easily reclassified as signs of disease or risk. Self-monitoring thus contributes to a situation in which individuals may come to see themselves as patients-in-waiting, obligated to act on numbers that have acquired diagnostic weight despite lacking clear clinical relevance (Timmermans & Buchbinder, 2010). The moral dimension is crucial. Yet, as we argued, acting on numbers does not necessarily lead to better health outcomes. On the contrary, it may expose individuals to unnecessary investigations, treatment, and the long-term consequences of living an overdiagnosed life.

Placebo and nocebo

Self-monitoring and numerical feedback can help individuals make sense of bodily sensations and symptoms (Pink & Fors, 2017). At the same time, such technologies may also undermine trust in embodied experience. When measurements produced by devices are interpreted as signs of risk or disease, individuals may begin to doubt their own sensory knowledge of the body. This dynamic is well illustrated in studies of osteoporosis, where patients describe how seeing scan images comes to replace bodily sensation as the primary explanatory model of their condition (Reventlow, 2008). What is felt in the body becomes secondary to what is seen on the screen. Dutch philosopher Annemarie Mol has shown how medical technologies do more than passively record bodily states. In her work on blood glucose measurement, Mol demonstrates how technology actively intervenes in everyday life, reshaping attention and directing focus away from bodily sensations and towards numerical values (Mol, 2000). Knowledge of the body that is not anchored in symptoms but instead produced through measurement introduces new forms of uncertainty. Individuals come to rely on technology to identify states of illness that they cannot otherwise feel, thereby making the body partially opaque without technological mediation (see also Chapter 7).

In medicine, the terms *placebo* and *nocebo* are used to describe how expectations shape bodily experience. A placebo effect occurs when positive expectations such as trust in a treatment or reassurance from a test result contribute to a perceived or measurable improvement in symptoms. Conversely, a nocebo effect arises when negative expectations, fear, or worry generate or exacerbate symptoms, even in the absence of physiological pathology.

Self-monitoring can have both placebo and nocebo effects. When numbers fall within what is defined as normal, they may generate confidence, security, and satisfaction. Conversely, unexpected or abnormal readings may provoke anxiety, doubt, and heightened bodily vigilance (Hortensius et al., 2012). Kate, a woman with epilepsy, uses sleep-tracking technology to assess her risk of having a seizure. She explains: 'If it says 78% sleep quality last night, that's pretty good for me … It's kind of self-manipulative. I feel like, "okay, I must have slept well, I'm going to have a good day today"' (Smith & Vonthethoff, 2017, p. 18). For Kate, favourable numbers generate reassurance and confidence. At the same time, poor sleep readings can trigger stress and anxiety, particularly because sleep deprivation is known to precipitate seizures. Here, numerical feedback does not merely reflect bodily states; it actively shapes expectations, emotions, and interpretations of risk.

The relationship between self-monitoring and placebo/nocebo effects remains underexplored. It is therefore difficult to assess the long-term health consequences of repeated exposure to worrying or ambiguous numerical feedback. Nevertheless, it is plausible that sustained nocebo responses may contribute to the development of physical or psychological symptoms over time. Such symptoms produced or amplified through anxiety, stress, and hypervigilance may subsequently become objects of medical attention and diagnosis. In this way, self-monitoring may indirectly contribute to overdiagnosis, as distress generated by numbers is reinterpreted as pathology, such as stress-related disorders or depression (Box 5.3).

Box 5.3 Definitions: placebo and nocebo

- **Placebo:** Positive expectations that contribute to perceived or actual improvement.
- **Nocebo:** Negative expectations that contribute to distress or adverse outcomes.

While placebo effects are well documented in medical research, nocebo effects have received less attention. Nocebo responses are typically associated with stress reactions and heightened activation of the amygdala, the brain's alarm system (Lunde, 2009).

Summary

Uncertainty is a fundamental condition of human life. With the rise of epidemiology and the expansion of biomedical knowledge, however, the concept of *risk* has shifted from being one expression of uncertainty to becoming a central object of management and intervention. Risk is no longer merely something one lives with, but something that can be calculated, acted upon, and at least in principle prevented through scientific means.

This shift is particularly visible in preventive medicine. Primary and secondary prevention encourage people to act upon quantified risks in order to avoid future disease. At the same time, the rapid development of medical and digital technologies has expanded the repertoire of risk management practices. Self-monitoring technologies, in particular, make it possible for individuals to continuously measure bodily states, identify deviations from statistical norms, and interpret these deviations as potential signs of illness.

These efforts to control risk are not without consequences. The expansion of screening, testing, and self-monitoring contributes to the identification of new risk groups and risk conditions, often in the absence of symptoms. In this context, overdiagnosis becomes more likely, as harmless bodily variations or transient states are interpreted by algorithms or by individuals themselves as disease. Such processes can generate anxiety, alter self-understanding, and, through mechanisms such as the nocebo effect, contribute to real suffering. Thus, attempts to manage uncertainty through risk-based prevention may paradoxically produce new forms of uncertainty, vulnerability and harm, also in the form of overdiagnosis.

6
Big Data, personalised medicine, and artificial intelligence

In June 2025, the *Telegraph* first reported plans that signal a profound shift in the future direction of the National Health Service (NHS) in the UK: within the next decade, every newborn baby is expected to undergo whole-genome sequencing shortly after birth. Framed as a cornerstone of a new ten-year health strategy, the initiative positions genomics, Big Data, and artificial intelligence (AI) at the heart of a move from reactive medicine towards prediction, prevention, and personalisation. According to government statements at the time, advances in genomic science and AI analytics are intended to enable the health service to anticipate disease risk long before symptoms emerge. By mapping each child's DNA, clinicians would be able to assess susceptibility to hundreds of conditions, paving the way for individualised monitoring, targeted interventions, and preventive treatments. Proponents argue that this approach could replace broad, population-level screening and standardised health checks such as routine measurements of blood pressure or cholesterol with tailored, personalised medicine. The proposed rollout builds on existing NHS pilot programmes that have already sequenced the genomes of up to 100,000 newborns, focusing on rare single-gene disorders that present in early childhood and for which effective treatments exist. Whole-genome sequencing represents a weighty expansion of current newborn screening practices, which rely on a heel-prick blood test to identify a small number of serious but uncommon conditions. In contrast, genomic sequencing produces enduring datasets that can be reanalysed over time as scientific knowledge and predictive algorithms evolve.

The policy illustrates part of a broader reconfiguration of healthcare delivery globally, which emphasises three major shifts: from hospital-based to community-based care; from analogue to digital systems; and from treating illness to preventing it. Alongside genomics, visions include widespread use of AI, predictive analytics, wearable devices, and virtual care platforms, supported by substantial public investment in life sciences and digital infrastructure. Large national genomic databases are expected to underpin this transformation, linking biological data with health records across the life course.

At the same time, the ambition to test all newborns has prompted ethical, social, and practical concerns. While genomic screening may offer life-saving opportunities for early intervention, it also means that children may grow up with probabilistic knowledge about future disease, a form of risk information they did not choose and may never wish to know. The interpretation and communication of such data require specialist expertise, sustained counselling, and careful attention to uncertainty. Questions about consent, data security, and the potential misuse of highly valuable genetic information have also been raised, particularly in light of recent high-profile data breaches in the commercial genomics sector (Høyer, 2023).

This chapter widens the lens to examine the broader landscape in which Big Data, personalised medicine, and AI are taking shape. In contemporary health policy and biomedical research, personalised medicine is frequently presented as a transformative paradigm that promises to match the right intervention to the right individual at the right time. Nowhere is this promise more visible than in oncology, where tailoring treatment to the molecular characteristics of a tumour is often described as a decisive break with standardised, population-based care. Yet the practical reach of such approaches remains more limited than the rhetoric suggests. Even in cancer care, where genomic technologies are most advanced, only a minority of patients are eligible for treatments informed by tumour sequencing, and fewer still benefit from therapies specifically adapted to their genetic profiles (Marquart et al., 2018). This gap between technological ambition and clinical applicability points to a recurring tension within personalised medicine: the expectation that increasingly fine-grained biological data will reliably translate into better outcomes for individuals.

A related assumption underpins much of the enthusiasm for predictive medicine more broadly. By linking large-scale genomic data with electronic health records, researchers and policymakers anticipate being able to identify who is likely to develop particular diseases in the future. While often framed as novel, this aspiration echoes much older ideas about knowledge, data, and prediction. Long before the advent of digital health infrastructures, social theorists argued that systematic data collection could reveal patterns that would allow societies to anticipate and manage future events (Høyer, 2023). What has changed is not the desire to predict, but the scale, speed, and authority now attributed to data-driven correlations. At the same time, a crucial dimension risks being sidelined. Disease does not emerge from genes alone. Behaviour, living conditions, social relations, environmental exposures, and broader structural factors play decisive roles in shaping health and illness. For instance, a Nordic nationwide cohort study from Denmark, Finland, and Sweden found that shared environment was the most important contributor to the heritability of getting colorectal cancer rather than genetic predisposition (Elmahdi et al., 2022). When predictive models privilege biological risk while downplaying these contexts, they risk narrowing the explanatory frame through which disease is understood and acted upon. This narrowing has important implications for prevention. Personalised medicine is often portrayed as enabling earlier and more precise interventions, but it may also expand the boundaries of who is considered at risk, drawing ever more people into regimes of monitoring, testing, and surveillance. In both primary and secondary prevention, such dynamics can contribute to overdiagnosis.

Big Data

When people speak about *Big Data*, they often invoke something abstract or futuristic. At its most basic level, however, the term simply refers to very large quantities of data. In this chapter, Big Data denotes the vast and growing collections of information that are assembled about people's bodies, lives, and behaviours. These data are heterogeneous in form and origin, and they are increasingly combined in ways that blur familiar boundaries between the biological and the biographical.

By *biological data* we refer to information generated from the human body itself. In health care, this includes laboratory values and medical images. This also includes data produced through so-called *omics* technologies, an umbrella term for methods that analyse large numbers of biological molecules, such as DNA, RNA, proteins, or metabolites. Whole-genome sequencing is perhaps the most well-known example, capturing the complete genetic code of an individual: roughly three billion base pairs organised into 23 pairs of chromosomes. In practice, biological Big Data rarely concerns the genome alone. It also encompasses epigenetic markers, patterns of gene expression, protein profiles, microbial compositions, and metabolic signatures, each offering a different window on to bodily processes and potential disease trajectories.

Alongside these molecular forms of data sit what we call *biographical data*: information generated through people's activities, movements, interactions, and institutional encounters (Vogt et al., 2019). In healthcare, this includes clinical notes and diagnostic codes. Beyond the clinic, biographical data are produced continuously through everyday life; depending on location, this could happen through municipalities and welfare systems, banks and insurers, social media platforms, smartphones, smartwatches, fitness trackers, apps, and other digital devices that record behaviour, location, and habits. Increasingly, such data are drawn into health-related analyses, sometimes with the explicit aim of predicting disease, sometimes as a by-product of digital infrastructures never designed with medicine in mind.

Additionally, commercial health data markets have become a quiet but powerful engine of Big Data. Direct-to-consumer DNA tests invite people to purchase genomic knowledge about ancestry, traits, and disease risk while simultaneously converting saliva samples into long-lived research assets that can be aggregated, reanalysed, and traded. This model 'uncouples' the production of health-related genetic data from the clinical encounter, relocating it into consumer marketplaces and platform infrastructures (Eissenberg, 2017). Once collected, genomic and behavioural data can be monetised through partnerships, licensing, and downstream analytics, making health data resemble a commodity whose value grows with scale, linkage, and reuse (Montori et al., 2025). Public attitudes research shows that commercial involvement matters: perceptions of legitimacy, trust, and willingness to share data shift when private actors are positioned as owners or beneficiaries of genomic repositories (Walshe et al., 2024). More broadly, social science analyses argue that digital health is increasingly shaped by 'surveillance capitalisms', where prediction and profit depend on continuous extraction of physiological and behavioural traces—exactly the kinds of traces produced by wearables, apps, and consumer testing (Rubeis, 2023). The commodification dynamic also has consequences for accountability: when corporate control changes (e.g. through mergers, acquisitions, or bankruptcy), the fate of donated data and the meaning of prior consent can become ethically and politically contested (LoTempio et al., 2025). With the commodification of health data, people do not merely contribute to Big Data, they increasingly *buy into it*, helping to expand the datasets that fuel AI risk models, personalised recommendations, and new markets for prediction.

It is tempting to assume that biological data are inherently more precise or trustworthy than biographical data, but this distinction is not as clear-cut as it may seem. Differences in validity and reliability do not follow automatically from whether data are biological or biographical; rather, they depend on why and how the data are produced. Biological data are typically collected for the explicit purpose of examining bodily processes or health states, often using standardised protocols, calibrated instruments, and regulatory quality controls. This does not make them error-free, but it does mean that their limitations are usually well described. Biographical data, by contrast, are often generated for reasons unrelated to health. A smartphone records steps to motivate exercise, a social media platform tracks engagement to optimise advertising, and administrative systems log interactions to manage services. Data collection procedures may be opaque, constantly changing, or poorly documented, and the devices involved may not be subject to formal quality standards. As a result, biographical data can range from highly reliable to deeply uncertain, sometimes within the same dataset.

What matters for Big Data in medicine is not simply the volume of information, but the assumptions made when different data types are combined and interpreted. When biological signals are read alongside behavioural traces and social indicators, the resulting analyses can appear richly detailed and objective. Yet they also inherit the ambiguities, gaps, and biases of their sources. Understanding Big Data, then, requires attention not only to what is measured, but to how data come into being—and to the lives and bodies they claim to represent.

From Big Data to spectrum bias

As health data grows in volume and variety, so too does the confidence placed in tests, algorithms, and predictive tools derived from them. Yet more data does not automatically produce more reliable knowledge. The way data is selected, grouped, and interpreted remains crucial. This brings us to *spectrum bias*, a classic, but increasingly relevant problem that sits at the intersection of diagnostic reasoning and data-driven medicine.

Spectrum bias is a well-established phenomenon in diagnostic research and clinical epidemiology (Ransohoff & Feinstein, 1978). It refers to the distortion that occurs when the apparent accuracy of a diagnostic test depends on the particular mix—or *spectrum*—of health and disease in the population in which the test is evaluated. The concept has long been central to assessing whether a diagnostic test is valid, useful, and appropriate for clinical practice, as well as to the principles of evidence-based medicine (Guyatt et al., 2015). When researchers evaluate a diagnostic test, they compare it against a reference standard; an agreed-upon method that stands in for 'truth'. A group of individuals is selected, all of whom undergo both the test and the reference standard. Measures such as sensitivity, specificity, predictive values, likelihood ratios, and the area under the receiver operating characteristic (ROC) curve are then used to quantify how well the test distinguishes between those with and without the disease (Guyatt et al., 2015). Crucially, these measures do not exist independently of context. They depend on both the reference standard chosen and the characteristics of the population being tested (see also Chapter 3).

The prostate-specific antigen (PSA) test provides a useful illustration. PSA levels tend to be very low in young men without prostate cancer and very high in men with advanced, metastatic prostate cancer. If we compare these two extreme groups of young, healthy men on the one hand, and older men with widely spread prostate cancer on the other, the PSA values form two distributions with very little overlap. In this situation, almost any reasonable threshold will separate the groups effectively. The test appears highly accurate: sensitivity, specificity, and predictive values are all high, and the likelihood ratios indicate a strong capacity both to rule out and to confirm prostate cancer (rule in). Correspondingly, the area under the ROC curve approaches its theoretical maximum, giving the impression of a highly accurate and discriminating diagnostic test (Figure 6.1)

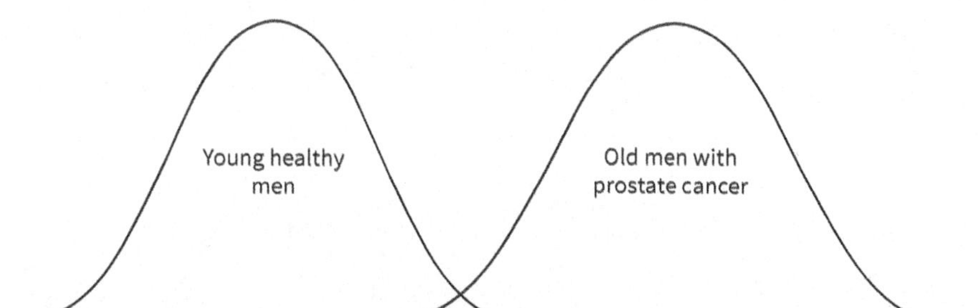

Figure 6.1 Prostate-specific antigen (PSA) levels in different groups of men: young healthy men and older men with prostate cancer, across two normal distribution curves. One curve represents young healthy men with generally low PSA values, while the other represents older men with prostate cancer with higher PSA values. The overlap illustrates that PSA levels alone cannot perfectly distinguish between men with and without prostate cancer.

Reproduced with permission from Samfundslitteratur.

However, this is not the situation clinicians encounter in everyday practice. Prostate cancer is common in older men, but most cases grow slowly and never cause symptoms or death. Many men live their entire lives with neoplastic cells in their prostate gland that meet diagnostic criteria for cancer but remain clinically harmless. If we instead compare men who will never develop prostate cancer with men who at some point are diagnosed with prostate cancer, some of whom will die from it and many of whom will not, the picture changes dramatically. In Figure 6.2, the group of healthy men now consists of men who never get prostate cancer, neither the harmless form nor the disease, and the group of sick men now consists of men who at some point in their lives are diagnosed with prostate cancer because they either develop symptoms of prostate cancer and/or die from prostate cancer (Figure 6.2).

When all men are tested at, say, age 65, PSA levels in these two groups overlap substantially. Where the threshold for a positive test is placed now becomes decisive. A low threshold will identify more men who will eventually develop clinically relevant cancer, but at the cost of many false positives among men who would never be harmed. A high threshold will spare healthy men unnecessary concern but miss many men who will go on to develop serious disease. If we place the threshold value between these two extremes, the diagnostic accuracy of the PSA test will be much less accurate than in Figure 6.1. This discrepancy is the essence of spectrum bias. When diagnostic tests are evaluated in populations with an artificially clear separation between health and disease, their performance appears better than it will be in real-world settings, where health and illness exist on a continuum. In such cases, tests calibrated on narrow or extreme spectra risk producing misleading confidence once they are applied broadly. In the context of Big Data, personalised medicine, and AI-driven diagnostics, spectrum bias becomes especially important: as datasets grow

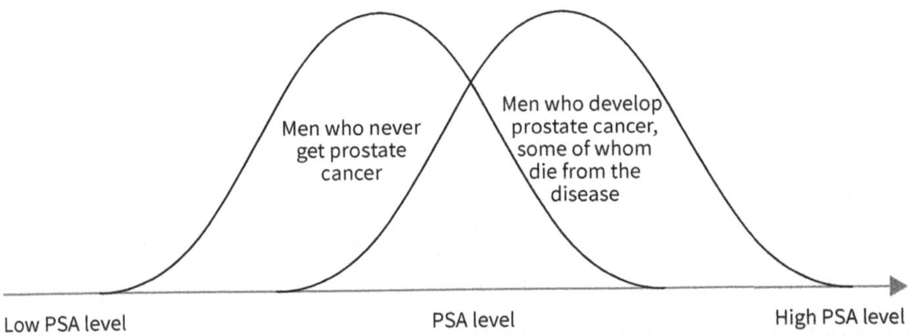

Figure 6.2 Prostate-specific antigen (PSA) levels in men who never develop prostate cancer and men who develop prostate cancer, some of whom die from the disease. One curve represents men who never develop prostate cancer, and the other represents men who will develop prostate cancer, some fatally. The overlap illustrates that PSA levels cannot clearly separate future cancer cases from non-cases.

Reproduced with permission from Samfundslitteratur.

larger, the temptation to overlook how populations are constructed and how disease is defined only increases.

Spectrum bias and overdiagnosis

Spectrum bias, as traditionally described in the clinical and epidemiological literature (see Guyatt et al., 2015; Ransohoff & Feinstein, 1978) rests on a simplified view of disease. Diagnostic test evaluation typically assumes that individuals fall into one of two categories: healthy or sick. This binary logic is built into the familiar 2 × 2 table that underpins calculations of sensitivity, specificity, and related measures of test accuracy (see also Chapter 3, Figure 3.2). What this framework leaves out is the possibility that a third group exists: people who are diagnosed with a condition that would never have caused them harm. When overdiagnosis occurs, the two-category model is no longer sufficient.

To account for this, the diagnostic landscape must be expanded conceptually from a 2 × 2 to a 2 × 3 table (see also Chapter 3, Figure 3.4). Figure 6.3 illustrates this shift by adding a third spectrum to the example introduced earlier: men who are overdiagnosed with prostate cancer. These men are neither clearly healthy nor clearly affected by life-threatening disease. They may receive a diagnosis through screening or as a result of investigations triggered by unrelated symptoms, for instance, lower urinary tract symptoms (LUTS) (see Chapter 4).

When this third group is included, the interpretive challenge becomes apparent. Assuming that all men are tested at the same age, the PSA distributions for healthy men, men with clinically consequential prostate cancer, and men who are overdiagnosed overlap extensively. Only at the very lowest and very highest PSA levels

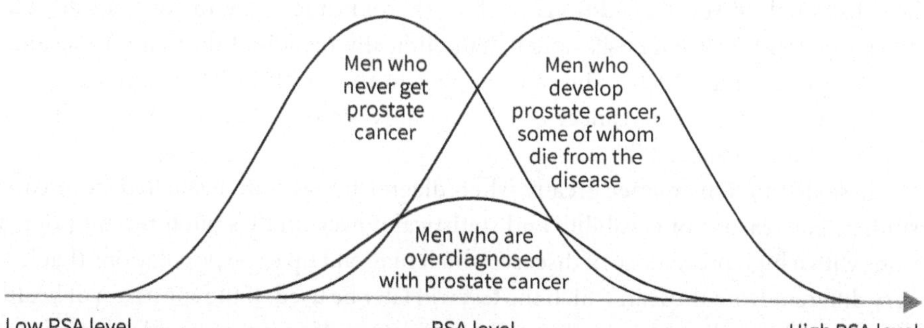

Figure 6.3 Spectrum bias and overdiagnosis.
Diagram with overlapping prostate-specific antigen (PSA) distributions showing three groups: men who never develop prostate cancer, men who develop prostate cancer (some fatally), and men who are overdiagnosed. This illustrates how PSA testing can detect cancers that would never have caused symptoms or harm.
Reproduced with permission from Samfundslitteratur.

can a small proportion of individuals be distinguished with some confidence. A low threshold may separate a fraction of men who will never develop prostate cancer from those who might be overdiagnosed or truly ill. A high threshold may isolate some men with advanced disease from the other two groups. Across most of the PSA range, however, these populations are indistinguishable at the individual level.

This is the crux of the problem: it is not possible to tell, for a given man with an elevated PSA and a cancer diagnosis, whether that diagnosis represents clinically relevant disease or harmless pathology. As Figure 6.3 shows, the distribution of men who are overdiagnosed overlaps almost entirely with both the healthy and the diseased spectra. Advances in data-intensive methods have helped narrow this uncertainty. Multi-parameter tests, such as the Stockholm 3 model developed in Sweden, combine biological markers, clinical variables, and statistical modelling to reduce unnecessary diagnoses (Grönberg et al., 2017). The same applies if magnetic resonance imaging (MRI)-directed targeted biopsy is used in men with abnormal PSA levels detected via screening (Hugosson et al., 2022). These tools can lower the proportion of overdiagnosis, but they cannot eliminate it: neither the Stockholm 3 PSA test, nor the MRI-directed targeted biopsy, can separate exactly the three spectra of men in Figure 6.3 from each other. Thus, as long as screening or diagnostic testing continues, some degree of overdiagnosis remains unavoidable.

The implications of this overlap differ depending on whether testing takes place in a screening or a diagnostic context. In population screening, the vast majority of those tested are healthy. Typically, fewer than one percent of screened individuals are sick or overdiagnosed, meaning that even small imperfections in test performance can translate into large numbers of false positives and overdiagnosis (Brodersen & Jørgensen, 2021). In diagnostic settings, where patients seek care because they have symptoms, the balance shifts. There are relatively more people with genuine disease and fewer who are entirely healthy, but the proportion who may be overdiagnosed can still be substantial. In some conditions, such as thyroid cancer, the majority of detected cases represent overdiagnosis rather than clinically meaningful disease (Vaccarella et al., 2016; Li et al., 2020). The same applies to men with LUTS, where the risk of overdiagnosis of prostate cancer is substantial (Østerø í Jákupsstovu & Brodersen, 2018; Widding et al., 2025).

These distinctions matter greatly when diagnostic tests are evaluated in research studies. For reasons of feasibility and statistical power, studies often recruit populations with a high prevalence of disease, which may end up to be populations that look very different from those in which the test will later be used. If the spectrum of health, disease, and overdiagnosis in the study population does not resemble that of real-world clinical practice, estimates of diagnostic accuracy may be misleading. The issue is not simply how many people in a study are healthy or sick, but whether the full spectrum of disease severity and the possibility of overdiagnosis is represented at all.

Assessing the validity of diagnostic accuracy studies therefore requires asking difficult questions about representativeness. Does the population included in the study reflect the range of health states, disease trajectories, and diagnostic uncertainties that clinicians will encounter? Are individuals who might be overdiagnosed part of the analysis, or are they rendered invisible by a binary framework? In an era of big data and AI-driven diagnostics, these questions become even more pressing, as increasingly sophisticated tools risk amplifying old biases while appearing to offer new precision.

When more data means more error: prediction models, complexity, and overdiagnosis

The promise of big data rests on the idea that more information leads to better predictions. Yet this intuition is only partly true. In prediction modelling, total error is not simply reduced by adding more data, more variables, or more sophisticated algorithms. On the contrary, under certain conditions, expanding data inputs can *increase* error. From a statistical perspective, total prediction error reflects a trade-off between *bias* and *variance*. Bias refers to systematic error: models that are too simple may miss important patterns and therefore make consistently wrong predictions. Variance, by contrast, reflects instability: highly complex models may fit the data they are trained on extremely well but perform poorly when applied to new individuals. The relationship between bias, variance, model complexity, and total error is well described in the methodological literature and is often illustrated as a U-shaped curve (Figure 6.4), where total error is minimised at an optimal level of complexity (Fortmann-Roe, 2012; Meland & Brodersen, 2016).

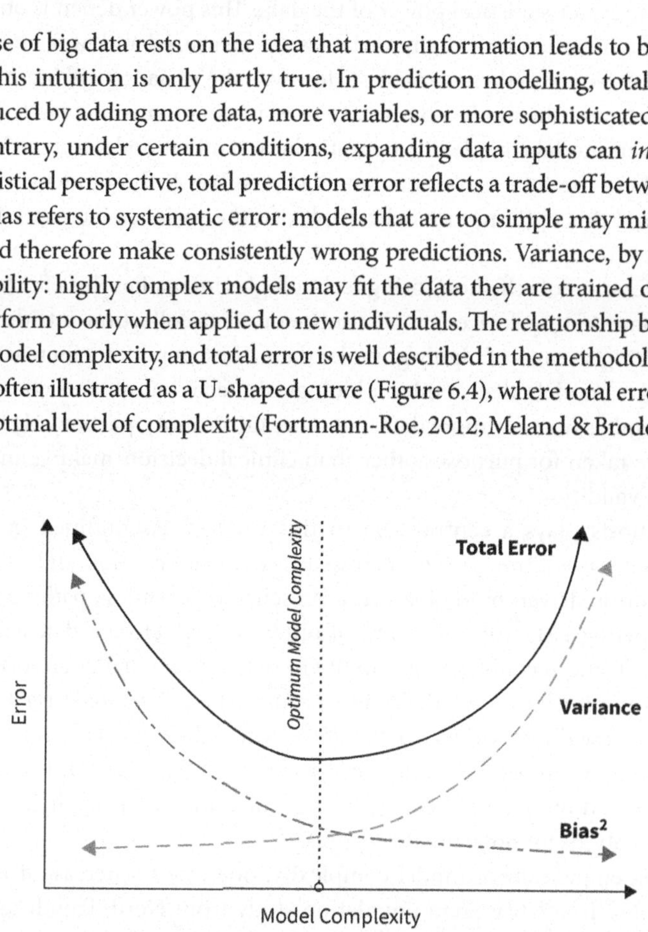

Figure 6.4 The relationship between bias, variance, increasing complexity and the degree of total error in a prediction model. Sources: Fortmann-Roe (2012); Meland and Brodersen (2016).
Graph illustrating the bias–variance trade-off in predictive models. As model complexity increases, bias decreases while variance increases. The total error curve forms a U-shape, with the lowest error occurring at an intermediate level of complexity, labelled the optimum model complexity.

Figure 6.4 illustrates the relationship between decreasing bias (dark grey dash-dotted line), increasing variance (light grey dashed line), increasing model complexity (x-axes), and total error (black U-shaped line). The vertical dashed line marks a trade-off where the optimum model complexity is defined in the figure. Big Data optimists (Høyer, 2019) tend to push models towards the right-hand side of this curve. As more variables are added, as measurements become more frequent, and as data sources become more heterogeneous, model complexity increases.

In classic quantitative and epidemiological research, it is well known that bias is reduced with greater statistical power of the data. This power depends on how many people a study includes, how many variables are measured and how often, and how many events there are in these variables. However, the variance will increase with the amount of data and the model complexity used in quantitative research. This means that for a given model complexity, the ratio between bias and variance has a model optimum where the total error is as small as possible. If the model complexity increases beyond this optimum model complexity, the variance increases and so does the total error.

The proliferation of self-monitoring technologies intensifies this effect. Wearables, apps, and home-testing devices enable continuous data collection outside clinical settings, producing streams of highly granular data. These inputs are increasingly folded into predictive models that combine biological, behavioural, and contextual variables. The result is not only more data, but more uncertainty, particularly when measurements are taken for purposes other than clinical decision-making and lack clear standards of validity.

Overdiagnosis plays a central role in this process. As outlined in Chapter 1, overdiagnosis arises through two main pathways: *overdetection* and *overdefinition*. Overdetection is driven by biology (the presence of harmless pathological conditions), competing risks (people dying of other causes before a detected condition would matter), and technology (the ability to detect ever smaller abnormalities and continuous monitoring). Overdefinition occurs when thresholds for treatment or risk are lowered without evidence of benefit, or when disease categories are expanded to include mild or ambiguous states (Brodersen et al., 2018a). All five mechanisms are activated, and often amplified, when Big Data (and AI) is applied to apparently healthy populations for preventive purposes.

If we look empirically at model complexity, one way to increase it is to include more variables. In a Norwegian population study from Nord-Trøndelag, Petursson and colleagues show that the variance (and thus the overdiagnosis rate) increases as more and more risk factors for cardiovascular disease are included in their model (Petursson et al., 2009). With one risk factor included, about 12% of participants were labelled at increased risk. Adding a second risk factor raised this by more than 20 percentage points and including three or more pushed nearly half of the population into a high-risk category. When individuals already diagnosed with cardiovascular disease or diabetes were accounted for, only a small fraction of the population remained

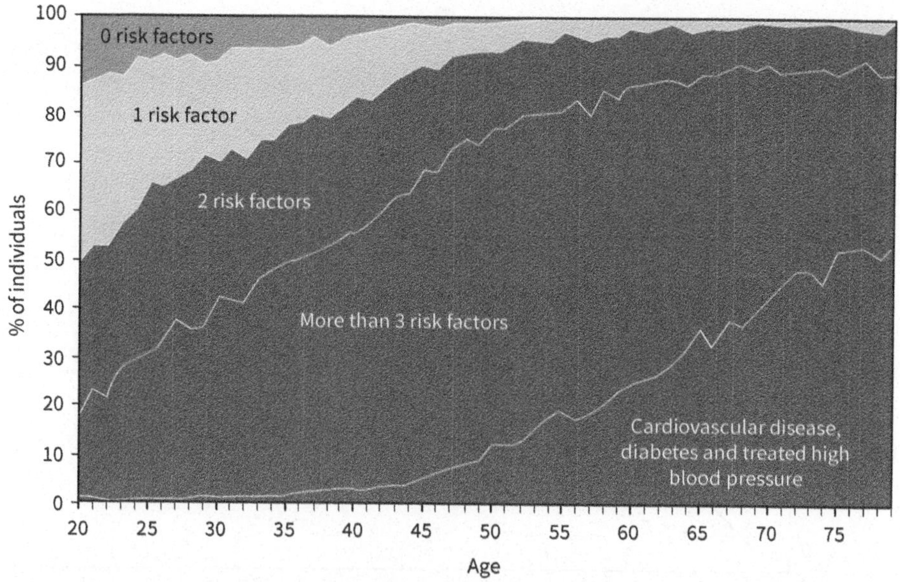

Figure 6.5 Prevalence of risk factors by age. By age, Figure 6.5 shows the prevalence among residents in Nord-Tröndelag of different conditions: 0, 1, 2, 3 or more risk factors for cardiovascular disease. Source: Petursson et al. (2009).
Stacked area chart showing accumulation of cardiovascular risk factors with age. The proportion of people with no risk factors decreases steadily, while the proportion with one or more risk factors increases. Older age groups show higher prevalence of multiple risk factors and related conditions.
Reproduced with permission from Samfundslitteratur.

classified as entirely healthy (Figure 6.5). As more variables entered the model, variance increased, and with it, the proportion of people likely overdiagnosed as at risk.

The problem with an increasing total error can also be illustrated in simulated data, where increasing model complexity varies according to different numbers of variables and different degrees of overdiagnosis (Figure 6.6). When the number of variables in a model increases, even very small rates of overdiagnosis within each variable accumulate. The implication is unsettling: complexity alone can turn large segments of a healthy population into patients-in-waiting (Timmermans et al., 2010). In Figure 6.6 the number of variables is set between 0 and 50, while the degree of overdiagnosis is set to 0.1%, 0.5%, 1%, 1.5%, or 2%.

Figure 6.6 demonstrates that the proportion of people who are overdiagnosed with at least one condition increases rapidly and non-linearly as both the number of variables and the degree of overdiagnosis rise. When 50 variables are included in a model and each carries an overdiagnosis rate of just 0.5%, approximately one-fifth of the population will be labelled with at least one unnecessary diagnosis. If the

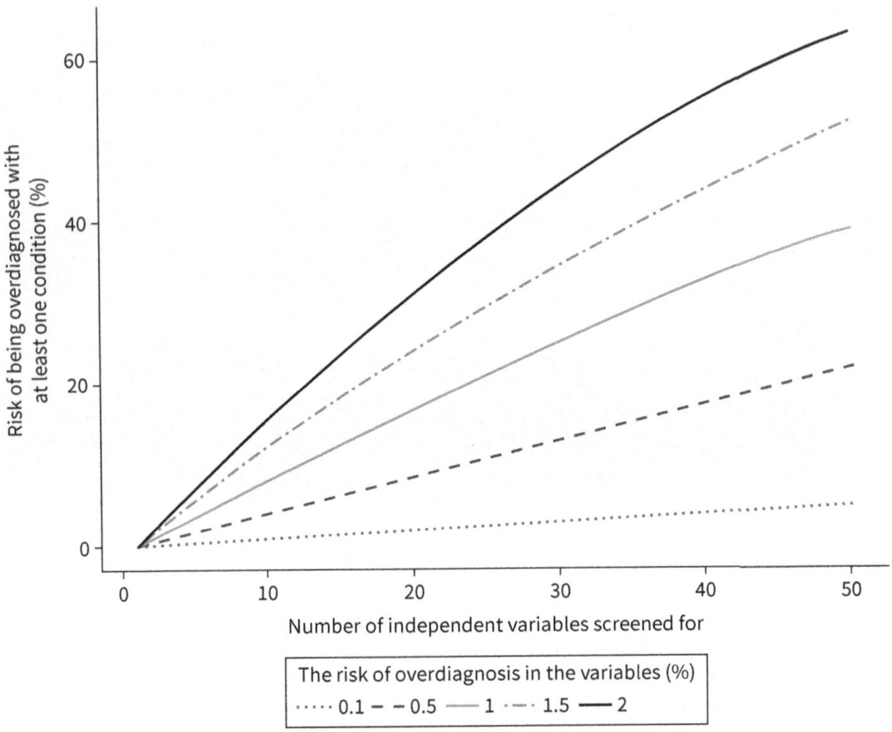

Figure 6.6 Correlation between the number of variables screened for, the degree of overdiagnosis in these variables, and the risk of being overdiagnosed with at least one condition (Vogt et al., 2019). The increasing risk of overdiagnosis is illustrated by both the five lines and the number of variables. The five lines illustrate: 0.1% overdiagnosis in the variables (dotted line), 0.5% overdiagnosis (dashed line), 1% overdiagnosis (grey line), 1.5% overdiagnosis (dash-dotted line), and 2% overdiagnosis (black line). The graph shows that the more overdiagnosis that occurs in the variables and the more variables that are examined in a model, the more people will be overdiagnosed. At very low levels of overdiagnosis, this relationship is almost linear (straight line), while the relationship increases exponentially when there is only 1% overdiagnosis in the variables.
Reproduced with permission from Samfundslitteratur.

overdiagnosis rate increases to 2% across the same 50 variables, more than 60% of individuals will be overdiagnosed. Even with a far more modest model comprising only 10 variables, an overdiagnosis rate of 2% per variable is sufficient to classify nearly 20% of the population as having at least one condition.

Crucially, real-world overdiagnosis rates are often far higher than those used in simulations. For common cardiovascular risk factors such as blood pressure, cholesterol, and body mass index, overdiagnosis rates may be closer to 20–50%. In cancer screening, overdiagnosis is frequently measured in two-digit numbers: around 25–30% in mammography, roughly 50% in lung cancer screening with low-dose CT, and similar levels in PSA-based prostate cancer screening (see Chapter 4). When such variables are incorporated into Big Data-driven preventive models aimed at healthy individuals, the logical endpoint is that almost everyone becomes abnormal in some way.

An illustrative case is the Pioneer 100 Wellness Project, which enrolled 108 apparently healthy adults aged 21–89 years and subjected them to extensive genomic sequencing, 218 clinical tests, including 643 metabolites, 262 proteins, and 4616 microbes, plus activity measurements from wearables (Price et al., 2017). Every participant received at least one abnormal result. Most received many. High cholesterol, vitamin D deficiency, elevated mercury levels, and pre-diabetes were widespread. While some findings may have been clinically meaningful, the fact that *no one* remained unlabelled strongly suggests that overdiagnosis was not an exception but a structural outcome of the model itself (Vogt et al., 2018).

In short, increasing the number of variables and refining prediction models may reduce bias, but at the cost of escalating variance and thus greater total error. In preventive contexts, that error often manifests as overdiagnosis. The challenge, then, is not merely technical. It is conceptual and ethical: deciding how much complexity is enough, what kinds of uncertainty are acceptable, and when prediction ceases to serve health and begins to medicalise everyday life.

Personalised medicine

As we have seen, prediction models are never neutral mirrors of reality. Measurement error, bias, variance, and model complexity shape what counts as risk, abnormality, or disease long before predictions are translated into clinical or preventive action. Yet despite these well-known limitations, contemporary data-driven health initiatives are rarely presented in cautious or conditional terms. Instead, they are framed through powerful promises about what prediction *will* deliver, how medicine *will* change, and why investment *must* happen now.

Promises lie at the heart of what sociologist Alan Petersen describes as the politics of digital health. According to Petersen (2019), digital and data-intensive health technologies are routinely advanced through *promissory discourses*: claims about future benefits that function as arguments in the present, not only to justify implementation, but to mobilise funding, infrastructure, and public support. In this sense, promises are not speculative add-ons to technological development; they are constitutive of it. Callahan (2009) has shown how such techno-optimism has historically acted as a driver of escalating healthcare costs, as each new innovation arrives framed as indispensable rather than optional. Science and technology studies (STS) scholars have long examined how expectations and promises circulate around emerging technologies. They emphasise that while promises point towards the future, their political and material effects are felt immediately reshaping priorities, reallocating resources, and redefining what counts as responsible action in the present (Høyer, 2023, p. 31).

It is within this promissory landscape that *personalised medicine* has emerged and gained traction. The concept is known under several labels including *personalised medicine, precision medicine*, and *P4 medicine* (predictive, preventive, personalised, participatory), but all share a common premise: that individuals are biologically unique, and that healthcare should therefore be tailored to the individual rather than the population average (Hood & Flores, 2012; Vogt et al., 2018; Green et al., 2020). Big Data and AI are positioned as the technical means through which this individualisation can finally be realised. In broad terms, personalised medicine operates in two distinct domains (Box 6.1). One targets people who are already ill: patients with symptoms, diagnoses, and established conditions. Here, data are used to refine treatment choices, adjust dosages, or stratify patients more precisely than traditional clinical categories allow. In this context, overdiagnosis is generally not the primary concern, unless data is explicitly used to search for additional diagnoses beyond those motivating care. For this reason, personalised medicine aimed at patients with manifest disease will not be further examined in this book.

The second domain targets people who are not ill or at least not known to be ill. Here, personalised medicine seeks to identify hidden risks and early deviations in apparently healthy individuals, often long before symptoms appear. It is in this preventive domain that overdiagnosis becomes unavoidable (Vogt et al., 2019).

Beyond the assumption of individual uniqueness, personalised medicine also rests on a strong belief in prediction: that future disease can be forecast with sufficient precision to enable effective primary prevention. If risks can be identified early enough, the argument goes, causal pathways can be altered through lifestyle changes, monitoring, or targeted interventions so that disease never occurs (Green et al., 2020). When this logic is applied to large datasets collected from asymptomatic populations, it closely resembles medical screening. The aim is early detection: identifying pathological conditions, risk factors, or deviations from statistical norms before they manifest as illness. For this reason, predictive personalised medicine among healthy individuals is best understood not as something fundamentally new, but as a novel form of screening that we might call *Big Data screening* (Vogt et al., 2019).

This form of screening differs from traditional medical screening in several important ways. First, traditional screening programmes usually focus on a single condition or variable, whereas Big Data screening simultaneously evaluates dozens,

Box 6.1 The two domains of Personalised medicine

- Personalised medicine targeting patients with symptoms, diseases, and conditions does not in itself lead to overdiagnosis.
- Personalised medicine that uses data to search for diagnoses or disease risks in apparently healthy individuals will inevitably produce some degree of overdiagnosis.

hundreds, or even thousands of variables (Vogt et al., 2019). Second, traditional screening is episodic, meaning that it is offered once or at fixed intervals over many years while Big Data screening can be repeated frequently or operate continuously as new data are generated. Third, participation in traditional screening typically requires physical presence and explicit enrolment, whereas Big Data screening often relies on data produced incidentally through everyday life, without any moment of clear entry or exit. In this context, it is argued that everyone has a *digital twin*; a fragmented, datafied digital representation of the individual made from biographical and biological data. Such a digital twin should therefore be seen as a more or less precise model of our behaviour, how we age, and what diseases we have or might get.

Perhaps most importantly, Big Data screening challenges established norms of informed consent. From a deliberative democratic perspective, traditional screening depends on individuals making an informed choice, having been told both the potential benefits and harms of participation (Jensen et al., 2021). In Big Data screening, much of the relevant data already exists, having been generated through interactions with health services, public institutions, financial systems, or digital platforms. It is therefore difficult to identify when or whether individuals meaningfully consent to being screened at all.

These differences are illustrated in Figure 6.7 and have led to various attempts to name the phenomenon: 'screening in absentia', 'screening incognito' or 'screening 2.0'. We adopt the term *screening incognito* to emphasise that it is often a person's *digital twin* that is being screened, rather than the living person themselves. This digital twin becomes the primary object of prediction and intervention. As we argue throughout this chapter, this fragmentation is a key driver of overdiagnosis: when health is decomposed into innumerable measurable components, it becomes increasingly unlikely that anyone will remain entirely 'normal'.

The promissory claim underpinning screening incognito is that individualised, participatory prevention often framed as lifestyle modification can meaningfully reduce morbidity and mortality (Price et al., 2017; Vogt et al., 2018; Green et al., 2020). Yet high-quality evidence consistently shows that individualised primary prevention has little or no lasting effect on hard outcomes, and that when effects do occur, they

Secondary prevention with screening	
Traditional medical screening	**Screening with big data**
Screening for one variable	Screening for many variables
Screening one or more times in life	Continuous screening throughout life
Screening is done by a physical presence	Screening is done without physical presence
Potential participants invited for screening are encouraged to make an informed choice about whether or not to be screened	Screening happens without invitation and without an informed choice

Figure 6.7 Differences between traditional medical screening and Big Data screening. Reproduced with permission from Samfundslitteratur.

tend to be small and transient (Krogsbøll et al., 2019; Jørgensen et al., 2024). The gap between promise and evidence is striking.

As with prediction models themselves, the issue is not simply whether personalised medicine *can* work, but what kinds of uncertainty, error, and unintended harm are produced when its promises are enacted at scale. Who is obliged to act on predicted risks? How much error is tolerable in the name of prevention? And at what point does anticipating disease become indistinguishable from medicalising everyday life? Proponents argue that integrating vast datasets, from molecular markers to digital self-tracking, will generate deeper insights into disease mechanisms, refine diagnostic categories, and even redefine wellness itself. Patients, in this vision, become active contributors, participating through digital platforms and data-sharing practices that promise both improved care and more sustainable health systems. Whether these promises can be realised without unintended consequences remains an open question.

Artificial intelligence (AI)

Following the discussion of personalised medicine, AI enters the scene as an often-praised tool to even more precise diagnostics. AI is, in technical terms, a machine-based intelligence: systems capable of performing tasks that would normally require human cognition. Within this broad field, *machine learning* refers to algorithms that improve their performance by learning from data rather than following explicitly programmed rules. What matters for our purposes, however, is less the formal definition than the role AI now plays in translating Big Data into predictions, recommendations, and decisions.

Recent years have seen a surge of interest in *generative AI*; systems able to process and produce human-like language, images, and patterns by training on vast datasets. In medicine, these models have attracted attention for their ability to summarise clinical records, interpret diagnostic images, retrieve medical knowledge, and even suggest possible diagnoses. A growing body of research highlights their speed and apparent accuracy in handling complex clinical information, positioning them as promising tools for decision support. At the same time, this research also documents important limitations, including sensitivity to data quality, lack of contextual understanding, and difficulty accounting for uncertainty.

At a more fundamental level, AI systems are built by looking backwards. Their first training datasets are almost always retrospective, drawing on historical records of people's lives, diseases, treatments, and outcomes. From such data, sometimes spanning the entire life course, algorithms identify statistical regularities and correlations. These patterns are then used to construct 'average' trajectories: typical sequences of risks, events, and outcomes associated with particular diagnoses or causes of death. When applied to new individuals, the algorithm compares them to these learned patterns and produces probabilistic predictions about what might happen next. Increasingly, these models are not static. They are continuously updated as new data arrives from electronic health records, wearables, apps, or administrative systems enabling predictions to be recalculated in near real time. This dynamic updating is often presented as bringing models closer to the 'truth' of the present moment. Yet it also means that predictions are constantly shifting, sensitive to small changes in inputs, measurement error, and evolving definitions of what counts as relevant data.

When AI and machine learning are combined with Big Data in personalised medicine aimed at apparently healthy individuals, a familiar set of problems in terms of overdiagnosis resurfaces now in algorithmic form (Phillips et al., 2022). As already discussed, prediction in this context resembles screening, and screening inevitably raises the risk of overdiagnosis. Spectrum bias is particular relevant in this context where the instability of prognostic factors over time, and the growth of total error as model complexity increases. AI does not remove these issues; it often intensifies them by scaling prediction across many variables and large populations.

AI is increasingly integrated into health systems, particularly in diagnostics, clinical decision support, patient triage, and health system management. Across the European Region, AI is most commonly used to support imaging interpretation, automate routine clinical tasks, and assist patient communication through chatbots, with the stated goals of improving efficiency, reducing workforce pressure, and enhancing care quality. These applications promise earlier detection, more consistent decision-making, and optimised resource allocation, especially in settings facing workforce shortages (World Health Organization (WHO), 2025).

At the same time, high-sensitivity algorithms may amplify the detection of incidental or clinically inconsequential findings, potentially increasing diagnostic cascades and low-value care. Uneven governance, limited health-specific AI strategies, and gaps in clinician training raise concerns about automation bias, erosion of clinical judgement, and overreliance on algorithmic outputs (WHO, 2025). Moreover, limited involvement of patients and the public in AI design and governance risks misalignment with lived experiences of illness and care. Addressing these challenges requires robust data governance, clear accountability, human oversight, and sustained attention to how AI-mediated diagnostics may reconfigure thresholds for disease and intervention.

A crucial point is that AI systems do not merely *analyse* data; they help determine what becomes visible as a problem in the first place. Data combined with models generate new forms of risk: scores, thresholds, and predictions that did not previously exist. In doing so, AI actively participates in defining what counts as abnormal, actionable, or in need of intervention. Risk is no longer simply discovered, it is co-produced by datasets, modelling choices, and algorithmic assumptions.

This has consequences for clinical judgement and responsibility. When AI systems deliver recommendations, rankings, or predictions, the role of professional judgement shifts. Clinicians may feel pressure to follow algorithmic outputs, even when these conflict with experiential knowledge or contextual understanding. Automation bias, the tendency to over-trust algorithmic outputs, further complicates this landscape (Dalsgaard, 2026).

More broadly, AI is never neutral (Zicari et al., 2021a; Dalsgaard, 2026). It embodies prior choices about which data matter, which outcomes are valued, ethical dilemmas, and which risks are prioritised. These choices shape practice, guide attention, and set boundaries for action often invisibly. In preventive contexts, this means that AI can quietly expand the population considered 'at risk', amplifying overdiagnosis while appearing to offer precision and personalisation (Zicari et al., 2021a). Understanding AI in personalised medicine therefore requires moving beyond questions of accuracy alone, to examine how prediction technologies actively reconfigure medical knowledge, clinical authority, ethical and societal implication, and the moral economy of prevention (Zicari et al., 2021a).

Prognosis, diagnosis, and the blind spot of overdiagnosis

A central difficulty in understanding overdiagnosis is that it cannot be identified in the moment of diagnosis. Neither the clinician nor the researcher can determine, here and now, whether a diagnosed individual is correctly diagnosed or overdiagnosed. This is because overdiagnosis is not defined by the presence of a pathological finding alone, but by its *prognosis*. The overdiagnosed person has a detectable pathological condition, yet that condition will never cause symptoms, illness, or death during their lifetime (Zicari et al., 2021b).

In everyday clinical practice, people can only be classified as healthy or sick in the present tense. To identify overdiagnosis, one must know the future. This requires access to longitudinal life-course data from following individuals from diagnosis until death or, for researchers, retrospective datasets that reconstruct complete life trajectories (Zicari et al., 2021b). Only then can one distinguish between those who would have benefited from diagnosis and treatment, and those who would have lived unaffected regardless.

Herein lies a structural problem. In most datasets, overdiagnosed individuals are not recognised as such. They are counted as correctly diagnosed unless clear evidence emerges to the contrary, for example through autopsy findings. As a result, they often receive treatment for conditions that would never have harmed them without this being visible as overtreatment. If a treatment genuinely prevents morbidity or mortality in a proportion of correctly diagnosed patients, then overdiagnosed individuals who receive the same treatment will appear indistinguishable from successfully treated patients. The absence of disease or death is interpreted as proof of effectiveness, even though the overdiagnosed would have had the same outcome without intervention. Treatment appears to 'work for everyone'.

This poses a profound challenge for personalised medicine based on Big Data using AI. In such datasets, it is not possible to separate those who were helped by treatment from those who never needed it in the first place (Zicari et al., 2021b). Even after death, the distinction remains blurred: some correctly diagnosed individuals will not die from the disease because treatment worked, while overdiagnosed individuals will not die from it because it was never a threat. Prognosis collapses into diagnosis, and prediction becomes contaminated by overdiagnosis (Zicari et al., 2021b).

A concrete illustration can be found in contemporary mammography screening. In a large population study of women aged 50–69 years undergoing biennial screening, Lauritzen and colleagues (2024) compared outcomes before and after the introduction of AI-assisted reading. Prior to AI, all mammograms were double-read by radiologists. With AI, scans classified as likely normal were single-read, while the remaining were double-read with AI support. The authors report that AI was highly effective at ruling out cancer and reduced false positives. They also note concerns about overdiagnosis of ductal carcinoma in situ (DCIS).

However, a closer look reveals something more troubling. Not only did DCIS diagnoses increase substantially after AI was introduced, but diagnoses of invasive breast cancer (IBC) also rose in absolute terms (see Table 6.1). At the same time, there was no reduction in the proportion of women diagnosed with lymph node metastases (lymph node positive), an outcome one would expect if earlier detection translated into meaningful prognostic benefit (Esserman et al., 2009). In effect, AI shifted the system towards detecting more cancer without improving indicators of disease severity (more women who were lymph node negative). What is being predicted, then, is no longer simply disease, but disease *plus* overdiagnosis. In their calculations, the authors report a decrease in the detection of IBC, but in fact, there is an increase in its detection, which, in absolute terms, is greater than the increase in DCIS cases. Table 6.1 provides the technical evidence to back this argument.

The MASAI study (Gommers et al., 2026) is the first ever randomised trial comparing AI-supported mammography screening with standard double reading without AI. Here, 76 additional women were diagnosed with screen-detected breast cancer in the intervention group, while 11 fewer women were diagnosed with breast cancer between two screening rounds (interval cancers). These findings might be interpreted as indicating that AI support enables radiologists to identify more women with clinically relevant breast cancer. However, they may also suggest that AI support leads to an increased number of diagnoses of breast cancers that may not be clinically relevant (overdiagnosis)—approximately in a ratio of 1:6 when comparing the reduction in interval cancers with the increase in overdiagnosis (Marinovich & Houssami, 2026). This interpretation is also consistent with the substantial increase in sensitivity reported by Gommers and colleagues (Gommers et al., 2026). Sensitivity will increase partly as a result of fewer interval cancers, but it will also increase with more overdiagnosis (Brodersen et al., 2014).

The same logic appears in other domains. In the Nord-Trøndelag population study, researchers were able to examine the natural history of untreated hypertension because a subgroup of participants had elevated blood pressure that was neither diagnosed nor treated (Jørgensen et al., 2017). Surprisingly, mortality did not differ

Table 6.1 Mammography screening with and without assistance from artificial intelligence (AI)

AI status, mammography	BC: IBC/DCIS	No BC	Total
Before AI			
Positive mammography	423: 359/64	1452	1875
Negative mammography	?	?	58,876
Total	?	?	60,751
With AI			
Positive mammography	480: 382/98	950	1430
Negative mammography	?	?	56,816
Total	?	?	58,246

Breast cancer (BC) includes both ductal carcinoma in situ (DCIS) and invasive breast cancer (IBC). For DCIS, 64 cases were detected among 60,751 women before AI was introduced, corresponding to about 1 case per 1000 women. After AI was introduced, 98 cases were detected among 58,246 women, or roughly 1.7 cases per 1000. This represents a relative increase of about 60%, which in absolute terms means 63 additional DCIS cases per 100,000 women screened. For IBC, 359 cases were detected before AI (about 5.9 cases per 1000 women), compared with 382 cases after AI (about 6.6 cases per 1000). This corresponds to a relative increase of around 11%, or 65 additional invasive cancer cases per 100,000 women screened. Importantly, these increases occurred without a corresponding reduction in advanced disease, such as lymph node metastases. As a result, AI-assisted screening does not simply improve the prediction of clinically meaningful cancer. Instead, it shifts detection towards identifying more cancers overall, including cases that would never have caused harm. In this way, prediction becomes blurred: it is no longer a prediction of disease alone, but a prediction of disease plus overdiagnosis.

between these individuals and those who had been diagnosed and treated for hypertension. This suggests that a substantial proportion of people labelled with hypertension are overdiagnosed. Moreover, being labelled as having high blood pressure was associated with worse self-rated health, indicating that diagnosis itself can cause harm, independent of physiological effects (Jørgensen et al., 2015).

Prognosis is further complicated because risk factors are not historically stable. Variables that once predicted disease and death may lose their predictive power over time as social conditions, treatments, and populations change. Body mass index (BMI, kg/m^2) provides a telling example. The BMI was first developed in 1832 by Belgian statistician Adolphe Quetelet, who sought to define the 'normal man' using statistical methods. In the 1950s, insurance companies began using weight tables to classify clients by body frame. The term *body mass index* was later introduced by physiologist Ancel Keys in 1972, who promoted its use in population studies. By 1997, the WHO had recognised obesity as a global epidemic (Pray & Riskin, 2023):

> Overweight and obesity are defined as abnormal or excessive fat accumulation that presents a risk to health. A body mass index (BMI) over 25 is considered overweight, and over 30 is obese. In 2019, an estimated 5 million noncommunicable disease (NCD) deaths were caused by higher-than-optimal BMI. (WHO, 2026)

Following this, a BMI between 18.5 and 25 has been defined as normal, with values <18.5 labelled as too low and values >25 as too high. In a similar way, cholesterol levels >5 mmol/L in otherwise healthy individuals have, in recent decades, been classified as abnormally high. These thresholds were not arbitrary. For people who died in the latter part of the twentieth century, epidemiological studies based on retrospective longitudinal data showed clear associations between higher BMI and cholesterol levels and an increased risk of morbidity and premature death. But this association has weakened or disappeared in more recent cohorts. When epidemiologists today look at data from people who died after 2000, these correlations are no longer seen (Petursson et al., 2011). Today, mortality risk increases clearly only at very high BMI levels, and even then, primarily among individuals with unhealthy lifestyles. Cardiorespiratory fitness, not body weight, is a far stronger predictor of survival (Petursson et al., 2011; Matheson et al., 2012; Weeldreyer et al., 2025). Similar patterns are observed for cholesterol, where higher levels in certain ranges appear neutral or even protective, particularly for women (Petursson et al., 2012).

These shifts raise uncomfortable questions. If risk factors and their thresholds change over time, what does it mean to label someone as abnormal today based on yesterday's data? Should categories such as normal, overweight, or high cholesterol be continuously revised or abandoned altogether? And what happens when AI systems, trained on historical data, project outdated risk patterns onto present and future populations? The distinction between diagnosis and prognosis thus becomes crucial. Big Data and AI excel at detecting patterns in the past, but overdiagnosis emerges precisely where prediction about the future is mistaken. Without careful attention to prognosis, prediction models risk transforming ever more people into patients accurately diagnosed in a technical sense, but misclassified in terms of the lives they will actually live.

Summary

This chapter has traced how personalised medicine, Big Data, and AI converge around a shared ambition: to know more about individuals in order to predict, prevent, and personalise healthcare. In practice, this ambition relies on the inclusion of a vast number of variables, drawn not only from biology, genomics, biomarkers, and imaging but also from people's lives, behaviours, and institutional encounters. Health data now flow from clinics, municipalities, banks, regions, digital platforms, and tracking technologies, producing dense, fragmented representations of human beings.

Each of these variables carries the possibility of identifying deviations, abnormalities, risk factors, or pathological findings that will never cause illness or death. Some variables may have only a small degree of overdiagnosis, while others such as certain risk factors or screening-derived findings may involve substantial overdiagnosis. As this chapter has shown, even modest levels of overdiagnosis in individual variables accumulate rapidly when many variables are combined. The more complex the prediction model, the greater the variance, the higher the total error, and the larger the pool of people who risk being overdiagnosed.

These problems are compounded by several structural features of Big Data-driven medicine. Biographical data vary widely in validity and reliability. Prognostic values of risk factors change over time as populations, treatments, and social conditions evolve. Predictions are typically built on retrospective data, even when they are continuously updated, meaning that future risks are inferred from past lives that may no longer resemble present ones. Under these conditions, what is often called 'precision' medicine can become deeply imprecise.

A particularly serious consequence arises when overdiagnosis is folded into the data used to define disease itself. If Big Data cannot distinguish between people who are correctly diagnosed and those who are overdiagnosed, then reference standards for disease, treatment success, and even death become contaminated. When AI is applied to such data, overdiagnosed cases are treated as true positives. With machine learning, systems can then amplify this error by learning to detect ever more of the same patterns, creating a self-reinforcing cycle. In this way, prediction drifts away from meaningful disease and towards the systematic production of patients.

These dynamics are not hypothetical. Commercial actors now explicitly market AI tools designed to extract additional 'diagnostic potential' from existing imaging and clinical data, including the identification of health risk factors and incidental findings. Such applications may appear efficient and innovative, but they also expand the diagnostic gaze in ways that almost inevitably increase overdiagnosis.

Finally, the chapter has raised a broader question about knowledge and responsibility. Personalised medicine produces vast amounts of information about who we are and who we might become. In a health culture that increasingly emphasises individual responsibility for future well-being, this knowledge can feel both compelling and burdensome. People are encouraged to act on risks that may never materialise, while living with labels and predictions whose meaning is uncertain. As we show in Chapter 7, the pursuit of ever more knowledge about ourselves and our bodies is not neutral. When knowing becomes an end in itself, the boundary between care and harm becomes increasingly difficult to draw and the potential for overdiagnosis grows accordingly.

7
Is it always good to know?

Clara's genetic risks

Clara was twenty when she consented to the test. The decision itself felt unremarkable; at the time it was nothing but one form signed among many, another sensible precaution taken in a year already defined by movement and transition. She was living in the United States as an au pair, staying with a family in which medicine structured both work and conversation. Their confidence in new technologies was quiet but total. Disease, the family believed, could be anticipated just as risk could be mapped. When the parents told Clara how they had all had genetic testing because it could reveal hidden risks long before illness appeared it felt less like a conversation and more like a suggestion and an invitation into adulthood. Knowledge, they said, was power. Prevention was responsibility. They spoke with the quiet certainty of people accustomed to being listened to, people for whom medicine had always been an ally rather than an intrusion. Clara noticed that no one asked whether she *wanted* to know, only whether she wanted to be prepared. At first, she hesitated. The idea of uncovering futures she had not yet imagined made her uneasy. But that unease was difficult to articulate. What argument could one make *against* knowledge? To decline felt vaguely irresponsible, almost childish, as if choosing ignorance over foresight. The test was framed as a sensible precaution, no different, it seemed, from wearing a seatbelt or buying insurance. When she called her parents back home, they were cautious but supportive. 'It might be good to know', her mother said. Clara heard in their voices a familiar mix of concern and trust in expertise. The decision slowly detached itself from emotion and began to feel administrative, a small step taken now to avoid regret later. She told herself she was doing it for her future self. She also sensed, though she would not have named it at the time, a subtler pressure. Everyone around her appeared so comfortable with prediction. The family offered to cover the relatively small fee for the test. To refuse would have marked her as different, perhaps ungrateful. No harm, she thought, could come from something so simple.

The results arrived a few weeks later, delivered not as prophecy but as numbers:

- An 8.5% lifetime risk of ovarian cancer, four times higher than average
- A reduced risk of lung cancer, whether she smoked or not
- A 30% increased risk of breast cancer, though the report admitted the evidence was still debated
- A markedly increased risk of salivary gland cancer, quickly dismissed as too rare to matter

- A 25% increased risk of heart disease
- A reduced risk of dying from influenza and pneumonia
- An increased risk of stroke
- A reduced risk of blindness, followed by a footnote about scientific uncertainty

Clara stared at the list, waiting to feel enlightened. Instead, she felt oddly hollow. Her host-mother, a neurosurgeon at a prestigious hospital, went through the results with her. She was kind, calm, and efficient. She explained percentages, uncertainty, the difference between risk and destiny. Clara nodded in all the right places. Still, when she left, a single question followed her out into the sunlight: *What am I meant to do with this?* The stroke risk made sense. Her mother had suffered one. So had her uncle. Clara began running in the mornings, swapped pastries for fruit, told herself this was how sensible people behaved. That part was manageable. But ovarian cancer and breast cancer lodged themselves firmly in her thoughts. These were not distant possibilities. These were words that carried weight. She asked about preventive surgery. The host-mother explained gently: removing her ovaries would force her body into menopause, raising the risk of osteoporosis unless she took oestrogen which might then increase her risk of heart disease. Clara listened, thinking of the children she cared for every day, of the children she had always assumed would one day be her own. Instead, the host-mother suggested annual ultrasound scans. A compromise, she called it. Reassuring. Proactive. She did not mention, perhaps she did not even know, that repeated scans in young, healthy women often discover things that never needed discovering.

Meanwhile, Clara's family back home had been disturbed by the results, and asked Clara to call the family physician. His response was different. Quieter. More cautious. 'You are healthy', the physician said after a pause. 'Try to enjoy your year. Come and see me when you're home. We'll talk then.'

Clara tried to take this advice. She tried to forget the numbers. But knowledge, once acquired, has a way of lingering. Late at night, she searched the internet. Breast cancer. Survival stories. Preventive mastectomies. Forums full of fear and certainty in equal measure. She began to notice her body more closely, perhaps too closely. Every unfamiliar sensation felt loaded with meaning. Gradually, she withdrew. She developed persistent stomach pain. Her laughter came less easily. Back home, Clara was eventually referred to a psychologist. They spoke not about cancer, but about fear. About uncertainty. About how to live without constantly rehearsing illness. Slowly, Clara learned to turn her attention back to the life she was actually living, rather than the many lives she might never have.

The genetic information remained accurate in the narrow technical sense. The risks were unchanged. What *had* changed was Clara's relationship to her body and her future. The test had not diagnosed disease, but it had altered the terms on which health was understood. Whether this constituted benefit or harm was not a question the test had been designed to answer.

This is a fictional case inspired by Welch et al. (2011) and drawing on an interview with a young Danish woman about her experiences with anxiety intended to illustrate just one possible way of living with the knowledge that follows from mapping one's genome and being presented with a catalogue of future risks. Others may react with relief, determination, or indifference. Some may feel empowered; others reassured. There is no single or correct response. What Clara's case brings into focus, however, is the more fundamental question of whether such knowledge is worth having when its consequences are so uncertain and ambiguous. Once risk information exists, it invites action but rarely specifies which action is appropriate. Should one intervene early or wait? Monitor the body more closely or try to ignore the numbers? Adjust everyday behaviour, pursue preventive treatment, or accept uncertainty as part of life? Should genetic information be shared with a potential partner before planning a pregnancy? Genetic risk does not exist in a vacuum. It enters lives that are already entangled in social relationships, cultural expectations, moral obligations, and personal aspirations. Clara's fears did not unfold in isolation but alongside her work with children, her dreams of having a family, her trust in medical authority, and her desire to be responsible without becoming consumed by vigilance. The question, then, is not only how much we can trust this kind of knowledge, but how much room we allow it to occupy in a human life that, for better or worse, is lived in the everyday world of family, friendships, careers, dreams, and fragile hopes for the future.

When the answer arrives

At some point, an answer arrives. It may come after a blood test, a scan, a screening programme, or after weeks of quietly collecting information about oneself in the form of sleep patterns, heart rhythms, genetic risks and so on. Sometimes the answer is clear. Sometimes it is tentative. Sometimes the answer is that no clear answer can be given at all. Yet something is always returned: a result, a number, a label, a statement that something has or has not been found. In this chapter, we are concerned with what happens *after* the answer arrives. Answers should not be understood as final truths about a person, but as forms of feedback, a type of temporary conclusions drawn from investigating fragments of a life, a body, or a future that is still unfolding. Being told that something is wrong is, of course, a serious and often distressing moment, particularly when the condition is life-threatening. In such cases, tests, scans, and symptom registrations are essential for initiating the right treatment at the right time. This is what we mean by timely diagnostics, and it is not the focus of our concern here. Even though overdiagnosis can occur in these situations, the psychological experience of receiving a diagnosis is largely the same at the moment it is given whether the diagnosis later proves to have been necessary or not. As we have shown earlier in the book, this distinction can only be made retrospectively.

The situation is different, and far more ambiguous, when the answer does not concern illness as such, but *risk*. Being told that one has an increased likelihood of developing a disease in the future, or that a deviation has been found that does not require treatment, places the individual in a much less defined position. On the one hand, knowledge about one's own body is often framed as a democratic right. We are repeatedly told that the more we know, the better we can act, that awareness enables prevention, and prevention enables control. On the other hand, this type of knowledge often becomes what we call *unintentional knowledge*. It is knowledge that creates concern, vigilance, and uncertainty rather than clarity or reassurance. It may have been obtained voluntarily through a test one actively chose but its consequences were not fully anticipated. The knowledge was not sought in order to worry, yet worry becomes its lasting effect.

This chapter looks at the psychological consequences of getting such answers. We begin with a discussion of how knowledge and evidence are constituted and show that there are limits to how much medical science can really know. From there, we turn to the forms of unintended knowledge that arise from overdiagnosis and risk-based information, and how these shape people's lives, choices, and sense of self. We argue that the effects of diagnoses and risk information extend far beyond the clinical encounter, carrying consequences not only for individuals, but for society as a whole.

What do we mean by knowledge?

All medical research sets out to produce information that, together with other forms of insight, may come to be understood as knowledge. Knowledge, in its broadest sense, includes both linguistically articulated understanding about everyday phenomena, other people, and ourselves and forms of embodied knowledge, such as knowing how to ride a bicycle or recognise a familiar face. Put simply, knowledge can be understood as organised information.

Yet knowledge is never neutral or complete. It is reductive, in the sense that it condenses complex empirical realities into limited statements about the world. And it is selective, because something must always be excluded, ignored, or set aside in order for something else to be known (Hastrup, 2004b, p. 9). Knowledge is therefore always *knowledge-about-something from a particular perspective*. It is produced in a context, shaped by assumptions, methods, and interests. What counts as knowledge in one period may later appear partial, misguided, or simply wrong when viewed from another time.

For knowledge to be recognised as *scientific*, however, additional criteria must be met. Scientific knowledge must be grounded logically or in natural laws, although the methods, theories, and epistemological foundations of science are continuously debated and revised. Like all other forms of knowledge, science is produced through negotiation within particular social, cultural, historical, and economic settings. As the philosopher and biologist Donna Haraway famously argued, knowledge is never neutral or universal; it is partial and situated (Haraway, 1988, p. 583). All knowledge emerges from a position and this position determines what it is possible for us to investigate and know about a particular phenomenon (Haraway, 1988, p. 583). Without acknowledging this, implicit assumptions and research traditions risk being mistaken for objective truths. It is this epistemological foundation that enables us to explain how we know, and without it, implicit biases and research traditions become entangled with research outcomes, leading to hypotheses and assumptions being mistakenly built upon them (Haraway, 1988, p. 583). In other words: scientific knowledge is not necessarily the expression of an eternally valid truth but must meet a number of scientific and scientific–ethical obligations that can be used as benchmarks for the validity of knowledge. Biomedicine, like all other knowledge systems, therefore means different things depending on where and when it is practised.

Biomedical knowledge is based on natural science, where nature and biology are used as explanatory models for disease, rather than, as in other medical systems, disease being explained by folklore, religion, morality, psychological, or social understandings. In a biomedical context, disease is a natural phenomenon in another natural phenomenon: the body. Organs, tissues, and biological processes are treated as causal systems that can be isolated, measured, and explained.

As medical anthropologist Hanne Mogensen has pointed out, biomedical knowledge is often regarded as universal and transferable. Bodies are measured against standardised norms, and deviations from these norms are treated as meaningful regardless of context (Mogensen, 2005). On the one hand, this has enabled standardised treatments aimed at providing equal care based on the best available evidence. On the other hand, the very idea of a 'normal' body has opened the door to medicalisation and pathologisation of variation (Lock & Nguyen, 2018 [2010], p. 39ff; see also Chapter 3).

From a social science perspective, several scholars have examined how biomedicine functions as an institutional system that exercises social control. Through professionalisation and bureaucratisation, human suffering, difference, and deviant behaviour may be redefined as disease, often with far-reaching consequences for individuals and societies alike (Box 7.1). These dynamics lie at the heart of contemporary health culture (Chapter 2).

Many biomedical researchers have long been critical of how biomedical knowledge is produced and used. The volume of scientific publications increases year by year, driven in part by academic incentive structures that reward productivity over reflection (Ingwersen & Larsen, 2014). For clinicians, policymakers, and citizens alike, it has become increasingly difficult to navigate what counts as reliable knowledge.

In response, frameworks for assessing the quality of medical research have been developed. One of the most influential was proposed by the Scottish physician Archie Cochrane, whose critique of healthcare systems and therapeutic effectiveness helped lay the foundations of the evidence-based medicine movement. Evidence, Cochrane insisted, is not proof, but substantiation of a hypothesis. Cochrane and his students were supporters of free and effective treatment for everyone with the same needs, and they founded the demand for documented efficacy of therapeutic efforts (Thorgaard et al., 2010, p. 8; Cochrane, 1972). This meant both stricter standards for knowledge within specialised medicine, and these have subsequently been used as an overarching management model for the distribution of resources in the healthcare system

Box 7.1 Case: Biomedicine as a political tool

A well-known illustration of the political use of biomedicine comes from anthropologist Nancy Scheper-Hughes' work with mothers of malnourished and starving children in north-eastern Brazil. At the time, Brazil was facing profound economic and political crisis. Poverty, food scarcity, and lack of clean water were central to children's suffering. Yet these structural causes were rarely addressed directly. Instead, malnourished children were treated with pills. As Scheper-Hughes observed, each pill the mother gave her child subtly reframed the problem. Hunger, inequality, and political neglect were transformed into a medical condition with a medical solution. Over time, she argued, this process obscured the true causes of suffering, replacing political responsibility with biomedical intervention (Scheper-Hughes, 1992).

(Thorgaard et al., 2010). Different understandings of evidence have given rise to criticism, especially when evidence-based medicine is used to create standards and templates, but does not take into account the individual preferences, needs, and values of each person (Greenhalgh et al., 2014).

Yet the most widely accepted definition of evidence-based medicine explicitly includes these dimensions. According to Guyatt and colleagues, evidence-based medicine rests on three principles: the use of the best available evidence; critical appraisal of that evidence's credibility; the clinical context; and clinical decision-making that balances benefit and harm while taking patient values, preferences, and life situations seriously (Guyatt et al., 2015).

Despite these critical reflections, biomedicine is often presented as objective and neutral. In practice, however, science today operates within dense networks of technology, politics, economics, and institutions, making it difficult to separate facts from values or knowledge from power (Latour, 1993). For laypeople, this blurring complicates the task of distinguishing robust scientific knowledge from speculation or pseudoscience (Hopf et al., 2019). When falsehoods are presented with scientific authority, the consequences can be severe (Box 7.2).

Still, biomedicine has maintained its status and managed to create an understanding that everything can, in principle, be known: with sufficient data, better technology, and enough time, uncertainty is assumed to shrink. This brings us back to the question raised by Clara's story: what happens when the pursuit of knowledge has no natural stopping point? What are the consequences of an endless search for answers, when knowing more does not necessarily mean understanding better or living well? This leads to what we call *unintentional knowledge*: information that is scientifically produced and formally valid, yet creates uncertainty, anxiety, and moral pressure once it enters a person's life. It is knowledge whose consequences were neither intended nor fully anticipated and it is to this form of knowledge that we now turn.

Box 7.2 Case: Scientific misconduct in medical research

One of the most damaging examples of scientific misconduct in modern medicine is the case of the British physician Andrew Wakefield. In 1998, Wakefield published a study in *The Lancet* claiming a link between the measles–mumps–rubella (MMR) vaccine and autism. More than a decade passed before it became clear that the data had been falsified and that no such link existed (DeStefano & Thompson, 2004). *The Lancet* eventually retracted the paper (Eggertson, 2010).

The damage, however, had already been done. Wakefield's claims fuelled widespread vaccine scepticism that persists to this day. Many individuals continue to refuse vaccination for themselves or their children, placing both individual and public health at risk on the basis of knowledge that was never true.

Unintentional knowledge

Unlike animals, humans do not merely possess knowledge; we know that we know. As Zygmunt Bauman writes, human consciousness allows us to relate reflexively to our own thoughts in much the same way as we relate to our bodies (Bauman, 1992). Knowledge therefore has an existential quality: once acquired, it cannot simply be undone. When we search for a forgotten word, we do so with the certainty that it exists somewhere in our mind; when we misplace our glasses, we know they are still there, just out of sight. Unwanted knowledge must be handled in a similar way. It cannot be erased, only suppressed, pushed aside, or lived with (Bauman, 1992; Jønsson et al., 2022a). This irreversibility is central to what we term unintentional knowledge. From an overdiagnosis perspective, unintentional knowledge refers to information that is scientifically generated and formally valid, but whose personal, psychological, or social consequences are unforeseen and undesirable. It is knowledge that, in hindsight, the individual would rather not have had. Importantly, this does not mean that the knowledge is false or produced in bad faith. On the contrary, it often emerges from well-intentioned medical practices such as screening, risk assessment, or preventive testing. Whenever a person undergoes an examination whether prompted by symptoms, participation in a screening programme, or voluntary testing they will receive some form of answer. But not all answers are equally meaningful, actionable, or bearable. Part of the overdiagnosis problem lies precisely here: once information has been transformed into knowledge about one's body or future health, it cannot be taken back, even if it offers no clear path for action or improvement. The individual may only realise too late that the knowledge has altered their relationship to their body, their future, or their sense of self.

Relating to overdiagnosis, unintentional knowledge tends to take one of two forms. The first is being told that you *have* a condition, often one that is asymptomatic, indolent, or unlikely ever to cause harm. The second is being told that you *carry a risk* of developing a condition in the future. While these categories may appear distinct, they often overlap in lived experience. Both can generate uncertainty, vigilance, and anxiety, particularly when no clear or proportionate response exists. Crucially, unintentional knowledge places individuals in a moral and practical dilemma. Should they act on the information or ignore it? Should they monitor their body more closely, change their behaviour, seek further tests, or accept uncertainty? Medical knowledge, especially when framed as risk, often comes without guidance on how much it should matter in a life that is embedded in everyday realities of family, relationships, work, ambitions, and hopes. In this way, unintentional knowledge does not merely inform; it transforms. It reshapes how people understand themselves and their futures, even when no disease ever materialises. In the next section, we explore how unintentional knowledge is experienced psychologically and socially, and why its harms are so difficult to recognise, measure, and legitimise within contemporary healthcare systems.

But isn't it good to know?

The idea that early diagnosis automatically leads to better survival is a remarkably simplistic and often misguided interpretation of a disease as heterogeneous and unpredictable as cancer. Disease does not necessarily develop in a constant or linear fashion. Some cancers progress so quickly, or are so aggressive, that no matter how early they are detected, nothing can be done to change the individual's prognosis. Even when the cancer is found in a screening programme before the woman had any symptoms, it may still be untreatable, because the prognosis also depends on the type of cancer and its biological behaviour. Importantly, it is always appropriate to respond to symptoms in the body. Detecting disease because something feels wrong is fundamentally different from detecting localised stages of cancer before symptoms arise. The latter can be problematic, because some of these early detected conditions never develop into disease at all. But if a diagnosis is given because of symptoms, such as a woman finding a lump in her breast, it is never overdiagnosis.

But research points out that there are often consequences of being told that there *might* be something wrong in the body or mind. And once a suspicion of a diseases or high risk of disease is raised, it is unethical and nerve-wracking for people, patients, relatives, and doctors not to react. To illustrate this, let us look at an extreme case (Box 7.3).

The neuroblastoma case is a particularly instructive example because it shows how intrusive and in some cases fatal the consequences of treatment can be, once an asymptomatic person has a condition or risk detected. It should be noted that neuroblastoma is a rare disease, and the harms described here should be attributed to screening and associated overdetection, not to the standard treatment of neuroblastoma.

The broader point about this form of unintentional knowledge is that knowledge and information are almost always assumed to be unequivocally good. Yet studies

Box 7.3 Case: Screening for neuroblastoma in children

Neuroblastoma is a very rare tumour that develops outside the brain and most commonly affects children aged <5 years. There are no known causes of the disease. Treatment has improved significantly over the past 30 years, particularly when the disease has not spread. Neuroblastoma is therefore a cancer that *may* benefit from early detection. At the same time, it can still be fatal, but because it can also regress spontaneously, some cases are monitored rather than treated to observe how the condition develops.

In the 1990s, a simple urine test was developed to detect neuroblastoma. Two large randomised studies were conducted in Canada and Germany, involving almost two million children. Among the screened children, twice as many cases of neuroblastoma were detected as among those who were not screened. However, there was no difference in mortality between the two groups. The conclusion was therefore that screening did not help.

Many parents when facing what would be the ultimate tragedy of losing a child would argue that it is better to know anyway and to be on the safe side. However, the German study suggests that 99 out of 149 detected cases were overdiagnosed. These children were diagnosed unnecessarily, but because this is a statistical calculation, it is impossible to determine retrospectively which children were affected. Once knowledge of a diagnosis is established, it cannot be withdrawn.

The increased findings in the screening must also be weighed against the harms caused by treatment. Of the 149 diagnosed children, three died: one from adverse effects of chemotherapy and two as a result of surgical complications. In the Canadian study, all 44 diagnosed children were alive five years later, but some had serious complications to the treatment. One child developed leukaemia as a result of chemotherapy and had to undergo further surgeries and transplants, leading to further complications. Another developed an intestinal blockage requiring repeated surgeries; these interventions resulted in complications that ultimately left the girl in a chronic vegetative state.

It is impossible to determine whether these children were correctly diagnosed or overdiagnosed. Because neuroblastoma can recur, this screening case illustrates a form of knowledge that can itself lead to harm. For this reason, the screening programme was not introduced (Schilling et al., 2002; Woods et al., 2002).

show that apparently healthy people do not become or stay reassured of their good health simply by being examined (Rolfe & Burton, 2013). On the contrary, many experience discomfort from examinations; a few experience more or less serious side-effects; and healthy people can experience psychosocial consequences of false-positive results, including anxiety, depression, behavioural changes, and shifts in existential values (Brodersen & Lunde, 2002; Brodersen et al., 2010a; Brodersen & Siersma, 2013; Gram et al., 2023b, 2024).

At the same time, a common lay attitude is that these detrimental effects are a small price to pay for finding disease early. Whether this price is worth paying depends not only on statistical outcomes, but also on individual values and the context of the disease in question. An older study shows that the risk of dying after lung cancer surgery for a person aged >65 years is 5% when part of the lung is removed and 10% when the entire lung is removed (Finlayson & Birkmeyer, 2001). These numbers may have changed with surgical and treatment development over the past decade, but hypothetically, let us stay with this example. It may be a risk a person is willing to take if they are at high risk for lung cancer and have symptoms. But what if there have been no symptoms and the cancer is, for example, an incidental finding (incidentoloma) discovered during an unrelated examination and therefore potentially overdiagnosed?

Adding to the argument, not all diagnosed diseases require immediate action. One example is localised, asymptomatic prostate cancer with a Gleason score ≤6, where the risk of metastasis and spread is very low. These patients are typically followed in an *active surveillance* programme, monitoring the 'disease' with PSA testing and urological or GP consultations every 6–12 months. An often-used argument is that these men do not feel sick and are not bothered by attending this programme, rather they feel safe in being monitored. To investigate if this holds water, a study interviewed a group of Danish men aged 68–81 years with this type of prostate cancer about their experiences of being diagnosed without experiencing symptoms (Nielsen et al., 2020). The men, who had been diagnosed for an average of four to five years, were surprised to learn that they had cancer at the time of diagnosis, which for most of them also caused great uncertainty about whether their cancer would develop. The men responded in different ways. Some began monitoring their bodies closely; one thought about his prostate cancer every time he urinated, another asked where the cancer would first spread and then regularly checked his lymph nodes. Others described feelings of helplessness or anxiety. Despite this, all the men said they were glad to have been informed of their diagnosis, because they believed that regular follow-up would detect any progression 'in time'. Still, it is reasonable to ask whether they would have been better off without this knowledge. One man described his cancer as a 'ticking time bomb', a metaphor that is misleading due to the very low risk of spread associated with this type of cancer, a fact all the men had been informed about. By exaggerating the danger to himself, he could justify having sought out this knowledge, based on a lay assumption that any progression would then be caught early (Nielsen et al., 2020). This becomes particularly relevant when weighing the pro's and con's of 'knowing', given that for localised prostate cancer with a Gleason score ≤6, it is estimated that at least 90% of cases are overdiagnosed (Loeb et al., 2016).

Another example of a diagnosis that does not necessarily require treatment is abdominal aortic aneurysm (AAA), a bulging of the abdominal artery. If the aneurysm ruptures, it is life-threatening, and around 80% of people who reach hospital with a ruptured AAA die (Basnyat et al., 1999). AAAs are more common in men than women, partly because men are more likely to develop atherosclerosis, which contributes to the rupture or an arterial blockage. In 80–85% of cases, atherosclerosis is caused by smoking. Preventive surgery is recommended when an aneurysm exceeds 5.5 cm in diameter or grows more than 1 cm per year. Smaller aneurysms are monitored over time. Again, the intuitive reaction is that it must be good to know. But the MASS study, which followed 67,500 men, shows on the one hand that if you screen for AAA, there is a relative reduction in the risk of dying from AAA of 42% (which is the same as an absolute risk reduction of about 0.3%). However, screened men were not found to live longer that those not screened. At the same time, the diagnosis introduces new concerns: attention to bodily sensations, uncertainty about appropriate behaviour, consideration for relatives, and fear of premature death. In a Swedish qualitative study, one man expressed that he would have preferred not to have this knowledge at all: 'I would have lived a better life without this information ... if I cannot do anything about it anyway, I would rather be without that knowledge.' (Hansson et al., 2012, p. 351, our translation).

For most people, the question of testing and treatment ultimately comes down to whether early diagnosis offers something to gain, which is only true in some cases. As shown, some cancer screening programmes detect cancers that would never cause symptoms or harm. Instead, the programme confers a new identity: that of a patient. The consequence is more years in patienthood, with all that entails (see also Chapter 4).

Patienthood

In the social sciences, *patienthood* refers not simply to having a disease, but to entering a social, institutional, and existential position shaped by medical knowledge, authority, and expectations. Building on work in medical sociology and anthropology, patienthood can be understood as a status that reorganises identity, social relations, and everyday practices through diagnosis, classification, and ongoing interaction with healthcare systems (Parsons, 1951; Mol, 2008; Jutel, 2011). Becoming a patient is therefore not only a biomedical event, but a social transition that carries normative assumptions about behaviour, responsibility, and risk management. We use *patienthood* to describe the condition people enter when they are diagnosed with a potentially long-term, debilitating, or life-threatening disease or are classified as being at increased risk of such a condition. When a person is diagnosed with breast cancer, for example, they move from being regarded as healthy to being recognised as a patient. They acquire patienthood. The concept is not intended to be value-laden. Every day, people receive diagnoses that are necessary and beneficial, and patienthood is often an unavoidable and appropriate consequence of medical care. Analytically, however, the concept is useful because it captures what happens in periods of life when one is no longer simply healthy, but lives under the social, institutional, and existential conditions of being a patient. *Patienthood* here refers to a state that encompasses both correctly diagnosed and overdiagnosed individuals. In most cases, it is not possible to distinguish between the two at the level of the individual. Once diagnosed, people must live with the consequences of that knowledge, regardless of whether the diagnosis later turns out to have been unnecessary. This is where Michel Foucault's insight becomes central: *man is shaped by the knowledge produced about him* (Foucault, 2002 [1966]). When an individual is diagnosed or categorised as being at risk following a health examination, this knowledge does not remain abstract. It affects psyche, identity, and sociality. Even diagnoses or risk classifications that do not require treatment can reshape how people understand themselves and their bodies. Individuals who are diagnosed with a condition that does not require immediate treatment occupy a particular and unstable position. They are made patients by virtue of diagnosis, yet they are not patients in the full sense of undergoing treatment. Instead, they are often placed under surveillance, invited back for regular check-ups, scans, or tests, while being told that there is 'nothing to worry about'. The message communicated is contradictory: *something has been found*, but *nothing should be done*. This produces a condition of being neither clearly healthy nor clearly ill. Such situations resemble what Gregory Bateson famously described as *double binds*: situations in which authority figures communicate conflicting messages that demand opposing responses (Bateson, 1972). The theory was developed in connection with Bateson and colleagues' study of schizophrenia (Bateson et al., 1956), but it is also a theory that he uses to illuminate a general dilemma of receiving conflicting messages from authority figures. We can see such double bindings in the health dogma of both 'going to the doctor on time' and 'not overloading the system'. For individuals positioned as not-quite-patients, this creates a situation in which any response risks being perceived as wrong. In continuation of the argument on unintentional knowledge, it is not only the access to unquestionable information, but the fact that the information provided is ambiguous and contains contradictory messages for action that makes up patienthood. Based on the research on men living with prostate cancer monitored in watchful waiting programmes (Nielsen et al., 2020), it is likely that in some cases the individual is told not worry but feels an urgency to reflect on things that can be interpreted as symptoms or increased risks. This ambiguous state can be fruitfully understood through the anthropological concept of *liminality*. First introduced by Van Gennep (1960) and later developed by Victor Turner, liminality refers to a transitional phase in which individuals are 'betwixt and between' established social categories (Turner, 1967, 1974). In classic anthropological studies, liminality describes the period between separation from a previous status and incorporation into a new one for example, between child and adult, or unmarried and married. The liminal phase begins with a separation from the previous social category (Turner, 1981 [1969], p. 154), a period that in tribal rituals is initiated by the elders of the tribe. The liminal phase itself, in which an individual is 'betwixt and between' is a symbolic phase where one is transformed into what the person will or can be (Turner, 1981 [1969], p. 159). Turner describes the state in which people find themselves here as 'ambiguous, neither here nor there, betwixt and between all fixed points of classification' (Turner, 1974, p. 232). Applied here, liminality helps illuminate the experience of individuals who acquire unintentional knowledge about disease or risk. An individual who was previously unaware of an AAA may have felt healthy. Once informed, that knowledge becomes embedded in everyday life and linked to bodily sensations, family histories, and imagined futures ('Have I been feeling dizzy lately?'; 'Didn't my grandfather die young from something related?'). The person no longer fully inhabits the category of 'healthy', but neither are they unequivocally sick. They exist in an in-between state, marked by uncertainty and anticipation.

In classical ritual contexts, liminality is initiated by elders or authorities and followed by reintegration into a new, stable social category. In contemporary healthcare, biomedical knowledge, technologies, and screening programmes function as the initiating authority. However, unlike ritual processes, healthcare often places individuals in an in-between state without providing a clear pathway out of it. Individuals may remain suspended between categories: monitored but untreated, labelled but not acted upon with no resolution as to whether they are legitimately ill or effectively healthy.

Importantly, this liminal state can coexist with other forms of patienthood. Many people diagnosed with AAA, for example, already live with other chronic conditions and may already identify as patients. Here, the in-between status applies not to the person as a whole, but to a specific organ or diagnosis. Lay understandings may nevertheless exaggerate the danger of the newly discovered condition relative to others, even when this is not supported by biomedical assessments.

Whether fully or partially inhabited, patienthood has consequences. You may not fully be a patient, but you are no longer 'not sick'. This position generates patient identification and often results in more years lived as a patient or near-patient under conditions of uncertainty and discomfort. Patients and almost-patients require monitoring, follow-up, and institutional attention; they may take sick leave, modify behaviour, or experience stress and depression in response to what they perceive as serious illness. These consequences incur both personal and societal costs, regardless of whether the diagnosis was correct or represented overdiagnosis (Haynes et al., 1978; Rasmussen et al., 2014; Jensen et al., 2020). Take congenital or acquired heart conditions as an example: conditions that are also subject to overdiagnosis (Pedersen et al., 2019). Receiving such a diagnosis requires individuals to make sense of a new bodily condition, reassess future prospects, and adapt to norms associated with being a patient, including expectations around 'optimal behaviour' such as dietary modification, physical activity, and ongoing monitoring. For patients and their families, patienthood often involves an ongoing process of renegotiating identity and social roles as new information about disease, treatment, and prognosis emerges. Everyday life must be reinterpreted in ways that render the situation meaningful and manageable (Stull et al., 1999). Patienthood, then, is a direct consequence of diagnosis. At this point, the central distinction is no longer between sick and healthy, but between patient and non-patient. Crucially, the social, psychological, and practical implications of patienthood are largely the same whether the diagnosis is timely, necessary, or the result of overdiagnosis. Once a person has been made a patient, the effects follow.

You are at risk

In his 1948 essay *The humanitarian theory of punishment*, C.S. Lewis writes:

> Of all tyrannies, a tyranny sincerely exercised for the good of its victims may be the most oppressive. It would be better to live under robber barons than under omnipotent moral busybodies. The robber baron's cruelty may sometimes sleep, his cupidity may at some point be satiated; but those who torment us for our own good will torment us without end for they do so with the approval of their own conscience.

Today it almost reads as a warning that interventions carried out 'for the good' of others may become particularly oppressive precisely because they are morally justified. Phenomena that were previously described as hazards or uncertainties are today more often framed as *risks* (Adelswärd & Sachs, 1996). Being told that one is 'at risk' is rarely the result of something felt or experienced in the body. Rather, it originates in epidemiological and statistical calculations that are transformed into clinical knowledge and then applied to individuals. Once translated into personal risk information, these calculations can have significant psychosocial consequences (Hansson et al., 2012).

Psychologist Svend Brinkmann describes this development as *risk pathologisation*: a process through which people are governed and govern themselves via statistical susceptibilities rather than symptoms or suffering (Brinkmann, 2010, p. 278; Rose, 2007, p. 137). Risk pathologisation is particularly pronounced in relation to screening and genetic testing, where individuals are classified according to probabilities rather than disease. Brinkmann further notes that this form of pathologisation tends to individualise what are often social or structural problems, placing responsibility for managing risk squarely on the individual (Brinkmann, 2010, p. 278). As Nikolas Rose has argued, this development must be understood within a broader neoliberal health culture (see Chapter 2), where individuals are expected not only to know their risks, such as implications of one's genome, but also to manage them responsibly (Rose, 2007).

The idea that knowing one's genome or genetic risk factors is inherently beneficial may seem intuitively reasonable. A well-known critique is offered by the physician and researcher Gilbert Welch in *Should I be tested for cancer? Maybe not and here's why* (2006). Welch's first argument is that genetic testing does not eliminate uncertainty about who will develop cancer. A 30-year-old woman who tests positive for the BRCA1 mutation has an estimated 50% risk of being diagnosed with breast cancer by age 70. If she tests negative, her risk is around 10%. In neither case is the answer definitive. Cancer develops through complex interactions between genes, heredity, environment, life circumstances, and chance.

For some women, the difference between a 10% and a 50% risk is meaningful and actionable. For others, the information has little practical value. Whether knowledge of a BRCA1 mutation is useful depends on whether the individual is willing and able to act on it. If no action is possible or acceptable, the knowledge may simply occupy consciousness without offering guidance or resolution. We would argue that such knowledge often creates unnecessary anxiety though this remains a matter of debate. What is less debatable is that risk knowledge leads to increased healthcare utilisation. Welch's second argument is precisely that genetic tests often provide information without clear advice on what to do next. The result is knowledge without direction.

Genetic testing is not the only way risk is made visible. Osteoporosis provides another example of a condition that is typically asymptomatic and can be revealed through opportunistic tests or screening. Osteoporosis is a progressive systemic condition characterised by low bone density and structural deterioration of bone tissue, resulting in an increased risk of fractures, particularly of the wrist, spine, and hip. According to the Danish patient organisation for osteoporosis, approximately one in three women and one in eight men aged >50 years will develop osteoporosis. These figures are likely influenced by overdiagnosis, but they nevertheless raise questions about what such widespread risk knowledge can actually be used for. Among 60-year-old women without osteoporosis, 2.3% will suffer a hip fracture within ten years. Among those diagnosed with osteoporosis, the risk increases to 7.8% (Reventlow et al., 2006). This means that most women diagnosed with osteoporosis will not experience a hip fracture, just as some women without osteoporosis will. Yet the diagnosis has consequences. A qualitative study shows that women diagnosed with osteoporosis reinterpret bodily sensations such as pain during everyday activities as signs of disease. They become more cautious in their everyday life and adjust their behaviour accordingly. Women who are not diagnosed but are informed about osteoporosis risk during menopause similarly report worry and anxiety about the future (Reventlow et al., 2006).

This shift in bodily understanding can be illuminated through the phenomenology of Maurice Merleau-Ponty, who emphasised that experience is always grounded in the lived body. According to Merleau-Ponty, it is the body that acts, suffers, learns, and ages; it precedes reflection and cognition. He describes this fundamental condition as *being-in-the-world* (Merleau-Ponty, 1997 [1945]). When testing, screening and examining asymptomatic individuals, statistical numbers based on population norms must be reconciled with a body that may feel healthy. In this process, scan images often become the dominant explanatory model for bodily experience, reshaping how sensations are interpreted and understood (Reventlow et al., 2006, p. 2729). Many people report that learning about 'hidden diseases' gives them a sense of control over their bodies. Yet, as the examples of osteoporosis, high blood pressure, and abdominal aortic aneurysm show, such diagnoses often create a feeling of being ill despite the absence of symptoms. Because both diagnosis and prognosis remain uncertain, this knowledge simultaneously creates dependency. From the moment of diagnosis, individuals require medical technologies and professional interpretation to understand their bodies.

One of the central challenges of unintentional knowledge is that it is difficult not to act on it even when no meaningful action is available. Healthcare professionals are ethically obliged to respond to risk findings, often leading to further investigations and the possibility of additional diagnoses. Individuals, in principle, have the freedom to decline further action. In practice, this freedom is constrained by health culture and a common, and reasonable, fear of premature death or severe disease. On the one hand, most people want to live long lives; on the other, they are morally expected to take responsibility for their bodies as citizens of the welfare state. Richard Deyo has described this dynamic as a *cascade effect* of biotechnology, where one test result leads to another, often exposing patients to unnecessary anxiety, radiation, or treatment-related harm (Deyo, 2002). When outcomes remain unclear, as in the case of untreatable conditions or risk factors, patients may 'strive tirelessly to resolve uncertainty' (Sah et al., 2013). In this way, scientific uncertainty derived from paraclinical tests is transformed into a form of risk that cannot be undone once it has been discovered (Meyer et al., 2005, p. 238).

Many individuals respond to risk by attempting to change their health behaviour or by seeking preventive treatment. From a biomedical perspective, however, such responses are not always appropriate. This can generate conflict between patients and healthcare professionals. One study shows that some patients in Norway put pressure on their GPs to pursue further examinations despite the absence of clinical indications and despite the risk of harm (Opdal et al., 2019). In settings where patients pay to see their doctor, it may even be the other way round, with physician self-referral (Chapter 8) encouraging more testing for financial gain of their clinic. Such situations may undermine trust between patient and doctor, with consequences for adherence and treatment prioritisation (Nilsen & Malterud, 2017).

If we take patienthood into account, modern medicine not only relates to health and illness, but actively produces new forms of responsibility, uncertainty, and moral pressure. Once knowledge about risk enters a person's life, it is difficult not to act on it even when action is impossible, inappropriate, or harmful.

Do you need to know everything?

Current society has been described as an *information society* and it is based on the Enlightenment idea that the more people know, the better they are able to control their destiny (Tsoukas, 1997, p. 828)—an idea that, as anthropologist Marilyn Strathern has written, continues to blind the information society from seeing what visibility conceals (Strathern, 2000, p. 310), and that more information does not necessarily lead to more understanding; it may just as easily generate confusion, distrust, and uncertainty (Tsoukas, 1997). A blessing and a curse of being human is our ability to imagine alternatives, possibilities, and *what ifs*. This constant 'what if' is rooted in a desire to alleviate or avoid suffering and disease, and it materialises in an ongoing search for knowledge about one's own body. Developments in biotechnology now give doctors and patients access to increasingly detailed information about bodily sub-elements: cysts in specific organs, biochemical markers, and risk factors localised in the genome. In some cases, such information can improve treatment and reduce morbidity or mortality. The challenge is not that this information is incorrect. The challenge is how it is *known*.

Anthropologist Gregory Bateson describes this problem as an *epistemological error*: the mistaken assumption that a living organism can be understood by analysing its parts in isolation. Bateson argues that the nature of a living system such as the human body is always more than the sum of its parts, and that meaning arises from the interaction between those parts as they unfold in a lived body and in relation to an environment (Bateson, 2005 [1972], p. 314 ff.). When medical knowledge isolates a bodily fragment and presents it as representative of the whole, a sub-element risks being mistaken for the person's health as such. This is why even findings that clinicians consider unlikely to cause illness are almost always interpreted by patients as indications of being potentially ill. A statistically defined deviation, detached from symptoms and lived experience, becomes meaningful precisely because it is communicated as medical knowledge. In Bateson's terms, this is an epistemological fallacy: a person who is otherwise healthy is made ill by knowledge about a bodily part that may never cause harm. Bateson further describes how such errors can develop into *cascading processes* (or runaway processes), in which epistemological mistakes become so deeply embedded that they reinforce themselves and become difficult or impossible to correct (Bateson, 1972, pp. 461, 479). One familiar example is the diagnostic cascade: a screening finding suggests possible disease; treatment or monitoring is initiated; secondary findings emerge; new investigations follow; and further interventions are set in motion. What begins as an attempt to secure health may end up producing illness. A PSA test that leads to treatment and results in impotence or urinary incontinence is a well-known illustration of this dynamic.

For Bateson, epistemology (how we know what we know) cannot be separated from ontology (how the world is experienced and organised in a given socio-cultural context) (Bateson, 1987, p. 19). Different epistemologies are more or less suited to the worlds they help produce. This makes it necessary to ask not only whether knowledge is correct, but what kinds of worlds it creates and whether those worlds generate more or less health. Bateson's thinking here is inspired by Alfred Korzybski's famous dictum that 'the map is not the landscape' (Bateson, 1979, p. 58). Korzybski argued that the human conceptual world is limited by our senses and our language, and our reality is therefore always a reflection of the brain's filtering of reality, which for Bateson also includes the culture's filtering of reality. Maps—models, measurements, test results—can be useful, but they are abstractions. Epistemological fallacies arise when the map is mistaken for the landscape itself, when numerical values or visualised deviations are treated as equivalent to lived health and suffering. Bateson argues that epistemological fallacies are part of everyday human life: We are surrounded by information that we somehow know to be untrue, but which nevertheless forms the basis of our thinking.

Together with Danish anthropologist Benedikte Møller Kristensen, we have examined how patients gaining digital and instant access to their own test results affects their understanding of health and illness (Kristensen et al., 2022). Both patients and healthcare professionals know that numerical measurements are not complete expressions of health. Nevertheless, these numbers are often treated *as if* they directly represent a person's bodily condition (Kristensen et al., 2022). In Bateson's terms, these epistemological errors are self-validating and potentially pathological: they contribute to creating a world that corresponds to the assumptions built into the knowledge systems themselves (Bateson, 1979; Bateson, 2005 [1972]). Bateson warns that when technological systems allow humans to act on such errors at scale, the consequences can be profound. Humans may end up living in a world structured by false premises that they themselves have created and must now navigate (Bateson, 1979). In the case of unrestricted access to medical test results, this often manifests as uncertainty, anxiety, and a compulsion to act. Patients know a great deal, but much of what they know concerns probabilistic deviations detached from lived experience and future certainty. Yet this knowledge feels morally binding and demands response (Kristensen et al., 2022).

One of Bateson's more provocative claims is therefore that humans need a degree of *non-knowledge*. He illustrates this with perception: we can only see because we trust our sensory apparatus. If we were fully conscious of every neurological and physiological process involved in vision, intuitive seeing would become impossible (Bateson, 1987, p. 95). Knowledge of parts enriches us, but understanding emerges from wholes. Too much knowledge of fragments can obscure pattern recognition, meaning, and coherence. Applied to health, this suggests that knowing everything about one's own risk factors may undermine the ability to experience the body as a whole. The self becomes dependent on fragments of biomedical knowledge to interpret sensations, actions, and futures. This problem is reinforced by a scientific discourse that rests on Cartesian dualism: a separation of mind and body combined with the assumption that knowledge directly produces rational action. This underpins preventive health models that presume individuals will change behaviour once informed (Yoder, 1997). Bateson explicitly challenges this assumption. Using the example of alcoholism, he argues that knowing what is harmful does not automatically translate into the ability to act differently (Bateson, 2005 [1972]). Human behaviour cannot be reduced to rational decision-making based on information, but neoliberalistic health culture intensifies this problem by framing responsibility as an individual moral obligation. A responsible person is one who acquires knowledge and acts on it. Yet, explanations that do not align with people's lived ways of being in the world may themselves be harmful (Sjørslev, 2017, p. 176). Despite critical awareness of the limits of knowledge, individuals are still expected to seek information about their health when invited to do so, for example, through age- and gender-based screening programmes such as osteoporosis assessments. Despite the fact, as we have shown in this chapter, that this kind of knowledge often has no medical significance because it cannot or should not be acted upon, it has major individual consequences, partly because we expect people with such knowledge to change their behaviour or be more careful. And for most people, this has negative psychosocial consequences such as stress, anxiety, worry and, in severe cases, depression, as well as affecting social relationships. The key point is that responsibility cannot reasonably be placed on the individual to decide whether the harms of knowing outweigh the benefits. The moral pressure to know and act is too strong, and behaviour change too difficult in lives shaped by competing values and obligations (Ørtenblad et al., 2018). This is therefore not an individual problem, but a structural one.

Summary

This chapter has examined how medical knowledge, far from being a neutral or unqualified good, can have profound and sometimes harmful consequences when translated into diagnoses, risk classifications, and expectations for action. In a healthcare system where information is increasingly equated with certainty, control, and moral responsibility, knowing more does not automatically lead to better health or to better lives.

Overdiagnosis cannot be understood as a problem of excess testing alone. Rather, it emerges from the complex interplay between bodies, minds, technologies, and epistemologies. Medical knowledge is inherently probabilistic and fragmentary, yet it is often communicated and experienced as definitive and actionable. For this reason, neither strict limitations on what may be examined nor unrestricted access to all possible tests offer a viable solution. Any meaningful response must remain grounded in clinical judgement, the best available evidence, and careful attention to the individual patient's situation.

Unintentional knowledge, knowledge that individuals did not seek but must nevertheless live with, can alter self-understanding, bodily experience, and social position. Diagnoses and risk labels may draw people into patienthood, suspend them in liminal states between health and illness, and subject them to contradictory demands to both worry and remain calm, to act and yet not overreact. Once such knowledge is introduced, it cannot be undone, and its consequences unfold regardless of whether the diagnosis ultimately proves necessary, beneficial, or representative of overdiagnosis.

Importantly, this is not a dilemma that can be resolved by shifting responsibility onto individuals. In a health culture that emphasises self-management and personal responsibility, people cannot reasonably be expected to navigate complex probabilities, uncertain futures, and competing moral expectations on their own. The expectation that individuals should simply make the 'right' choices obscures the power of medical knowledge and underestimates the difficulty of living with uncertainty.

The central challenge, then, is not whether knowledge should be produced, but how medical knowledge is generated, communicated, and acted upon. Addressing overdiagnosis requires structural, ethical, and epistemological reflection on what kinds of knowledge actually contribute to health, and on when knowing more ceases to be beneficial. The question is not how much we can know, but when knowledge helps and when it quietly does harm.

8
Soon we will all be patients

Case: screening for 'myoletraxia'

An expert committee at a national health authority has been convened to reassess a screening programme; here we will use the case of the fictitious disease 'myelotraxia'. The programme targets 'myoletraxia' and has, for decades, been promoted as an unambiguous public good. Uptake is high, survival statistics for screened individuals are favourable and advocacy groups continue to push for broader eligibility and earlier initiation. But prior to this meeting, the committee has been presented with new analyses suggesting that a substantial proportion of detected myoletraxia would never have caused symptoms or death, even if left undiscovered. At the same time, artificial intelligence (AI)-assisted image analysis and increasingly sensitive biomarkers are identifying ever smaller abnormalities, accelerating diagnostic cascades without clear evidence of improved outcomes. The committee members are experts in their fields and generally well-informed. They know that early detection can reduce mortality. But they are also aware that technologies drive optimism for genomics, Big Data, and machine learning while the very same technologies also reshape what counts as disease. The members of the committee have been presented to international evidence showing that overdiagnosis is not a marginal phenomenon, but a structural feature of modern screening programmes, observed across healthcare systems as different as those of the USA, Canada, Europe, and East Asia (Welch et al., 2011; J.L. Carter et al., 2015a; World Health Organization (WHO), 2022). They know that guideline decisions are increasingly contested, politicised, and subject to pressure from professional societies, industry actors, patient organisations, and the media. Outside the meeting room, the pressure is palpable. Neighbouring countries have recently expanded their screening programmes, and newspaper headlines frame hesitation as negligence. Patient stories circulate widely on social media, often following a familiar script: 'Screening saved my life—why deny others the same chance?' Meanwhile, medico-tech companies promise to 'unlock hidden diagnostic potential' in existing tests, arguing that failing to adopt their tools means leaving disease undetected. The implicit moral logic is hard to resist: more detection must be better than less.

The committee faces a dilemma that has become increasingly common in contemporary medicine. If the programme is expanded, more people will be labelled as having 'myoletraxia' or 'pre-myoletraxia', subjected to surveillance, treatment, and lifelong patienthood despite never being at risk of becoming sick. If it is restricted, some future deaths may not be prevented, and responsibility for those deaths will be publicly attributed. There is no neutral option. As international screening debates have shown, from mammography to prostate cancer to lung cancer, decisions about prevention are no longer simply technical. They are ethical, political, and deeply entangled with how societies understand risk, responsibility, and the future.

This case is fictional, but versions of it are unfolding every day in health systems around the world. Experts, stakeholders, and policymakers are repeatedly confronted with similar dilemmas as they assess existing public health programmes and consider new ones. These are not simple technical decisions. They are complex questions that take shape within a landscape marked by competing interests, divergent aims, and fundamentally different perceptions of risk, benefit, and responsibility. In principle, there is broad agreement that evidence should take precedence over personal attitudes, professional preferences, or political agendas when healthcare services are implemented or evaluated. In practice, however, this ideal is difficult to realise. Evidence does not speak for itself. It must be interpreted, weighed, and translated into action, and this process is shaped by a wide range of drivers that influence what is seen as relevant, convincing, or urgent. What counts as good evidence, how uncertainty is tolerated, and which outcomes are prioritised are all matters of judgement as much as measurement.

This chapter differs deliberately from the preceding ones. Rather than relying primarily on large-scale quantitative studies or established social science theories, it adopts a more explicitly reflective and debating tone. The aim is to lay out the incentives, causes, mechanisms, and drivers that contribute to overdiagnosis, and to situate them within the political and organisational contexts in which modern healthcare operates. Some of these drivers are well documented through empirical research. Others emerge from clinical experience, policy practice, and everyday encounters with health systems, and are therefore more speculative or hypothetical in nature. Still others are plausible in theory but have yet to be studied empirically.

This heterogeneity is not a weakness of the analysis but a reflection of the problem itself. Overdiagnosis is not produced by a single mechanism or actor, and it cannot be addressed by isolated interventions. If the number of people who are overdiagnosed is to be reduced or, ideally, if overdiagnosis is to be avoided altogether then all potential incentives and drivers must first be made visible. Only by identifying and scrutinising these forces, including those that are uncomfortable, poorly measured, or politically inconvenient, can meaningful action be taken.

Overdiagnosis in society

At a general level, there is little disagreement about the overarching goals of healthcare: patients should be diagnosed in a timely manner and receive the best possible treatment. These aims are widely shared across professions, institutions, and political systems. Yet consensus quickly dissolves when we ask what timely diagnosis means, what counts as the best treatment, and for whom. Engaging critically with overdiagnosis whether from a clinical, research, or practice-oriented perspective does not imply opposition to early diagnosis or effective care. On the contrary, attention to overdiagnosis is motivated by a concern for doing better medicine, not less. At the same time, healthcare systems across high-income countries are under sustained and growing pressure. Demographic changes, particularly ageing populations and rising prevalence of chronic disease, have led economists and policymakers to predict that difficult prioritisation decisions will become unavoidable. Questions about how to balance health benefits against costs are no longer theoretical but structural features of contemporary health systems (Pedersen, 2015). Within this context, evidence from Australia, the UK, and the USA (primarily from secondary care) suggests that only around 60 percent of clinical activities can be classified as high-value care. Roughly 30 percent constitute low-value care (see Figure 8.1), while approximately 10 percent are directly harmful, including practices that lead to overdiagnosis and overtreatment (Braithwaite et al., 2020).

This waste is particularly troubling given that it coexists with persistent underprioritisation elsewhere. While some people are exposed to excessive medical attention, others, often from socially disadvantaged groups, remain undiagnosed, underdiagnosed, or inadequately treated for conditions that genuinely affect their health and quality of life (Rozing et al., 2021). Still, on a global scale, overdiagnosis is no longer only present in affluent settings, but is affecting also mid-level and lower-level income countries, leading to even more unjust resource allocation for underserved communities (Albarqouni et al., 2022). Overutilisation and underutilisation are not opposing problems but interconnected outcomes of the same system, shaped by how priorities are set and resources distributed.

Within clinical and research communities, awareness of overdiagnosis has increased markedly over the past decade. Journals, conferences, and professional debates increasingly acknowledge the issue. Yet it is equally important that those

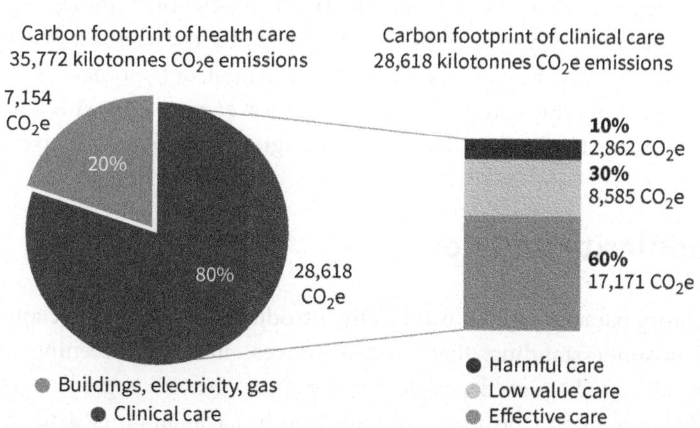

Figure 8.1 The carbon footprint of healthcare and the share of its carbon emissions attributable to harmful, low value, and effective care.
Source: Barratt et al. (2022).

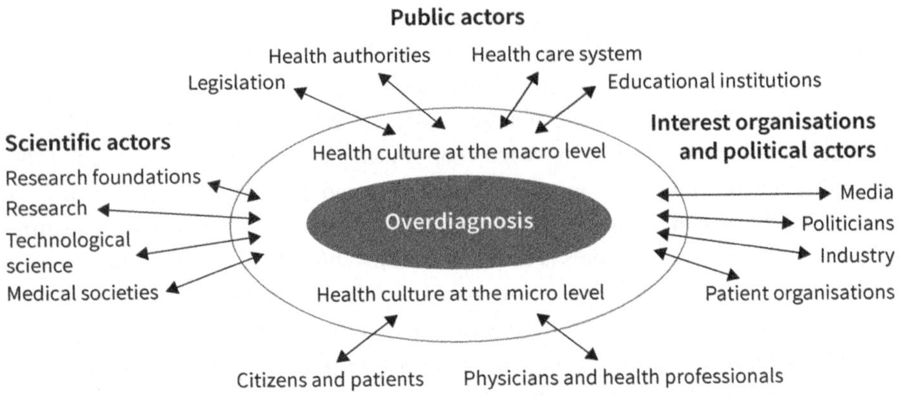

Figure 8.2 Possible incentives, causes, mechanisms of action and drivers of overdiagnosis.
At the centre is overdiagnosis within health culture at macro and micro levels. Surrounding actors include public institutions, scientific actors, interest organisations, media, industry, patient groups, physicians, and citizens, illustrating how multiple societal forces influence overdiagnosis.
Reproduced with permission from Samfundslitteratur.

responsible for organising, managing, and governing healthcare systems, who are often trained in social science, economics, management, or the humanities, engage with the problem. This raises an uncomfortable question: if overdiagnosis is so consequential, why is there not more literature addressing it outside medical research? Why does it attract relatively little sustained political attention, and why are public debates so limited?

Figure 8.2 attempts to map this terrain. It illustrates the incentives, causes, mechanisms, and drivers of overdiagnosis identified in scientific studies, encountered through research and clinical experience, or proposed as theoretically plausible. Some are well documented; others are less visible, experiential, or hypothetical.

Before unpacking this complex landscape, however, we begin with what we consider the single most influential driver of overdiagnosis: the popularity paradox.

The popularity paradox

The popularity paradox (which was briefly introduced in Chapter 5) captures a fundamental misunderstanding: that survival proves effects of screening. But as per definition, all overdiagnosed people survive their 'disease', regardless of whether they receive treatment. Consider a woman who has a small lump detected through screening mammography. Further tests and a biopsy led to a diagnosis of breast cancer. She undergoes treatment and later describes herself as having survived breast cancer. It remains possible, likely indeed, for a substantial proportion of cases, that such a lump would never have progressed, or would have grown so slowly that the woman would have lived to die from other causes. In such a case, she would have 'survived' the cancer even if it had never been detected. Still, for many people it remains deeply counterintuitive. Most of us know someone who perceives themself as saved by screening or early detection. And even if we do not, the media offer an abundance of such stories: grateful patients who credit the healthcare system with finding their disease 'just in time'. We even have a powerful rhetoric for these individuals: cancer survivors.

Throughout this book, we have presented examples of overdiagnosis across a wide range of conditions, including prostate cancer, thyroid cancer, breast cancer, melanoma, hypertension, hypercholesterolaemia, and osteoporosis. The paradox lies in the fact that most people who are overdiagnosed with these conditions will never know and therefore see themselves as survivors. At the population level, however, the overdiagnosis becomes visible. Australian data suggest that around one in five women and one in four men diagnosed with cancer are overdiagnosed (Glasziou et al., 2020). From this perspective, it would be more accurate to recognise that some people counted as survivors are, in fact, individuals who have been harmed by the healthcare system by being unnecessarily labelled as patients and exposed to interventions they did not need.

But survival narratives are powerful. Frequently mobilised by healthcare professionals, authorities, politicians, patient organisations, journalists, and patients themselves they are compelling arguments for more screening, earlier diagnosis, and easier access to testing. Such stories function as a form of evidence, regardless of what systematic medical research may show, because they resonate with intuition and emotion. Scientifically, however, these narratives are rarely documented in a way that allows us to distinguish benefit from harm. Many may, in fact, be indicators of overdiagnosis rather than proof of effective prevention. When intuitively persuasive stories are translated directly into political action, the result is often expanded testing and screening, leading to even more overdiagnosis. This, in turn, generates more survival stories, which further reinforce calls for early detection. Raffle and Gray illustrated this dynamic as a vicious circle, which we reproduce here as Figure 8.3, showing that, ironically, this process becomes self-perpetuating and harmful, driven by popular narratives rather than evidence.

The consequences of the popularity paradox extend far beyond individual cases. By using survival stories to justify allocating ever more resources to screening and early detection, healthcare systems channel resources towards people who are currently healthy. Unless additional funding is provided, this necessarily means that resources are diverted from other areas. Prioritisation becomes unavoidable. The outcome may be increased health inequality, where those who need care least receive more, and those who need it most receive less. Julian Tudor Hart described this mechanism more than fifty years ago as the Inverse Care Law (Hart, 1971). Closely related is what Brody and Light later termed the Inverse Benefit Law: the more an intervention is expanded to low-risk populations, the smaller the average benefit and the greater the overall harm (Brody & Light, 2011).

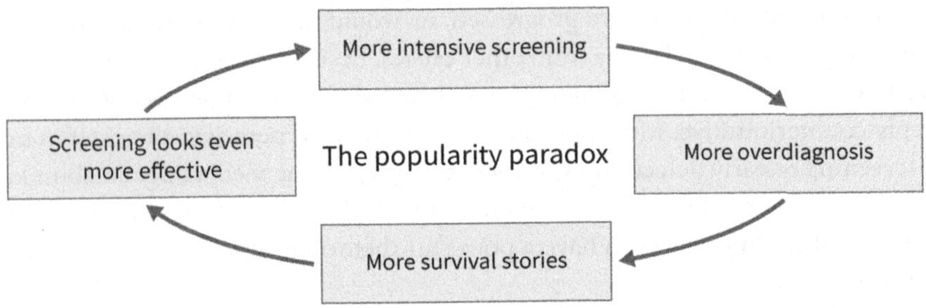

Figure 8.3 The popularity paradox: survival stories drive screening to more overdiagnosis. Source: Raffle and Gray (2007).
More intensive screening leads to more overdiagnosis, which produces more survival stories. These stories make screening appear more effective, encouraging even more screening and reinforcing the cycle.

Empirical studies support these concerns. Research from Denmark, the USA, and China shows that people with higher socioeconomic position are more likely to be overdiagnosed with cancers such as melanoma, breast cancer, prostate cancer, and thyroid cancer (Karlsen et al., 2013; Welch & Fisher, 2017; Lin et al., 2026). Overdiagnosis, in other words, is not randomly distributed; it follows existing social gradients and risks reinforcing inequality through unjust allocation of resources.

The popularity paradox may be one of the main reasons why overdiagnosis is on the rise, because it is so difficult to speak out against 'survival stories'. Unlike these, overdiagnosis is not an easy story to sell to journalists or patient organisations (McCaffery et al., 2016). It is not an easily digestible political message and can also, unintentionally, be perceived as a criticism of medical doctors and healthcare. At the same time, the more people you overdiagnose, the more people you designate and proclaim to be 'survivors'. The most valid measure of a screening programme would therefore be to report on mortality, not survival (see Chapter 4). The popularity paradox permeates the understanding of both public and private actors, individuals and organisations, because it intuitively seems like the right thing to do: to diagnose more people when so many are 'surviving'.

However, another paradox is that if the overtesting, overexamination, or overtreatment that overdiagnosed people are getting can lead to increased morbidity and mortality, there can actually be an overmortality among those who are overdiagnosed, which can lead to, on average, an increased mortality but at the same time also an increase in average survival rate.

The popularity paradox is not the only driver of overdiagnosis, but it is among the most influential. In the sections that follow, we examine these forces one by one, situating them within the political, organisational, and cultural contexts that allow overdiagnosis to flourish.

Health cultures

Health cultures (see Chapter 2) operate on at least two interconnected levels: the individual and the societal. At the individual level, contemporary understandings of health in the Global North are deeply shaped by what has been described as neoliberal governmentality. Citizens are encouraged implicitly and explicitly to view 'taking care of oneself' and 'living healthily' not merely as personal choices, but as moral obligations. Health becomes a value in itself, and responsibility for managing future illness is increasingly placed on the individual. Uncertainty about potentially developing serious disease is something one is expected to anticipate, monitor, and control.

This responsibility is exercised through participation in state-led prevention initiatives, such as screening programmes, but also through self-surveillance: paying attention to bodily signals, tracking symptoms, and using digital tools to monitor health indicators. All of this is grounded in the powerful normative idea that earlier is always better. As technologies evolve and diagnostic tools become more sensitive, trusting one's own bodily sensations becomes more difficult, especially when X-rays, blood tests, or algorithms suggest that something may be wrong (see Chapter 7). For most people without medical training, disease is understood in linear terms: once present, it progresses in a single direction unless interrupted by medical intervention. The possibility that pathological changes may regress, remain harmless, or never cause illness sits uneasily with this everyday understanding of disease (Brodersen et al., 2018b; Damhus et al., 2024).

Assumptions about disease and prevention are continually reinforced by the popularity paradox. Survival stories, early detection narratives, and moral appeals to responsibility are intuitively persuasive and notoriously difficult to challenge. Even when individuals are presented with robust medical evidence about overdiagnosis and limited or no benefits of certain preventive interventions, pre-existing beliefs often prevail (Røssel et al., 2023). Dominating beliefs frame how evidence is received, particularly when that evidence conflicts with deeply held ideas about health, control, and prudence (Petersen et al., 2020, 2025).

At the societal level, health culture is reflected in broader processes of medicalisation. Everyday experiences and common human conditions are increasingly framed in medical terms, while diagnostic thresholds, including in the field of mental health, have gradually been lowered or expanded (Frances, 2013; Brinkmannn & Petersen, 2015; Paris, 2015). At the same time, there is widespread enthusiasm for technological solutions, including personalised medicine and predictive analytics, often without sustained attention to their unintended consequences. This optimism is visible in political discourse, media coverage, professional debates, and advocacy work, where innovation is frequently equated with progress. In countries governed by neoliberal rationalities, these values are institutionalised. Individual responsibility for health and the prioritisation of prevention is embedded in legislation, healthcare organisation, educational systems, and public authorities. Health culture thus becomes a powerful backdrop against which decisions about screening, diagnosis, and prevention are made in ways that often appear self-evident and difficult to contest.

In the following sections, we therefore turn our attention to the actors, assumptions, and phenomena that constitute contemporary health culture, and to their role in producing and potentially reducing overdiagnosis.

Patients and seemingly healthy people

Most people are unfamiliar with the concept of overdiagnosis (Moynihan et al., 2015). It is therefore not surprising that many people find it difficult to grasp the difference between improved survival and reduced mortality, or to understand that increased survival rates signal overdiagnosis if mortality numbers remain stable. Likewise, it is not common knowledge that all human bodies contain deviations, abnormalities, risk factors, and pathological conditions that will never cause illness or death. In everyday thinking, such findings are interpreted as signs of latent disease requiring medical attention. Cancer, for example, is often perceived as a single disease with a uniformly poor prognosis (Elsass, 1992). However, cancer can be entirely harmless pathological conditions or aggressive diseases with high mortality. A 'late' diagnosis is therefore equated with a poor prognosis, and diagnosis itself tends to be conflated with outcome. Prognosis, by contrast, receives far less attention. Yet clinically, the relationship is often reversed. When patients present with clear alarm symptoms of cancer, diagnosis is typically made rapidly. Such symptoms are strong signals that prompt immediate investigation and referral. However, the prognosis for these patients is often poor, because cancers that produce clear alarm symptoms tend to have aggressive biological characteristics, high growth rates, and high mortality. By contrast, patients who present with general, vague, and non-specific symptoms such as fatigue or malaise are less likely to receive a diagnosis at the first consultation, and sometimes not even after several visits. In rare cases, these diffuse symptoms may mask an underlying cancer, which is then diagnosed only after some time, once symptoms have evolved or intensified. Such diagnostic trajectories are often experienced by patients as delayed or unsatisfactory. Yet, the prognosis for these patients is frequently better, because cancers that present with vague symptoms often have a slower progression and a more benign biological course (Tørring et al., 2011). This relationship between symptoms, diagnostic timing, and prognosis is not only poorly understood by the general population. It is also insufficiently recognised by politicians, health authorities, and some healthcare professionals. As a result, public and political discourse tends to equate speed of diagnosis with benefit, regardless of biological variability and prognostic diversity.

Most people also place great trust in screening and early diagnosis, a trust that is strongly reinforced by the popularity paradox (Hansson et al., 2012; Lindberg et al., 2013; Damhus et al., 2018; Gram et al., 2023b). Numerous studies show that people substantially overestimate the benefits of screening while either neglecting the possibility of harm or markedly underestimating the unintended negative effects (Henriksen et al., 2015; Hoffmann & Del Mar, 2015). This creates a persistent gap between evidence-based information provided to the public and the public's deeply held beliefs about screening as an almost risk-free good. When expectations of benefit are high and perceived harms are minimal, the conditions for genuinely informed choice are undermined (Petersen et al., 2020). This raises fundamental questions about whether informed and voluntary participation in screening is achievable in practice (Gram et al., 2023; Jensen et al., 2025).

In this context, it is unsurprising that citizens and patients often request more tests and more treatment, convinced that these will improve their prognosis. In societies with publicly funded healthcare, providers frequently encounter expectations from apparently healthy but concerned individuals who ask for paraclinical tests or comprehensive health check-ups.

Yet robust, high-quality evidence shows that inviting the general population to general health checks offers no benefit, including when the aim is to screen for cardiovascular risk factors (see also Chapter 4) (Krogsbøll et al., 2019; Jørgensen et al., 2024). On the contrary, such practices are associated with harm, including overtreatment and overdiagnosis, low-value and harmful care, increased healthcare costs, and higher carbon emissions (Andersen et al., 2022; Barratt et al., 2022; Braithwaite et al., 2020). There are even signals suggesting increased mortality among women exposed to health checks (Bender et al., 2019).

In insurance-based or market-oriented healthcare systems such as in the USA and other countries with weighty private provision, citizens and patients encounter additional pressures that shape demand for tests and treatments, often in ways that exacerbate overdiagnosis and overuse. In these settings, healthcare is not just a public good; it is also a commodity. Individuals may be encouraged to pursue more testing because insurers, providers, and commercial actors have financial incentives to promote diagnostic services. The same goes for private clinics advertising services not offered in publicly funded healthcare systems.

Another well-documented mechanism driving overuse and thus risking overdiagnosis is *physician self-referral*, in which clinicians order tests that they or their institutions stand to profit from, intentionally or unintentionally increasing test volume without clear benefit to the patient. Such practices were recognised in US policy debates around the Stark Law, which attempts but does not always succeed to limit financial incentives for unnecessary testing (Adashi & Kocher, 2015). In insurance-based settings, the interplay between consumer demand and provider incentives can thus create a feedback loop similar to that seen in public systems, but with additional commercial amplification. Patients may request tests because marketing and cultural narratives suggest that more information equals better health, while providers may be financially rewarded for performing those tests.

Seemingly healthy peoples' and patients' strong trust in treatment, early detection, and prevention thus plays an active role in driving further examinations. Evidence from systematic analyses shows that overuse of diagnostic testing is widespread across healthcare systems, with substantial variation in the prevalence of low-value tests. Overuse is not limited to imaging or laboratory tests; it is present across settings and contributes substantially to healthcare costs and potential patient harm (Müskens et al., 2022). Each additional test increases the likelihood of finding something abnormal, thereby contributing to the continuous creation of new patients, many of whom would never have benefited from being labelled as such.

Physicians and healthcare professionals

All physicians, regardless of specialty or country, practise under some degree of uncertainty and most carry a latent fear of missing something clinically important. This fear can lead clinicians to order paraclinical tests such as blood analyses or imaging even when their clinical suspicion of serious disease is very low, sometimes close to zero (Opdal et al., 2019). Such behaviour is often triggered by prior experiences, for example a complaint case, a malpractice claim, or a critical incident in which a diagnosis was perceived by patients, colleagues, or authorities to have been made 'too late'. When tests are ordered primarily to protect against blame rather than to benefit the patient, this practice is commonly described as *defensive medicine* (Hvidt et al., 2017).

Defensive medicine is a well-documented international phenomenon and a recognised driver of overdiagnosis (Berra et al., 2014; Berlin, 2017; Kainberger, 2017). It is particularly prevalent in healthcare systems characterised by litigation risk, performance monitoring, and public reporting of outcomes, but it is by no means limited to those contexts. Across settings, clinicians know that no diagnostic test is perfectly accurate since there are always false positives and false negatives. However, this probabilistic understanding of diagnostics is not always shared by politicians, health authorities, patient organisations, or the general public. The COVID-19 pandemic may have slightly altered this landscape. During the pandemic, extensive media attention was paid to the accuracy, sensitivity, and specificity of different coronavirus tests, potentially increasing public awareness of diagnostic uncertainty (Schneider et al., 2022). At the same time, the pandemic normalised large-scale testing of asymptomatic populations, which may have reinforced expectations that more testing is inherently beneficial even though overtesting increases the risk of overdiagnosis and overtreatment (Jensen & Stensballe, 2025).

A persistent challenge among healthcare professionals and decision-makers is a limited appreciation of how diagnostic performance depends on context. When pretest probability is low, as it is in asymptomatic populations or in patients with vague complaints, the risk of false positives and overdiagnosis increases substantially. In such situations, what may later be interpreted as a missed diagnosis can just as plausibly reflect the poor diagnostic accuracy of a test in a low-risk population, or the natural history of a disease with non-specific, fluctuating symptoms. Yet these nuances are rarely acknowledged in retrospective assessments of clinical decisions. Another internationally relevant driver of overdiagnosis among professionals is technological enthusiasm. New technologies, and in particular those with higher resolution or greater sensitivity, are often assumed to be superior simply because they detect more (Andersen et al., 2022). This assumption is widespread, from imaging to genomics and AI-assisted diagnostics. However, as discussed throughout this book, improved detection does not necessarily translate into improved prognosis. On the contrary, it may expand the pool of clinically inconsequential findings. This points to the importance of regulatory frameworks that require new medical technologies to be evaluated not only for potential benefits, but also for unintended harms, including overdiagnosis and overtreatment (Andersen et al., 2025).

It may not be surprising that decision-makers find it difficult to interpret the medical evidence showing overdiagnosis, because even physicians struggle to assess whether screening programmes actually work as intended. In a classic study, Wegwarth et al. (2012) demonstrated that most doctors interpreted increased survival rates and a higher proportion of 'early-stage cancer' as evidence that screening is effective despite the fact that both outcomes can be artefacts of overdiagnosis. And this is not a single trend. More recent research confirms big variations in how healthcare professionals perceive overdiagnosis: some see it as a serious harm, while others regard it as negligible or unavoidable. These views are closely linked to clinicians' broader beliefs about screening and strongly influence whether they encourage participation and whether they inform people about the risk of overdiagnosis (Piessens et al., 2025).

Along these lines, several scientific studies also show that physicians have difficulty understanding, and thus translating, evidence in their clinical practice (Ioannidis et al., 2017). For example, physicians overestimate the beneficial effects of screening and underestimate the harmful effects of screening (Hoffmann & Del Mar, 2017). Similarly, physicians have difficulty distinguishing between absolute and relative effects, which can affect their clinical behaviour (Gigerenzer et al., 2008; Nexøe et al., 2002). These cognitive and educational challenges are not individual failings, but systemic issues shaped by medical training, professional norms, guideline cultures, and performance pressures.

Politicians and policymakers

Most politicians, whether operating at national, regional, or local levels, share a basic structural condition: they want to be re-elected. Political success is therefore measured over relatively short time-horizons of a few years whereas meaningful improvements in public health typically unfold over decades. From a public health perspective, this mismatch in time-scales creates a persistent problem. Long-term investments in housing, education, working conditions, or social inequality rarely deliver visible results within a single election cycle. By contrast, initiatives that promise quick action, visible outputs, and immediate reassurance are far easier to communicate and far more politically attractive: doing more tends to look better than doing less. Acting faster tends to look better than waiting. In this context, policies that expand testing, screening, early diagnosis, and access to new technologies often appear as unequivocal progress especially when framed in language that resonates with everyday experiences of illness. Slogans such as 'The sooner the better' or 'Early detection saves lives' are politically powerful because they align with lay understandings of disease and with the popularity paradox described earlier in this chapter.

Policymakers including civil servants, senior administrators, and advisers working within ministries and agencies operate under a different but closely related set of incentives. Unlike elected politicians, they are not accountable to voters directly, but they are accountable to political leadership, performance indicators, and institutional mandates. Policymakers are often tasked with translating political visions into operational programmes, budgets, and measurable outcomes. This creates a strong preference for interventions that can be monitored, counted, and reported: numbers screened, numbers tested, numbers diagnosed, waiting times reduced. Outcomes that are difficult to measure such as avoided overdiagnosis, reduced medicalisation, or preserved quality of life tend to be neglected. In many health systems, policymakers also rely heavily on modelling, forecasting, and expert consensus to guide decisions. While these tools are indispensable, they often prioritise benefits that are easier to quantify, such as detection rates or projected lives saved, over harms that are more diffuse, delayed, or ethically complex, such as overdiagnosis and overtreatment. As a result, the balance between benefit and harm is frequently assumed rather than explicitly debated.

New technologies are particularly appealing in this policy environment. Personalised medicine, AI, digital self-monitoring, and population-level data infrastructures promise efficiency, modernisation, and sustainability, which are key policy goals in health systems under pressure. These technologies also fit neatly into narratives of innovation and competitiveness, especially in countries positioning themselves as leaders in life sciences and digital health (Topol, 2019; WHO, 2023; Zicari et al., 2021b). What tends to receive less attention is that when these tools are deployed among apparently healthy populations, they function as large-scale screening programmes in disguise, with a substantial risk of overdiagnosis. Prevention occupies a particularly ambiguous place in both political and policy discourse. Phrases such as 'It's better to prevent than to cure' are widely used yet rarely clarified. Prevention can refer to structural interventions (such as improving housing or reducing poverty), behavioural interventions (lifestyle modification), or biomedical interventions (screening and early detection). These approaches differ profoundly in their evidence base, ethical implications, and potential for harm. When prevention is left undefined, policy tends to drift towards biomedical solutions, because they are actionable within the healthcare system and easier to govern administratively. A striking illustration of how evidence-based policy advice can be overridden by political considerations is the recent case involving the Canadian Task Force on Preventive Health Care. When the Task Force declined to recommend lowering the starting age for routine breast cancer screening from 50 to 40 years, citing increased harms without clear mortality benefit, it faced intense political and public pressure. The subsequent decision by the federal Minister of Health to pause the Task Force's work effectively sidelined an independent scientific advisory body (Canadian Task Force on Preventive Health Care, 2024; Goel, 2025). In this landscape, politicians and policymakers are often caught between scientific uncertainty, political urgency, media narratives, and advocacy pressure. Restraint is difficult to defend, even when it is evidence-based. Overdiagnosis rarely produces immediate scandals or headlines, whereas a missed diagnosis can quickly become a political liability.

Legislation

Legislation sets the formal rules of the game. It defines responsibilities, obligations, and sanctions, and it tells citizens, professionals, and institutions what is expected of them and what will happen if those expectations are not met. In healthcare, Health Acts and related legislation determine who is responsible for treatment, prevention, and health promotion. They also define when something is considered a mistake. In most countries, physicians and other healthcare professionals can be sanctioned if errors are made in diagnosis or treatment.

At first glance, this seems reasonable. Patients should be protected, and professional accountability matters. The problem is that diagnostic medicine does not, and cannot, operate with certainty. Almost no diagnostic test is 100% accurate. Uncertainty is not an exception in clinical work; it is the rule. Every diagnostic decision involves judgement. For instance, the clinician must estimate the patient's pretest probability: how likely it is—given the patient's symptoms, signs, history, and context—that a particular disease is present. This estimation is not binary. It lies on a continuum between clearly healthy and clearly sick, and the interpretation of any test result depends on where along that continuum the patient is located.

Legislation, however, tends to struggle with this kind of uncertainty. Legal frameworks and clinical guidelines often imply a more algorithmic form of medicine: if symptom A is present, test B should be ordered; if result C appears, action D must follow. Such logic sits uneasily with the probabilistic nature of diagnosis. Because overdiagnosis is almost impossible to identify at the individual level, it rarely figures explicitly in legal or regulatory frameworks. Instead, attention is directed towards what can be measured and documented: missed diagnoses, delayed diagnoses, underdiagnosis, and misdiagnosis. These outcomes are turned into indicators of professional quality and patient safety.

From the clinician's perspective, this creates a powerful incentive structure. Being accused of missing a diagnosis is visible, documentable, and potentially sanctionable. Overdiagnosing someone, by contrast, is rarely recognised as an error precisely because it is so difficult to prove for any individual patient. Faced with this asymmetry, the safest course of action is often defensive medicine: ordering blood tests, scans, and other investigations at the slightest suspicion of disease, even when the clinical likelihood is very low. This strategy may protect the clinician, but it comes at a cost. When tests are used in patients with a pretest probability close to zero, the likelihood of false positives, incidental findings, and overdiagnosis increases substantially especially when high-resolution imaging or highly sensitive biomarkers are involved. At that point, diagnostic practice begins to resemble screening rather than targeted investigation. And as discussed in Chapter 4, screening low-risk or asymptomatic individuals is precisely where the risk of overdiagnosis is highest.

In this way, legislation designed to ensure quality and accountability can unintentionally push clinical practice towards more testing, more findings, and more diagnoses many of which do not benefit patients. Overdiagnosis is rarely written into the law, but it is quietly produced in its shadow.

Health authorities

Health authorities occupy a powerful and often ambivalent position in modern healthcare systems. They are typically responsible for administering health legislation and translating political intentions into concrete policies, guidelines, and programmes. Their formal mandates usually include promoting public health, preventing disease, organising diagnosis and treatment, and ensuring access to rehabilitation and palliative care. In practice, this places health authorities at the intersection of medicine, politics, and administration. Across countries, health authorities tend to operate within a broadly utilitarian framework. Their primary concern is whether an intervention appears to produce more benefit than harm at the population level. Decisions about screening programmes, preventive initiatives, and diagnostic pathways are therefore often framed as questions of balance: do the expected benefits outweigh the expected harms? Yet this balance is rarely made explicit. How benefits and harms are defined, weighted, and compared is often left implicit, embedded in technical reports or modelling assumptions rather than openly debated (Brodersen et al., 2010a; Jensen et al., 2025). This lack of transparency is problematic. Benefits and harms are not symmetrical or directly comparable (see also Chapter 4). Reduced mortality, earlier detection, psychological reassurance, and extended survival are measured in different units than are overdiagnosis, overtreatment, anxiety, complications, and lifelong labelling. Treating these as commensurable outcomes risks obscuring ethical trade-offs rather than clarifying them. In some cases, health authorities do not even apply an explicit utilitarian calculus, focusing instead almost exclusively on potential benefits while downplaying or omitting unintended harms altogether.

A key question rarely articulated in relation to overdiagnosis is where the threshold lies. How much benefit is enough to justify harm? For example: how large must a reduction in mortality be to justify one case of overdiagnosis in a screening programme? From a strictly utilitarian perspective, one might argue that preventing one death could outweigh the fact that a healthy individual is unnecessarily turned into a patient. From other ethical perspectives, however, the answer looks very different.

Deontological ethics, ethics of proximity, and the principle of *primum non nocere* (first, do no harm) raise serious concerns about causing avoidable harm to healthy individuals through overdiagnosis and overtreatment. This includes not only physical complications, but also psychological distress, social consequences, and the enduring effects of disease labelling. After all, while specific causes of death may be postponed, the mortality rate for all living beings remains 100%.

Health authorities do not make decisions in a political vacuum. They are often subject to intense pressure from elected officials, professional organisations, patient advocacy groups, and the media. These pressures can push decision-making in directions that are only loosely connected to scientific evidence. Screening expansions, lowering of age thresholds, and one-off 'catch-up' programmes are often politically attractive, symbolising action and care. But when health authorities prioritise visibility and responsiveness over careful consideration of harms, overdiagnosis becomes a predictable outcome.

Healthcare organisation

The level of activity in a healthcare system depends not only on professional indications and evidence-based practices, but also on financial incentive structures. Overuse, overtesting, overtreatment and thus overdiagnosis are therefore also more common in a privately funded healthcare system than in a publicly funded system (Docking et al., 2025). The logic is simple, if uncomfortable: if doctors are paid to do more, they will do more. Financial incentives not only affect healthcare professionals; they also shape patient behaviour. In insurance-based systems, individuals generally consume less healthcare when they are required to pay more out of pocket. Conversely, when services are heavily subsidised or fully covered, utilisation increases. This phenomenon is well described as moral hazard in health economics: insurance reduces the incentive to prevent or minimise loss, leading people to take risks they might otherwise avoid or to demand more extensive and more expensive care once illness is suspected (Einav & Finkelstein, 2018). While insurance protects against catastrophic costs and improves access to care, its unintended downside is an increase in healthcare expenditure and, in some cases, unnecessary medical activity.

Money, however, is not the only driver of behaviour. Increasingly, clinical practice is governed by performance metrics and so-called quality indicators. These indicators are intended to improve care, but they can also distort priorities. For example, if an objective of a healthcare system is that diagnoses are made fast, so that the time between the patient's first symptom and diagnosis is as short as possible, this emphasis on earlier diagnosis might lead to overdiagnosis (Damhus et al., 2024).

In much of the Global North, healthcare systems are fundamentally disease-oriented. Their primary task is to identify and treat diseases, and organisational structures reflect this aim. Hospitals are divided into specialties and subspecialties based on organs, diagnoses, and procedures. This fragmentation can be efficient for treating well-defined conditions, but it also increases the risk of overdiagnosis by encouraging narrow diagnostic focus rather than holistic assessment. In contrast, primary care and community-based services have traditionally attempted to adopt a more patient-centred or citizen-centred approach, considering the whole person rather than isolated diseases. Even in primary care, however, this ideal is under pressure. Clinical guidelines often focus on single diseases or organs and are difficult to apply to patients with multiple chronic conditions. For people with multimorbidity, following several disease-specific guidelines simultaneously can lead to excessive testing, polypharmacy, and medicalisation of everyday life (Jønsson, 2018). In such settings, overdiagnosis does not arise from error or negligence, but from well-intentioned adherence to fragmented standards of care.

The consequences of a disease-oriented approach are perhaps best illustrated by a simple clinical scenario. Imagine a 48-year-old man, Peter, visiting his local doctor because of persistent back pain. If the doctor practises within a disease-oriented framework, attention is directed primarily toward physical pathology. The consultation may focus on identifying a structural cause rather than exploring broader contextual factors such as Peter's sedentary job as a long-distance truck driver, his lack of movement, or the stress he experiences due to fear of losing his job. In this imagined scenario, Peter is referred for imaging, and the X-ray reveals an incidental finding. This finding has little or no relevance to his pain and would never have caused symptoms, yet it triggers further investigation or even treatment. Peter leaves not only with back pain, but with a diagnosis he never needed. In Peter's case overdiagnosis can emerge naturally from routine practice when healthcare systems prioritise diseases over people. Financial incentives, performance metrics, and organisational structures all push in the same direction: towards doing more, finding more, and diagnosing more. In such a system, restraint, watchful waiting, and contextual understanding are harder to justify even when they would serve the patient better.

Educational institutions

Physicians and other healthcare professionals are shaped long before they enter clinical practice. Their habits, assumptions, and professional instincts are formed during their education at universities and university colleges. At most medical faculties in the Global North, teaching is dominated by a biomedical model rooted in the natural sciences and positivist traditions. Disease is approached as something that can be located, classified, and treated, and learning is organised around organs, specialties, and diagnostic categories. If students are trained to think in silos from early on, they risk gaining a fragmented, disease-oriented understanding of medicine. What is largely missing from many curricula is a systematic engagement with evidence-based medicine including evidence-based diagnostics (Guyatt et al., 2015). While evidence-based treatment is often mentioned, far fewer programmes, to our knowledge, teach students how to think critically about diagnostic testing, pretest probability, false positives, and overdiagnosis. As a result, only a minority of medical students and physicians are formally trained in what evidence-based diagnostics actually entails, and, just as importantly, what it does not entail. Some encounter these ideas later, during specialist training or continuing medical education, but many never do.

Our own experiences from countless tutorials, lectures, workshops, conferences, and training sessions with medical students, nursing students, public health students, physicians, and other healthcare professionals across Europe suggest a consistent pattern. When diagnostics are taught, the emphasis is typically on identifying the correct diagnosis, not on understanding prognosis or weighing whether making a diagnosis will meaningfully benefit the patient. Again and again, students describe 'getting the diagnosis' preferably as early as possible as a good outcome in itself.

We should be clear: these observations are experiential rather than systematically studied. They are shaped by our own positions and interactions and therefore come with uncertainty and potential bias. However, we argue that one important driver of overdiagnosis may lie in medical education itself. Students are trained to master disease categories within their chosen specialties, but they receive far less training in understanding the whole person, living with uncertainty, or caring for patients with multiple chronic conditions. Multimorbidity, context, and prognosis sit uneasily within a curriculum built around single diseases. When future clinicians are taught to think primarily in terms of diseases rather than people, overdiagnosis becomes not an exception, but an almost inevitable outcome of good intentions applied within a narrow frame.

Commodification of health

Alongside institutional and professional drivers of overdiagnosis, a powerful and rapidly expanding force operates outside traditional healthcare systems: the commodification of health. Over the past two decades, health has increasingly become something that can be bought, optimised, monitored, and upgraded through consumer markets. Private actors now advertise health services directly to citizens, often bypassing clinicians altogether. These services include commercially marketed general health checks, vitamin and hormone panels, microbiome analyses, genetic risk profiles, and an expanding range of wellness screenings. They are typically promoted through persuasive narratives of empowerment, personal responsibility, and control over future health, inviting individuals to take action now in order to avoid illness later.

What unites these offerings is the promise of early detection and personalised insight, despite limited or entirely absent evidence that such tests improve meaningful health outcomes in asymptomatic individuals. Researchers have repeatedly warned that many direct-to-consumer tests enter the market without adequate evaluation of benefits, harms, or downstream consequences (Moynihan et al., 2019; Brodersen et al., 2023). Advertising materials tend to foreground potential benefits while omitting or downplaying information about false positives, uncertainty, overdiagnosis, and overtreatment. This imbalance mirrors and often amplifies the popularity paradox described earlier in this chapter, where survival narratives and early detection are celebrated while harms remain largely invisible.

The growing market for direct-to-consumer testing also reflects a profound shift in how responsibility and risk are distributed. Individuals are increasingly encouraged to monitor themselves continuously, often outside clinical oversight, and to interpret test results without the contextual framing that healthcare professionals are trained to provide. Empirical research shows that such testing can lead to overtesting, unnecessary follow-up investigations, psychological distress, and inappropriate use of supplements or treatments, particularly when results are ambiguous or of unclear clinical significance (McCartney, 2017; Green et al., 2020). Rather than preventing disease, these pathways frequently create new patients—people who feel unwell, worried, or labelled—without ever deriving tangible health benefits.

An emerging and particularly concerning trend is the repurposing of clinical tests for consumer markets. Biomarkers originally developed for use in clearly defined clinical contexts such as prostate-specific antigen, hormone assays, or inflammatory markers are now marketed directly to healthy individuals as indicators of 'biological age', 'hormonal balance', or 'hidden cancer risk'. When such tests are applied to populations with very low pretest probability of disease, false positives and incidental findings become the norm rather than the exception (Welch et al., 2011; Ioannidis, 2018). These findings can trigger diagnostic cascades that yield little or no health gain, but considerable harm in the form of anxiety, labelling, invasive follow-up testing, overdiagnosis and overtreatment.

From a sociological and anthropological perspective, the commodification of health blurs the boundary between health promotion and medicalisation of normal human variation. Ordinary fluctuations in biomarkers, age-related changes, or benign deviations are reframed as risks requiring surveillance and intervention. As scholars have long argued, this transformation is not value-neutral. It embeds normative assumptions about what constitutes a 'good' body, a 'responsible' citizen, and an acceptable level of uncertainty in everyday life (Rose, 2007; Petersen, 2019). Markets do not merely respond to health anxieties; they actively produce and amplify them.

Commodified health services also interact with broader health cultures and political discourses. In neoliberal contexts, where individuals are expected to take responsibility for their own health, purchasing tests can feel less like a choice and more like a moral obligation. Choosing not to test may come to be seen as irresponsible or reckless. This dynamic further shifts decision-making away from healthcare professionals who are trained to weigh benefit against harm and towards individuals acting on marketing cues, testimonials, and social media influence rather than evidence.

The role of industry in this development cannot be ignored. The concept of disease mongering has been used to describe how medical conditions are expanded or newly constructed in ways that create markets for treatments, often pharmacological ones (Moynihan & Cassels, 2005). Disease mongering typically involves redefining normal life experiences or mild symptoms as medical problems, exaggerating prevalence or severity, and promoting early intervention where the balance between benefit and harm is uncertain and unfavourable.

Beyond overt marketing, industry also supports professional societies, research initiatives, and guideline development that document statistically significant benefits when treatment thresholds are lowered or disease classifications expanded (overdefinition) (Moynihan et al., 2019). However, statistically significant effects do not necessarily translate into clinically meaningful benefits. In many cases, the absolute effects are so small that neither patients nor clinicians would consider them important if they were presented transparently (Copp et al., 2017; Bell et al., 2018). Recognising this problem, a group of researchers has proposed a checklist of evidence requirements that should be met before lowering treatment thresholds or expanding disease definitions, with particular emphasis on explicitly assessing the balance between potential benefit and potential harm (Doust et al., 2017).

Industry, of course, has a legitimate interest in selling its products. In a market economy, growth, innovation, and expansion are expected goals. Yet healthcare is not an ordinary market. When pharmaceutical and medical device industries contribute to overdiagnosis, whether through disease mongering, overdetection, or overdefinition the consequences are not merely economic. They affect real people, who become patients unnecessarily and may be harmed by interventions they never needed. In this context, treating healthcare purely as a market may risk sacrificing ethical responsibility for commercial gain. Expanding markets by inventing questionable diseases or redefining normality is not a neutral business strategy; it is a practice with profound implications for individuals, public health, and trust in medicine.

Research funding

Research funding plays a decisive role in shaping what we know about health, disease, and medicine but it also quietly shapes what we don't know. Around the world, the landscape of research investment has shifted markedly over the past two decades. Basic, curiosity-driven inquiry once formed the backbone of academic science, supported by core public funding for independent research at universities and research institutes. Today, such funding is under pressure in many countries, with governments, charities, and private foundations increasingly prioritising strategic, framework-driven, and innovation-oriented research. This means that projects promising technological breakthroughs, patents, commercialisation, or strong links with industry often fare better in competitive funding processes than work aiming to critically examine existing practices, including harms associated with overdiagnosis. Such trends reflect broader shifts in science policy toward excellence, impact, and economic growth, often measured through short-term outputs rather than long-term societal benefit (PwC, 2025).

The bias towards innovation and growth creates a challenging environment for research that questions prevailing assumptions. Projects focused on overdiagnosis, especially those that might cast doubt on high-profile screening programmes or widely adopted technologies, are less likely to attract funding because they do not align with narratives of progress or commercial opportunity. As argued by Moynihan and colleagues, research that spotlights harms, low-value care, or negative outcomes rarely fits neatly into funding priorities that are dominated by disease-targeting, novel therapies, and technological solutions; yet such work is critical to understanding and reducing harm in health systems (Moynihan et al., 2019).

Beyond structural bias, conflicts of interest are a persistent concern. Industry sponsorship, whether from pharmaceutical companies, device manufacturers, or health technology firms, has been shown repeatedly to correlate with research outcomes that favour sponsors' interests. Such funding arrangements can skew research agendas toward product development and marketable innovations, at the expense of independent evaluations of harms, cost-effectiveness, or unwelcome side-effects of medical interventions. Attempts to manage and mitigate conflicts of interest through disclosure policies are widespread, but empirical work suggests that such policies alone do not reliably prevent bias in research design, conduct, or reporting (Graham et al., 2025). The current international funding ecosystem tends to reward big, predictable, and commercially appealing research programmes while giving less support to work that challenges the status quo or investigates unintended harms like overdiagnosis.

Research

At the same time as basic funding for independent research is shrinking, the conditions under which research is carried out at universities are changing in ways that matter for what knowledge is produced. Across countries, permanent academic positions are becoming rarer. Short-term contracts, project-based employment, and fixed-term appointments are now the norm for many researchers, particularly early- and mid-career scholars. With less job security and limited time-horizons, researchers are under pressure to produce results quickly—ideally results that align with the priorities, policy frameworks, and strategic goals set out by funding bodies. In this environment, everyone wants a success story. Funders, institutions, and policymakers tend to favour research that demonstrates that something works, that a problem can be solved, that an intervention is effective or beneficial. Studies showing positive effects are easier to promote, easier to defend, and easier to translate into policy. This preference is reinforced by a well-known phenomenon in evidence-based medicine: publication bias (Guyatt et al., 2015). Research showing no effect (or worse: harm) is less likely to be published than research reporting positive findings. The scientific literature therefore tends to overrepresent benefits and underrepresent failures and harms. But publication bias is only part of the story. A deeper problem arises when certain research questions are not asked at all. If research systematically focuses on benefits while neglecting potential harms including overdiagnosis, then the knowledge base itself becomes skewed. This has been clearly documented in relation to cancer screening programmes, where early studies often failed to investigate or even acknowledge overdiagnosis as a possible outcome (Heleno et al., 2013). When harms are not studied, they cannot inform decision-making. This is not merely a technical oversight; it is a structural problem in how research agendas are set.

There are broader implications. Research that avoids uncomfortable questions threatens more than scientific balance. Free inquiry, critical reflection, and the willingness to challenge dominant practices are cornerstones of both science and democracy. When funding structures, career incentives, and institutional pressures make it difficult to pursue research that questions prevailing assumptions, this undermines free research, free thought, and, ultimately, freedom of expression—values that underpin democratic societies. On a practical level, studying harms is also harder. Measuring potential benefits of a health intervention is often quicker and more straightforward than documenting its unintended consequences (Zorzela et al., 2016). In countries with strong population registries such as the Nordic countries it is relatively easy to determine when people die and what they die from, thanks to comprehensive registries and unique personal identifiers. Mortality outcomes can therefore be assessed with reasonable efficiency. Overdiagnosis, however, is a different matter. Because it is impossible to determine at the individual level whether a person has been correctly diagnosed or overdiagnosed, identifying overdiagnosis requires long-term follow-up at the population level. In practice, this means randomised studies that follow participants until death, sometimes decades later, to observe who benefits and who is harmed. Such studies are costly, slow, and unattractive in a funding climate that prioritises rapid results. As an illustration, less than half of the participants in the Danish lung cancer computed tomography screening trial had died 11 years after the first participant was screened (Heleno et al., 2018). Drawing robust conclusions about overdiagnosis in such contexts can easily take 20 years or more.

Technological development

Technological science is advancing at a remarkable pace. Medical technologies are becoming cheaper, more accessible, more sensitive, and capable of producing ever higher resolution images and measurements. What once required specialised equipment and trained professionals is increasingly migrating into everyday life. Tests that were previously performed once, perhaps during a clinical encounter, can now be carried out repeatedly or even continuously through wearable devices, home-based self-tests, and diagnostic apps. This shift fundamentally changes not only how data are produced, but also how health and disease are perceived.

New technology is often introduced with an implicit assumption of improvement: higher sensitivity is equated with better care, more data with better knowledge, and continuous measurement with better prevention. These assumptions are rarely scrutinised. In contrast to pharmacological treatments, which must pass through extensive regulatory processes demonstrating efficacy and safety before approval, new medical technologies and digital health tools are often subject to far less stringent evaluation. In many countries, health apps, diagnostic devices, and self-tests can enter the market with limited evidence of benefit and minimal assessment of potential harm. Several scholars have therefore argued that regulatory frameworks for medical technology, particularly digital and AI-based tools, should be strengthened to reflect their capacity to cause harm, including overdiagnosis and overtreatment (Topol, 2019; Babic et al., 2021; WHO, 2023; Zicari et al., 2021b).

The risk is not hypothetical. A clear example can be found in breast cancer screening. The transition from analogue to digital mammography increased image resolution, allowing radiologists to detect smaller abnormalities. However, evidence from population-based studies shows that digital mammography has led to increased overdiagnosis compared with analogue technology, without corresponding reductions in advanced disease or mortality (Farber et al., 2021, 2024a, 2024b, 2025). If AI is added to digital mammography and flags even subtler screening findings, the risk of overdiagnosis appears to increase (Gommers et al., 2026; Lauritzen et al., 2024). Nevertheless, mammography screening programmes across the Global North have almost universally transitioned to digital technology, and an increasing number of countries are implementing AI systems to support or partially replace human reading of mammograms. These decisions are often framed as inevitable progress. Rarely is the question asked whether detecting more abnormalities necessarily improves outcomes for women, or whether it simply expands the pool of people labelled as having cancer or pre-cancer. A similar dynamic may unfold as diagnostics move beyond clinical settings into everyday life. Self-tests for biomarkers, hormones, infections, and genetic risks are becoming increasingly available, often marketed directly to consumers. Diagnostic apps promise early detection, personalised risk assessment, and continuous monitoring. As tests become cheaper and easier to access, thresholds for testing fall, and measurements multiply. The combination of high sensitivity, frequent testing, and low pretest probability creates ideal conditions for false positives, incidental findings, and overdiagnosis.

What is striking is how little evidence exists to guide these developments. There is virtually no robust scientific basis for determining whether the rapid expansion of medical technology leads to more benefit, more harm, or both at the population level. Most evaluations focus on technical performance: accuracy, sensitivity, or user engagement, rather than on downstream consequences such as overdiagnosis, psychological burden, unnecessary treatment, or inequitable resource use. Long-term outcomes, including effects on morbidity, mortality, and quality of life, are rarely studied.

Medical colleges and societies

Most medical colleges and professional societies are organised around a single organ or a single diagnosis, for example, the European Society of Cardiology (an organ) and the American Epilepsy Society (a diagnosis). These societies play an important role in their work to ensure that national and international clinical guidelines establish a high and uniform level for all types of treatments. The development of clinical guidelines often happens in collaboration with national authorities or international bodies such as the Cochrane Collaboration, the US Preventive Services Task Force, or the Canadian Task Force on Preventive Health Care. Organ- and diagnosis-specific guidelines tend to view patients through narrow clinical lenses. People with multimorbidity are effectively split into multiple silos, one for each diagnosis or organ system. What is lost in this process is an understanding of the whole person: how conditions interact, how treatments accumulate, and how risks and benefits compound over time. As several studies have shown, this siloed approach makes it difficult to apply guidelines meaningfully to patients with complex health profiles, who are increasingly the norm rather than the exception (Kristensen et al., 2017, 2018a, 2018b). One notable exception is the National Institute for Health and Care (NICE) guideline on multimorbidity published in 2016, which explicitly addresses this gap and remains relatively unique in the international guideline landscape (Kernick et al., 2017). The dominance of organ- and diagnosis-specific thinking has consequences for overdiagnosis. When abnormalities, risk factors, or deviations are detected within a single organ, they are easily interpreted as disease, especially when found through increasingly sensitive technologies in people who feel entirely well. Similarly, specialist societies often advocate for expanding disease definitions or lowering treatment thresholds, particularly for risk factors, in the hope of improving prognosis. As we have shown throughout this book, these mechanisms are central drivers of overdiagnosis.

At the clinical level, most organ specialists have encountered patients diagnosed at very advanced stages of disease. In such cases, it is tempting to assume that earlier diagnosis would necessarily have led to a better prognosis. This linear understanding of disease progression is widespread, not only among the public but also within the medical profession (Damhus et al., 2024). Healthcare workers often report being confronted by patients or relatives who believe that a delayed diagnosis reflects a professional failure, even when the disease biology was aggressive and the outcome unlikely to have changed. These narratives can damage trust, strain professional relationships, and unintentionally promote more testing and earlier diagnosis regardless of whether this benefits future patients. Underlying this is a limited appreciation of the natural history of disease. Some conditions progress rapidly and unpredictably; others remain indolent or never cause harm at all. Not every abnormality becomes disease, and not every disease becomes clinically meaningful. Yet the focus by specialists on 'their' organ or diagnosis can create what might be described as an intellectual conflict of interest: a strong inclination to see clinical significance where, from a broader perspective, there may be little or none.

Finally, professional behaviour does not exist in a vacuum. Financial incentives also shape clinical practice. Specialists who are reimbursed for procedures, tests, or consultations are more likely to deliver more of them. Relationships with industry as consultants, advisors, or researchers have been shown to influence prescribing patterns, guideline recommendations, and clinical decision-making (Lundh & Bero, 2017; Mintzes et al., 2018; Nejstgaard et al., 2020). While financial conflicts of interest are now routinely disclosed in scientific publications, their impact on overdiagnosis remains difficult to quantify and even harder to address.

Patient organisations

International research has consistently shown that many patient organisations receive substantial financial support from industry, including pharmaceutical and medical device companies. This support may take the form of unrestricted grants, project-based funding, sponsorship of campaigns or conferences, or direct donations (Rose et al., 2017; Fabbri et al., 2019, 2020; Mulinari et al., 2020; Pashley et al., 2022; Gentilini & Parvanova, 2023). Industry is a well-documented driver of overdiagnosis through mechanisms such as disease expansion, lowered treatment thresholds, and promotion of early detection. Financial ties therefore create a structural risk that patient organisations—though often unintentionally—become aligned with agendas that increase overdiagnosis.

Patient organisations are, by their very nature, organised around specific diseases or diagnostic categories. Their core mission is to advocate for people affected by these conditions, to improve care, raise awareness, and secure political attention and resources. In health systems across the Global North, this advocacy has become increasingly influential. Health is one of the most salient political issues for voters, and patient voices carry strong moral authority. As a result, healthcare has become a central battleground where patient organisations seek to influence politicians, health authorities, clinicians, researchers, and the media, often in close collaboration with medical societies and, at times, industry partners.

A recurring focus of patient advocacy is the call for more and faster diagnosis. For example, in Northern Europe and the UK, national cancer patient organisations have been strong proponents of national cancer plans, fast-track diagnostic pathways, and expanded screening programmes. These initiatives have often been framed around the goal of achieving cancer survival rates comparable to those in neighbouring countries or international benchmarks (Damhus et al., 2024). Survival, in this context, becomes a powerful and emotionally compelling metric.

When patient organisations argue for expanded screening, easier access to testing, or faster diagnostic pathways for 'their' disease, be it cancer, sclerosis, osteoporosis and so on, these initiatives will very likely increase overdiagnosis in cases where patients can be diagnosed without symptoms and with the chance of never developing symptoms or dying from the disease, even when untreated. In this way, patient organisations can become central actors in the popularity paradox: more diagnosis leads to more survivors and more members that can advocate for awareness and earlier diagnostics. However, it is important to note that awareness and earlier diagnostics are not inherently harmful, but they can become so when they unintentionally lead to overdetection and the lowering of diagnostic or treatment thresholds.

This dynamic is rarely driven by ill intent. Patient organisations speak from lived experience, often shaped by encounters with severe disease, delayed diagnosis, or loss. Yet the collective effects of their advocacy can differ markedly from the intentions of individual members. When overdiagnosis is not acknowledged, and when prognosis is conflated with diagnosis, advocacy efforts risk prioritising visibility and speed over proportionality and evidence. The result is a political and cultural environment in which restraint becomes difficult to defend and caution can be misinterpreted as indifference.

The media

Health has become one of the most dominant storylines in contemporary media landscapes. It is now difficult to find a newspaper, news website, television channel, or social media feed that does not feature one or more health-related stories every single day. This is not only a matter of public service or journalistic responsibility. Health stories attract attention, clicks, and emotional engagement and therefore advertising revenue. Illness, risk, and survival are universally relatable, and they lend themselves particularly well to storytelling. But media coverage of health varies greatly in quality. Some journalists are highly skilled at communicating complex scientific evidence, uncertainty, and nuance. Others, often constrained by deadlines, formats, or editorial priorities, lean more heavily on personal stories and dramatic narratives. This is where the popularity paradox reappears. Individual cases, especially stories of survival following early detection, are powerful and memorable. They put a face to disease. They also resonate strongly with lay understandings of illness, even when they are poor representations of population-level evidence. Overdiagnosis, by contrast, is deeply resistant to media logic. It cannot be seen in the individual case. It has no clear protagonist. It unfolds over time and only becomes visible at the population level. Explaining it requires probability, counterfactual reasoning, and an uncomfortable acknowledgment that some diagnoses and even treatments were never needed. This makes overdiagnosis difficult to communicate through the traditional narrative tools of journalism (Moynihan et al., 2015; McCaffery et al., 2016). As a result, media coverage tends to privilege detection, diagnosis, and survival, while harms such as overdiagnosis and overtreatment remain largely invisible.

Recent research confirms that this imbalance is not incidental. A systematic analysis of health reporting across multiple countries found that media coverage overwhelmingly emphasises benefits of screening and testing while rarely mentioning harms, false positives, or overdiagnosis. A study showed that news stories frequently rely on press releases that themselves overstate benefits and downplay uncertainty, creating a cascade of exaggeration as research moves from journals to headlines (Yavchitz et al., 2022). This dynamic is not confined to traditional media; it is amplified in digital environments such as social media where speed, shareability, and emotional impact are rewarded. And the rise of social media and influencer culture has intensified these dynamics further, particularly in insurance-based and private healthcare contexts. Influential accounts with millions of followers routinely promote health checks, genetic tests, hormone panels, full-body magnetic resonance imaging, and multi-cancer blood tests as tools for 'taking control' of one's health or 'catching disease early'. Empirical analyses of influencer content show that such posts almost never mention potential harms, including false positives, anxiety, downstream testing, or overdiagnosis, while commercial ties are often opaque or disclosed only minimally (Nickel et al., 2025). In this setting, medical tests are reframed as lifestyle choices rather than clinical interventions, further detaching them from evidence-based decision-making.

A concrete example of how media narratives can fuel overdiagnosis comes from a widely circulated story about the Vancouver Canucks' equipment manager, who was diagnosed with melanoma after a spectator at a hockey game pointed out a mole on his neck. The story went viral internationally and was republished by major outlets, including *The New York Times*, under the headline 'Hockey Fan Spots Cancerous Mole at Game and Delivers a Lifesaving Note' (Smith, 2022). The narrative is compelling, generous, and emotionally satisfying. It also subtly promotes the idea that vigilant observation of other people's bodies and unsolicited advice is not only acceptable but morally commendable. The ripple effects of such stories are difficult to predict but potentially far-reaching.

Media ecosystems are also shaped by financial structures. Many outlets depend on advertising revenue from pharmaceutical companies, medical device manufacturers, and private healthcare providers. These relationships can subtly influence which stories are told and how they are framed, even in the absence of overt editorial interference. While some journals, conferences, and media organisations have chosen to limit or exclude industry advertising, this remains the exception rather than the rule.

Conclusion

Ours is a world increasingly preoccupied with health, risk, and the prevention of disease. Across political arenas, healthcare systems, patient organisations, professional societies, and industry, the shared ambition is to do more: detect earlier, intervene faster, and optimise health before illness appears. Yet in this crowded and well-intentioned landscape, one group is strikingly absent from the conversation, namely the apparently healthy citizens who stand to bear the unintended consequences of these efforts.

Throughout this book, we have shown how overdiagnosis emerges not from a single decision or actor, but from the cumulative effects of many interacting forces: health cultures that equate action with care; screening programmes evaluated through misleading outcomes; technological developments that increase sensitivity without proportional benefit; personalised medicine and AI that fragment the person into risk variables; commercial interests that expand disease definitions; media narratives that privilege survival stories; and political incentives that reward visibility over restraint. None of these forces are inherently malicious. Most arise from a sincere desire to help. Yet together, they create a system that steadily transforms healthy people into patients often without improving prognosis, quality of life, or longevity.

Overdiagnosis is particularly difficult to confront because it lacks a clear victim in the present. The overdiagnosed individual feels healthy, is often grateful, and may even identify as a survivor. The harm unfolds quietly: through unnecessary treatments, lifelong labels, anxiety, side-effects, opportunity costs, and the diversion of resources away from those who need care most. Consequently, overdiagnosis remains politically invisible, ethically uncomfortable, and culturally hard to acknowledge.

At the beginning of this book, we referred to Jules Romains' satirical play *Doctor Knock* from 1923, in which the doctor declares that 'healthy people are sick people who do not yet know it'. What was once a caricature of medical excess now reads uncomfortably like a diagnosis of our own time. When health becomes a moral obligation, when uncertainty is no longer tolerated, and when every deviation is framed as a risk demanding action, the category of the healthy begins to disappear.

This book is not an argument against medicine, prevention, or diagnostics. Awareness and timely diagnostics are not inherently harmful. The harm arises when they are used often unintentionally to justify overdetection, lowered thresholds, and the expansion of disease into ever larger parts of everyday life. Nor is this a call for inaction. It is a call for proportionality, humility, and a renewed focus on what medicine is ultimately for: improving patient's lives, not merely finding more abnormalities.

If we fail to take a more critical and reflective approach to our health culture, our screening programmes, early diagnostics, personalised medicine, prevention strategies, patient advocacy, and political priorities we risk creating societies in which everyone is a patient, but fewer people are truly healthier.

References

Aagaard, M., á Rogvi, J., Modin, F., Nicolaisdóttir, D., Siersma, V., & Brodersen, J.B. (2025). Short term complications of conisation and long term effects on fertility related outcomes in Denmark: Register based nationwide cohort study. *BMJ*, 388, e078140.

Aarre, T.F. (2018). *En mindre medisinsk psykiatri [A smaller medical psychiatry]*. Universitetsforlaget.

Aberle, D.R., Adams, A.M., Berg, C.D., Black, W.C., Clapp, J.D., Fagerstrom, R.M., Gareen, I.F., Gatsonis, C., Marcus, P.M., & Sicks, J.D. (2011). Reduced lung-cancer mortality with low-dose computed tomographic screening. *New England Journal of Medicine*, 365(5), 395–409.

Abraham, E. (2008). Erratum: Correction of conflict of interest statement. *American Journal of Respiratory and Critical Care Medicine*, 178(5), 542.

Adamu, I., Lambert, A., Bello, S., Abdulmalik, F.A., & Marshall, T. (2025). The effects of antibiotic prescribing for respiratory tract infection on future consultations in primary care: A systematic review and meta-analysis. *medRxiv*, 2025.2001.2015.25320600.

Adashi, E.Y., & Kocher, R.P. (2015). Physician self-referral: Regulation by exceptions. *JAMA*, *313*(5), 457–458.

Adelswärd, V., & Sachs, L. (1996). The meaning of 6.8: Numeracy and normality in health information talks. *Social Science and Medicine*, 43, 1179–1187.

Ahn, H.S., Kim, H.J., & Welch, H.G. (2014). Korea's thyroid-cancer 'epidemic'—Screening and overdiagnosis. *New England Journal of Medicine*, 371(19), 1765–1767.

Albarqouni, L., Arab-Zozani, M., Abukmail, E., Greenwood, H., Pathirana, T., Clark, J., Kopitowski, K., Johansson, M., Born, K., Lang, E., & Moynihan, R. (2022). Overdiagnosis and overuse of diagnostic and screening tests in low-income and middle-income countries: A scoping review. *BMJ Global Health*, 7(10), e008696. https://doi.org/10.1136/bmjgh-2022-008696

Andersen, C.A., Guetterman, T.C., Fetters, M.D., Brodersen, J., Davidsen, A.S., Graumann, O., & Jensen, M.B. (2022). General practitioners' perspectives on appropriate use of ultrasonography in primary care in Denmark: A multistage mixed methods study. *Annals of Family Medicine*, *20*(3), 211–219.

Andersen, C.A., Brodersen, J.B., Mainz, J., Thomsen, J.L., Graumann, O., Løkkegaard, T., & Jensen, M.B. (2025). Does point-of-care ultrasound examination by the general practitioner lead to inappropriate care? A follow-up study. *Scandinavian Journal of Primary Health Care*, 43(3), 613–625.

Andersen, M., Munck, A., & Lykkegaard, J. (2019). *Audit om defensiv medicin i almen praksis*. APO.

Anderssen, I. (2000). Men du har jo den angsten i dæ . . . 'Om å leve med risiko som diagnose'. In E. Swensen (Ed.), *Diagnose: Risiko* (pp. 86–97). Universitetsforlaget.

Andriole, G.L., Crawford, E.D., Grubb, R.L., Buys, S.S., Chia, D., Church, T.R., Fouad, M.N., Gelmann, E.P., Kvale, P.A., Reding, D.J., Weissfeld, J.L., Yokochi, L.A., O'Brien, B., Clapp, J.D., Rathmell, J.M., Riley, T.L., Hayes, R.B., Kramer, B.S., Izmirlian, G., . . . & Berg, C.D. (2009). Mortality results from a randomized prostate-cancer screening trial. *New England Journal of Medicine*, 360(13), 1310–1319.

Babic, B., Gerke, S., Evgeniou, T., & Cohen, I.G. (2021). Direct-to-consumer medical machine learning and artificial intelligence applications. *Nature Machine Intelligence*, *3*, 283–287.

Bae, J.M. (2015). Overdiagnosis: Epidemiologic concepts and estimation. *Epidemiology and Health*, 37, e2015004.

Bakken, R. (2020). *Alle vil leve længe, men ingen vil blive gamle*. Samfundslitteratur.

Barratt, A., & McGain, F. (2021). Overdiagnosis is increasing the carbon footprint of healthcare. *BMJ*, 375, n2407.

Barratt, A., Bell, K., Charlesworth, K., & McGain, F. (2022). High value health care is low carbon health care. *Medical Journal of Australia*, 216(2), 67–68.

Barton, M.B., Moore, S., Polk, S., Shtatland, E., Elmore, J.G., & Fletcher, S.W. (2001). Increased patient concern after false-positive mammograms: Clinician documentation and subsequent ambulatory visits. *Journal of General Internal Medicine*, 16(3), 150–156.

Basnyat, P.S., Biffin, A.H., Moseley, L.G., Hedges, A.R., & Lewis, M.H. (1999). Mortality from ruptured abdominal aortic aneurysm in Wales. *British Journal of Surgery*, 86(6), 765–770.

Bateson, G. (1972). *Steps to an ecology of mind: Collected essays in anthropology, psychiatry, evolution, and epistemology*. University of Chicago Press.

Bateson, G. (1979). *Mind and nature: A necessary unity*. Bantam Books.

Bateson, G. (1987). *Angels fear: Towards an epistemology of the sacred*. Hampton Press.

Bateson, G. (2005). Mentale systemers økologi, Part III. Akademisk Forlag. [Originally published as: Bateson, G. (1972). *Steps to an ecology of mind: Collected essays in anthropology, psychiatry, evolution, and epistemology*. Chandler Publishing Company]

Bateson, G., Jackson, D.D., Haley, J., & Weakland, J. (1956). Toward a theory of schizophrenia. *Systems Research*, 1, 251–264.

Bauman, Z. (1992). *Mortality, immortality, and other life strategies*. Polity Press.

Bauman, Z. (1999). *Culture as praxis*. SAGE Publications.

Beck, U. (1997). *Risikosamfundet—på vej mod en ny modernitet*. Hans Reitzels Forlag.

Beer, D. (2014). The biopolitics of biometrics: An interview with Btihaj Ajana. *Theory, Culture & Society*, 31(7–8), 329–336.

Beich, A. (2017). Fokus på overdiagnostik gør os til bedre læger—ikke dårligere. *Dansk Selskab for Almen Medicin*, 6 April. dsam.dk/dsam_mener/holdninger_og_politikker/fokus-paa-overdiagnostik-goer-os-til-bedre-laeger-ikke-daarligere/ (accessed 14 May 2021).

Bekele, D., & Martínez-Hernáez, A. (2025). Qualitative studies on men with prostate cancer: A systematic meta-synthesis. *International Journal of Qualitative Studies on Health and Well-being*, 20(1), 2436720. https://doi.org/10.1080/17482631.2024.2436720

Bell, K.J.L., Del Mar, C., Wright, G., Dickinson, J., & Glasziou, P. (2015). Prevalence of incidental prostate cancer: A systematic review of autopsy studies. *International Journal of Cancer*, 137(7), 1749–1757.

Bell, K.J.L., Doust, J., & Glasziou, P. (2018). Incremental benefits and harms of the 2017 American College of Cardiology/American Heart Association high blood pressure guideline. *JAMA Internal Medicine*, 178(6), 755–757.

Bender, A.M., Jørgensen, T., & Pisinger, C. (2019). Higher mortality in women living in high-participation areas of a population-based health check and lifestyle intervention study. *International Journal of Public Health*, 64(1), 107–114.

Berlin, L. (2017). Medical errors, malpractice, and defensive medicine: An ill-fated triad. *Diagnosis*, 4(3), 133–139.

Berra, A., Pira, E., & Romano, C. (2014). Overdiagnosis and defensive medicine in occupational medicine. *Giornale italiano di medicina del lavoro ed ergonomia*, 36, 448–456.

Bibbins-Domingo, K., Grossman, D.C., Curry, S.J., Barry, M.J., Davidson, K.W., Doubeni, C.A., Epling Jr, J.W., Kemper, A.R., Krist, A.H., Kurth, A.E., Landefeld, C.S., Mangione, C.M., Phipps, M.G., Silverstein, M., Simon, M.A., Siu, A.L., & Tseng, C.W. (2017). Screening for thyroid cancer: US Preventive Services Task Force Recommendation Statement. *JAMA*, 317(18), 1882–1887.

Bie, A.K.L., Martiny, F.H.J., Jauernik, C.P., Rahbek, O.J., Nielsen, S.B., Gram, E.G., Kindt, I., & Brodersen, J.B. (2025). Physical harms in colorectal cancer screening: An overview of the reporting in systematic reviews and randomised controlled trials. *PLoS One*, 20(9), e0331104.

Biesheuvel, C., Barratt, A., Howard, K., Houssami, N., & Irwig, L. (2007). Effects of study methods and biases on estimates of invasive breast cancer overdetection with mammography screening: A systematic review. *Lancet Oncology*, 8(12), 1129–1138.

Bøker, T.L., Brodersen, J., & Sandøe, P. (2018). A study of anti-fat bias among Danish general practitioners and whether this bias and general practitioners' lifestyle can affect treatment of tension headache in patients with obesity. *Obesity Facts*, 11(6), 501–513.

Bond, M., Pavey, T., Welch, K., Cooper, C., Garside, R., Dean, S., & Hyde, C.J. (2012). Psychological consequences of false-positive screening mammograms in the UK. *BMJ Evidence-Based Medicine*, 18(2), 54–61.

Bonney, A., Malouf, R., Marchal, C., Manners, D., Fong, K.M., Marshall, H.M., Irving, L.B., & Manser, R. (2022). Impact of low-dose computed tomography (LDCT) screening on lung cancer-related mortality. *Cochrane Database of Systematic Reviews*, 8(8), Cd013829.

Braithwaite, J., Glasziou, P., & Westbrook, J. (2020). The three numbers you need to know about healthcare: The 60–30–10 Challenge. *BMC Medicine*, 18(1), 102.

Bretthauer, M., Wieszczy, P., Løberg, M., Kaminski, M.F., Werner, T.F., Helsingen, L.M., Mori, Y., Holme, Ø., Adami, H.O., & Kalager, M. (2023). Estimated lifetime gained with cancer screening tests: A meta-analysis of randomized clinical trials. *JAMA Internal Medicine*, 183(11), 1196–1203.

Brinkmann, S., & Petersen, A. (2015). *Diagnoser—perspektiver, kritik og diskussion*. Klim.

Brinkmann, S. (2010). *Det diagnosticerede liv. Sygdom uden grænser*. Klim.

Brinkmann, S. (2014). *Stå fast. Et opgør med tidens udviklingstvang*. Gyldendal Business.

Brkljačić, B., Karoussou-Schreiner, A., Sosna, J., Foley, S., Bly, R., Brady, A., Ebdon-Jackson, S., Demuth, F., Singer, C., Saban, M., Bergovoy Yellin, L., Hierath, M., & Szucsich, M. (2024). European co-ordinated action on improving justification of computed tomography – Results and recommendations from a first-time multi-national study on CT justification in the EU. Publications Office of the European Union. https://op.europa.eu/en/publication-detail/-/publication/dc071d95-7179-11ef-a8ba-01aa75ed71a1/language-en

Brodersen, J. (2017a). How to conduct research on overdiagnosis. A keynote paper from the EGPRN May 2016, Tel Aviv. *European Journal of General Practice*, 23(1), 78–82.

Brodersen, J. (2017b). Overdiagnosis: An unrecognised and growing worldwide problem in healthcare. *Zdravstveno varstvo*, 56(3), 147–149.

Brodersen, J., & Jørgensen, T. (2021). Screening. In B.B. Jensen, M.K. Grønbæk, & S. Reventlow (Eds.), *Forebyggende sundhedsarbejde*. 7. udgave (pp. 539–565). Munksgaard.

Brodersen, J., & Lunde, I.M. (2002). Konsekvenser af usikkerheder og overdiagnosticering ved screening. *Ugeskrift for læger*, 164(2), 181–187.

Brodersen, J., & Siersma, V.D. (2013). Long-term psychosocial consequences of false-positive screening mammography. *Annals of Family Medicine*, 11(2), 106–115.

Brodersen, J., & Thorsen, H. (2008). Consequences of screening in breast cancer (COS-BC). Development of a questionnaire. *Scandinavian Journal of Primary Health Care*, 26(4), 251–256.

Brodersen, J., Thorsen, H., & Cockburn, J. (2004). The adequacy of measurement of short and long-term consequences of false-positive screening mammography. *Journal of Medical Screening*, 11(1), 39–44.

Brodersen, J., Jørgensen, K.J., & Gøtzsche, P.C. (2010a). The benefits and harms of screening for cancer with a focus on breast screening. *Polish Archives of Internal Medicine, 120*(3), 89–94.

Brodersen, J., Thorsen, H., & Kreiner, S. (2010b). Consequences of screening in lung cancer: Development and dimensionality of a questionnaire. *Value in Health*, 13(5), 601–612.

Brodersen, J., Siersma, V.D., & Ryle, M. (2011). Breast cancer screening: 'Reassuring' the worried well? *Scandinavian Journal of Public Health*, 39(3), 326–332.

Brodersen, J., Schwartz, L., & Woloshin, S. (2014). Overdiagnosis: How cancer screening can turn indolent pathology into illness. *Acta Pathologica et Microbiologica Scandinavica*, 122(8), 683–689.

Brodersen, J., Schwartz, L.M., Heneghan, C., O'Sullivan, J.W., Aronson, J.K., & Woloshin, S. (2018a). Overdiagnosis: What it is and what it isn't. *BMJ Evidence-Based Medicine*, 23(1), 1–3.

Brodersen, J., Siersma, V.D., & Thorsen, H. (2018b). Consequences of screening in cervical cancer: Development and dimensionality of a questionnaire. *BioMed Central Psychology*, 6(1), 39.

Brodersen, J., Hansson, A., Johansson, M., Siersma, V., Langenskiöld, M., & Pettersson, M. (2018c). Consequences of screening in abdominal aortic aneurysm: Development and dimensionality of a questionnaire. *Journal of Patient-Reported Outcomes*, 2(1), 37.

Brodersen, J., Voss, T., Martiny, F., Siersma, V., Barratt, A., & Heleno, B. (2020). Overdiagnosis of lung cancer with low-dose computed tomography screening: Meta-analysis of the randomised clinical trials. *Breathe*, 16(1), 200013.

Brody, H., & Light, D.W. (2011). The inverse benefit law: How drug marketing undermines patient safety and public health. *American Journal of Public Health*, 101(3), 399–404.

Brownlee, S., Chalkidou, K., Doust, J., Elshaug, A.G., Glasziou, P., Heath, I., Nagpal, S., Saini, V., Srivastava, D., Chalmers, K., & Korenstein, D. (2017). Evidence for overuse of medical services around the world. *Lancet*, 390, 156–168.

Buys, S.S., Partridge, E., Black, A., Johnson, C.C., Lamerato, L., Isaacs, C., Reding, D.J., Greenlee, R.T., Yokochi, L.A., Kessel, B., Crawford, E.D., Church, T.R., Andriole, G.L., Weissfeld, J.L., Fouad, M.N., Chia, D., O'Brien, B., Ragard, L.R., Clapp, J.D., ... & Berg, C.D. (2011). Effect of screening on ovarian cancer mortality: The Prostate, Lung, Colorectal and Ovarian (PLCO) Cancer Screening Randomized Controlled Trial. *Journal of American Medical Association*, 305(22), 2295–2303.

Bynum, W., & Porter, R. (1993). *Companion encyclopedia of the history of medicine*. Routledge.

Cai, J., Vonder, M., Pelgrim, G.J., Rook, M., Kramer, G., Groen, H.J.M., de Bock, G.H., & Vliegenthart, R. (2024). Distribution of solid lung nodules presence and size by age and sex in a Northern European nonsmoking population. *Radiology*, 312(2), e231436.

Callahan, D. (2009). *Taming the beloved beast: How medical technology costs are destroying our health care system*. Princeton University Press.

Canadian Task Force on Preventive Health Care. (2024). *Breast cancer (update)—Draft recommendations*. https://canadiantaskforce.ca/guidelines/published-guidelines/breast-cancer-update-2024/?lang=fr

Carr, D., Kent, D., & Welch, G.H. (2022). All-cause mortality as the primary endpoint for the GRAIL/National Health Service England multi-cancer screening trial. *Journal of Medical Screening*, 29, 3–6.

Carter, J.L., Coletti, R.J., & Harris, R.P. (2015a). Quantifying and monitoring overdiagnosis in cancer screening: A systematic review of methods. *BMJ*, 350, g7773. doi: 10.1136/bmj.g7773.

Carter, S.M., Rogers, W., Heath, I., Degeling, C., Doust, J., & Barratt, A. (2015b). The challenge of overdiagnosis begins with its definition. *BMJ*, 350, h869.

Castel, R. (1991). From dangerousness to risk. In G. Burchell, C. Gordon, & P. Miller (Eds.), *The Foucault effect: Studies in governmentality* (pp. 281–298). University of Chicago Press.

Centers for Disease Control and Prevention. (CDC). (2012). Real stories. Tips From Former Smokers. https://www.cdc.gov/tobacco/campaign/tips/stories/index.html

Claridge, R., Arnold, S., Morrison, N., & van Rij, A.M. (2017). Measuring abdominal aortic diameters in routine abdominal computed tomography scans and implications for abdominal aortic aneurysm screening. *Journal of Vascular Surgery*, 65(6), 1637–1642.

Cochrane, A.I. (1972). *Effectiveness & efficiency: Random reflections on health services.* The Nuffield Trust.

Collaborative Group on Hormonal Factors in Breast Cancer. (2019). Type and timing of menopausal hormone therapy and breast cancer risk: Individual participant meta-analysis of the worldwide epidemiological evidence. *Lancet*, 394(10204), 1159–1168.

Commission on Chronic Illness. (1956). *Chronic illness in the United States.* Published for the Commonwealth Fund by Harvard University Press.

Conrad, P. (1975). The discovery of hyperkinesis: Notes on the medicalization of deviant behavior. *Social Problems*, 23(1), 12–21.

Conrad, P. (2007). *The medicalization of society: On the transformation of human conditions into treatable disorders.* Johns Hopkins University Press.

Conrad, P., Schneider, J., & Gusfield, J. (1992). A theoretical statement on the medicalization of deviance. In P. Conrad & J.W. Schneider (Eds.), *Deviance and medicalization: From badness to sickness* (pp. 261–276). Temple University Press.

Copp, T., Jansen, J., Doust, J., Mol, B.W., Dokras, A., & McCaffery, K. (2017). Are expanding disease definitions unnecessarily labelling women with polycystic ovary syndrome? *BMJ*, 358, j3694.

Crawford, R. (1980). Healthism and the medicalization of everyday life. *International Journal of Health Services*, 10(3), 365–388.

Crawford, R. (2006). Health as a meaningful social practice. *Health*, 10(4), 401–420.

Dalsgaard, P. (2026). Tænkepauser: AI. Aarhus Universitetsforlag.

Damhus, C., Brodersen, J., & Jønsson, A.B.R. (2026). Does information inform? Societal dynamics of cancer screening: Building on Perception Gap Theory. *Health, Risk & Society*, 28(1–2), 63–80.

Damhus, C.S., Risør, M.B., Brodersen, J.B., & Jønsson, A.B.R. (2025). Rethinking the logic of early diagnosis in cancer. *Health*, 29(1), 3–22.

Damhus, C.S., Byskov, G.P., Ploug, T., & Brodersen, J. (2018). Informed or misinformed choice? Framing effects in a national information pamphlet on colorectal cancer screening. *Health, Risk & Society*, 20(5–6), 241–258.

Damhus, C.S., Quentin, J.G., Malmqvist, J., Siersma, V., & Brodersen, J. (2021a). Psychosocial consequences of a three-month follow-up after receiving an abnormal lung cancer CT-screening result: A longitudinal survey. *Lung Cancer*, 155, 46–52.

Damhus, C.S., Siersma, V., Hansson, A., Bang, C.W., & Brodersen, J. (2021b). Psychosocial consequences of screening-detected abdominal aortic aneurisms: A cross-sectional study. *Scandinavian Journal of Primary Health Care*, 39(4), 459–465.

Danish Health Authority. Sundhedsstyrelsen. (2004). *Mammografiscreeningen i Fyns Amt 1993–1997. En medicinsk teknologivurdering.* Medicinsk Teknologivurdering – puljeprojekter 2004; 4(1). København: Sundhedsstyrelsen, Center for Evaluering og Medicinsk Teknologvurdering. https://www.sst.dk/udgivelser/2004/mammografiscreeningen-i-fyns-amt-1993-1997-en-medicinsk-teknologivurdering

Darwood, R., Earnshaw, J.J., Turton, G., Shaw, E., Whyman, M., Poskitt, K., Rodd, C., & Heather, B. (2012). Twenty-year review of abdominal aortic aneurysm screening in men in the county of Gloucestershire, United Kingdom. *Journal of Vascular Surgery*, 56(1), 8–13.

DaSilva, P., & Gray, J.A. (2016). English lessons: Can publishing an atlas of variation stimulate the discussion on appropriateness of care? *Medical Journal of Australia*, 205(10), S5–S7.

Daskivich, T.J., Luu, M., Heard, J., Thomas, I.C., & Leppert, J.T. (2025). Overtreatment of prostate cancer among men with limited longevity in the active surveillance era. *JAMA Internal Medicine*, 185(1), 28–36.

Daston, L., & Park, K. (1998). *Wonders and the order of nature, 1150–1750*. Zone Books.

Davies, E. (2024). Informed by research, transformed by research. *BMJ Evidence-Based Medicine*, 29(1), 62–63.

Degeling, C., Carter, S.M., & Rychetnik, L. (2015). Which public and why deliberate?—A scoping review of public deliberation in public health and health policy research. *Social Science & Medicine*, 131, 114–121.

Degeling, C., Thomas, R., & Rychetnik, L. (2019). Citizens' juries can bring public voices on overdiagnosis into policy making. *BMJ*, 364, 1351.

Denis, B., Gendre, I., Sauleau, E.A., Lacroute, J., & Perrin, P. (2013). Harms of colonoscopy in a colorectal cancer screening programme with faecal occult blood test: A population-based cohort study. *Digestive and Liver Disease*, 45(6), 474–480.

DeStefano, F., & Thompson, W.W. (2004). MMR vaccine and autism: An update of the scientific evidence. *Expert Review of Vaccines*, 3(1), 19–22.

Deyo, R.A. (2002). Cascade effects of medical technology. *Annual Review of Public Health*, 23(1), 23–44.

Docking, S., Lacy-Nichols, J., Hensher, M., & Buchbinder, R. (2025). Corporatisation and ownership concentration in diagnostic imaging: An audit of Australian practices. *Australian Health Review*, 49(4), AH25073. https://doi.org/10.1071/AH25073

Douglas, M. (1992). *Risk and blame: Essays in cultural theory*. Routledge.

Doust, J., & Glasziou, P. (2013). Is the problem that everything is a diagnosis? *Australian Family Physician*, 42, 856–859.

Doust, J., Vandvik, P.O., Qaseem, A., Mustafa, R.A., Horvath, A.R., Frances, A., Al-Ansary, L., Bossuyt, P., Ward, R.L., Kopp, I., Gollogly, L., Schunemann, H., & Glasziou, P. (2017). Guidance for modifying the definition of diseases: A checklist. *JAMA Internal Medicine*, 177(7), 1020–1025.

DSAM. (2022). *Pejlemærker for faget almen medicin*. Dansk Selskab for Almen Medicin. dsam.dk/pejlemaerker/

Duffy, S.W., & Wald, N.J. (2022). When primary prevention replaces screening. *Journal of Medical Screening*, 29(2), 67.

Dumit, J. (2012). *Drugs for life: How pharmaceutical companies define our health*. Duke University Press.

Editorial. (2024). Direct-to-consumer medical testing: An industry built on fear. *Lancet*, *404*(10457), 991.

Edwards, A.G., Naik, G., Ahmed, H., Elwyn, G.J., Pickles, T., Hood, K., & Playle, R. (2013). Personalised risk communication for informed decision making about taking screening tests. *Cochrane Database of Systematic Reviews*, (2), Cd001865.

Eggertson, L. (2010). Lancet retracts 12-year-old article linking autism to MMR vaccines. *Canadian Medical Association Journal*, 182(4), E199–E200.

Einav, L., & Finkelstein, A. (2018). Moral hazard in health insurance: What we know and how we know it. *Journal of the European Economic Association*, *16*(4), 957–982.

Eissenberg, J.C. (2017). Direct-to-consumer genomics: Harmful or empowering? It is important to stress that genetic risk is not the same as genetic destiny. *Missouri Medicine*, *114*(1), 26–32.

Elmahdi, R., Wennerström, E.C.M., Andersson, M., Wohlfahrt, J., Melbye, M., Pukkala, E., Hortlund, M., Silander, K., Sutinen, K., Jess, T., & Dillner, J. (2022). Shared environment and colorectal cancer: A Nordic pedigree registry-based cohort study. *International Journal of Cancer*, 151(8), 1261–1269.

Elsass, P. (1992). *Sundhedspsykologi*. Gyldendal.

Esserman, L., Shieh, Y., & Thompson, I. (2009). Rethinking screening for breast cancer and prostate cancer. *JAMA*, 302(15), 1685–1692.

Estes, C.L., & Binney, E.A. (1989). The biomedicalization of aging: Dangers and dilemmas. *The Gerontologist*, 29(5), 587–596.

European Commision. (2020). *Policy mHealth*. ec.europa.eu/digital-single-market/en/mhealth

European Organization for all Occupational Therapists (COTEC). (2020). Prevent overdiagnosis in health care and overmedicalisation of society. Written statement on agenda item 5 (C), Advancing public health in the WHO European Region for sustainable development. https://www.woncaeurope.org/resources/view/overdiagnosis-in-health-care-and-overmedicalisation-of-the-society-%E2%80%93-68th-session-of-the-who-regional-committee-for-europe

Evans-Pritchard, E.E. (1976 [1937]). *Witchcraft, oracles and magic among the Azande*. Oxford University Press.

Ewald, F. (1991). Insurance and risk. In G. Burchell, C. Gordon, & P. Miller (Eds.), *The Foucault effect: Studies in governmentality* (pp. 197–210). Harvester Wheatsheaf.

Fabbri, A., Swandari, S., Lau, E., Vitry, A., & Mintzes, B. (2019). Pharmaceutical industry funding of health consumer groups in Australia: A cross-sectional analysis. *International Journal of Health Services*, *49*(2), 273–293.

Fabbri, A., Mosconi, P., Barbara, G., Frattaruolo, M.P., Lau, E., Kroeger, C.M., Lunny, C., Salzwedel, D.M., & Mintzes, B. (2020). Industry funding of patient and health consumer organisations: Systematic review with meta-analysis. *BMJ*, *368*, 16925.

Fagt, S., Matthiessen, J., Meinilä, J., Christensen, A.I., Ólafsdóttir, T., Lund, M., & Krokstad, S. (2025). Smoking, snuff, nicotine pouches, and e-cigarettes. In Nordic health and well-being 2025. Nordic Council of Ministers.https://pub.norden.org/nord2025-026/smoking-snuff-nicotine-pouches-and-e-cigarettes.html

Farber, R., Houssami, N., McGeechan, K., Barratt, A., & Bell, K.J.L. (2024a). Breast cancer stage and size detected with film versus digital mammography in New South Wales, Australia: A population-based study using routinely collected data. Cancer Epidemiology, Biomarkers & Prevention, 33(5), 671–680.

Farber, R., Houssami, N., McGeechan, K., Barratt, A., & Bell, K.J.L. (2024b). Systematic review and meta-analysis of prognostic characteristics for breast cancers in populations with digital vs film mammography indicate the transition may have increased both early detection and overdiagnosis. *Journal of Clinical Epidemiology*, *171*, 111339.

Farber, R., Houssami, N., McGeechan, K., Barratt, A.L., & Bell, K.J. (2025). The impact of the BreastScreen NSW transition from film to digital mammography. *Medical Journal of Australia*, 222(2), 82–90.

Farber, R., Houssami, N., Wortley, S., Jacklyn, G., Marinovich, M.L., McGeechan, K., Barratt, A., & Bell, K. (2021). Impact of full-field digital mammography versus film-screen mammography in population screening: A meta-analysis. *Journal of the National Cancer Institute*, 113(1), 16–26.

Feinstein, A.R., Sosin, D.A., & Wells, C.K. (1984). The Will Rogers phenomenon: Improved technologic diagnosis and stage migration as a source of nontherapeutic improvement in cancer prognosis. *Transactions of the Association of American Physicians*, 97, 19–24.

Feinstein, A.R., Sosin, D.M., & Wells, C.K. (1985). The Will Rogers phenomenon. Stage migration and new diagnostic techniques as a source of misleading statistics for survival in cancer. *New England Journal of Medicine*, 312(25), 1604–1608.

Finlayson, E.V., & Birkmeyer, J.D. (2001). Operative mortality with elective surgery in older adults. *Effective Clinical Practice*, 4, 172–177.

Fitzpatrick, M. (2001). *The tyranny of health: Doctors and the regulation of lifestyle*. Routledge.

Fortmann-Roe, S. (2012). *Understanding the bias–variance tradeoff*. scott.fortmann-roe.com/docs/BiasVariance.html

Foucault, M. (1982). The subject and power. *Critical Inquiry*, 8(4), 777–795.

Foucault, M. (1991). Governmentality. In G. Burchell, C. Gordon, & P. Miller (Eds.), *The Foucault effect: Studies in governmentality* (pp. 87–104). Harvester Wheatsheaf.

Foucault, M. (2002 [1966]). Videnskaberne om mennesket. In M. Foucault (Ed.), *Ordet og tingene. En arkæologisk undersøgelse af videnskaberne om mennesket* (pp. 387–422). Gyldendal.

Foucault, M. (2003 [1963]). *The birth of the clinic*. Routledge.

Foucault, M. (2009 [1979]). *Biopolitikkens fødsel. Forelæsninger på Collège de France 1978–1979*. Hans Reitzels Forlag.

Frances, A. (2013). *Saving normal: On insider's revolt against out-of-control psychiatric diagnosis, DSM-5, Big Pharma, and the medicalization of ordinary life*. William Morrow & Co.

Fugelli, P. (2006). The Zero-vision: Potential side effects of communicating health perfection and zero risk. *Patient Education and Counseling*, 60(3), 267–271.

Fulton, B.D., Scheffler, R.M., Hinshaw, S.P., Levine, P., Stone, S., Brown, T.T., & Modrek, S. (2009). National variation of ADHD diagnostic prevalence and medication use: Health care providers and education policies. *Psychiatric Services*, 60(8), 1075–1083.

Furuya-Kanamori, L., Bell, K.J.L., Clark, J., Glasziou, P., & Doi, S.A.R. (2016). Prevalence of differentiated thyroid cancer in autopsy studies over six decades: A meta-analysis. *Journal of Clinical Oncology*, 34(30), 3672–3679.

Gabis, L.V., Attia, O.L., Goldman, M., Barak, N., Tefera, P., Shefer, S., Shaham, M., & Lerman-Sagie, T. (2022). The myth of vaccination and autism spectrum. *European Journal of Paediatric Neurology*, *36*, 151–158.

Gannik, D.E., & Schmidt, D. (1990). Sygdom—fra et lægevidenskabeligt til et samfundsmæssigt anliggende. In P. Gundelach, N. Mortensen & J.C. Tonboe (Eds.), *Sociologi under forandring* (pp. 415–447). Gyldendal.

Gao, W., Wen, C.P., Wu, A., & Welch, H.G. (2022). Association of computed tomographic screening promotion with lung cancer overdiagnosis among Asian women. *JAMA Internal Medicine*, 182(3), 283–290.

Gentilini, A., & Parvanova, I. (2023). Industry funding of patient organisations in the UK. *BMJ Open*, *13*(6), e071138.

Getz, L., Kirkengen, A.L., Hetlevik, I., Romundstad, S., & Sigurdsson, J.A. (2004). Ethical dilemmas arising from implementation of the European guidelines on cardiovascular disease prevention in clinical practice. A descriptive epidemiological study. *Scandinavian Journal of Primary Health Care*, 22(4), 202–208.

Giddens, A. (1998). Risk society: The context of British politics. In J. Franklin (Ed.), *The politics of risk society* (pp. 23–34). Polity Press.

Gigerenzer, G., Gaissmaier, W., Milcke-Kurz, E., Schwartz, L.M., & Woloshin, S. (2008). Helping doctors and patients make sense of health statistics. *Psychological Science*, 8(2), 53–96.

Glasziou, P.P., Jones, M.A., Pathirana, T., Barratt, A.L., & Bell, K.J. (2020). Estimating the magnitude of cancer overdiagnosis in Australia. *Medical Journal of Australia*, 213(4), 189–189.

Glasziou, P.P., Moynihan, R., Richards, T., & Godlee, F. (2013). Too much medicine, too little care. *British Medical Journal*, 347, f4247.

Goel, V. (2025). Evidence, not ideology, must guide preventive health care policy recommendations. *Canadian Medical Association Journal*, 197(28), E872–E873.

Goffman, E. (1963). *Stigma: Notes on the management of spoiled identity*. Prentice Hall.

Gommers, J., Hernström, V., Josefsson, V., Sartor, H., Schmidt, D., Hjelmgren, A., Larsson, A.M., Hofvind, S., Andersson, I., Rosso, A., Hagberg, O., & Lång, K. (2026). Interval cancer, sensitivity, and specificity comparing AI-supported mammography screening with standard double reading without AI in the MASAI study: A randomised, controlled, non-inferiority, single-blinded, population-based, screening-accuracy trial. *Lancet*, 407(10527), 505–514.

Gøtzsche, P., & Jørgensen, K. (2013). Screening for breast cancer with mammography. *Cochrane Database of Systematic Reviews*, (6), CD001877.

Gøtzsche, P.C., Hartling, O.J., Nielsen, M., Brodersen, J., & Jørgensen, K.J. (2009). Breast screening: The facts—or maybe not. *BMJ*, 338, 446–448.

GOV.AU. (2025). Eating well. Australian Government Department of Health, Disability and Ageing. https://www.health.gov.au/topics/food-and-nutrition/about/eating-well

GOV.UK. (2026). https://nationalscreening.blog.gov.uk/2025/11/28/uk-nsc-opens-consultation-on-draft-prostate-cancer-screening-recommendation/

GRADE Working Group: https://www.gradeworkinggroup.org/

Graham, S.S., Grundy, Q., Sharma, N., Edward, J.S., Barbour, J.B., Rousseau, J.F., Majdik, Z.P., & Bero, L. (2025). Research on policy mechanisms to address funding bias and conflicts of interest in biomedical research: A scoping review. *Research Integrity and Peer Review*, *10*(1), 6.

Gram, E.G., Jønsson, A.B.R., Brodersen, J.B., & Damhus, C.S. (2023a). Questioning 'informed choice' in medical screening: The role of neoliberal rhetoric, culture, and social context. *Healthcare (Basel)*, 11(9).

Gram, E.G., Knudsen, S.W., Brodersen, J.B., & Jønsson, A.B.R. (2023b). Women's experiences of age-related discontinuation from mammography screening: A qualitative interview study. *Health Expectations*, 26(3), 1096–1106.

Gram, E.G., Siersma, S., & Brodersen, J.B. (2023c). Long-term psychosocial consequences of false-positive screening mammography: A cohort study with follow-up of 12–14 years in Denmark. *BMJ Open*, 13(4), e072188.

Gram, E.G., Siersma, V., Nicolaisdóttir, D.R., & Brodersen, J.B. (2024). Downstream healthcare use following breast cancer screening: A register-based cohort study. *Journal of Epidemiology and Community Health*, 79(4), 242–248.

Gram, E.G., Haas, R., Niklasson, A., Woloshin, S., Kramer, B., Brodersen, J., Jørgensen, K.J., Johansson, M., Wilt, T., Bell, K., & Preventing Overdiagnosis Research Day group. (2025). Less is more for patients, practitioners, public and planet: A taxonomy for the harms of too much medicine. *BMJ Evidence Based Medicine*, 10.1136/bmjebm-2025-113874 [online ahead of print].

Green, S., Vogt, H., & Brodersen, J.B. (2020). De raske patienter i personlig medicin: Sygdomsforebyggelse og overdiagnosticering. In S.H. Klausen, & K. Christiansen (Eds.), *Personlig medicin* (pp. 181–212). Munksgaard.

Greenhalgh, T., & S. Wessely. (2004). 'Health for me': A sociocultural analysis of healthism in the middle classes. *British Medical Bulletin*, 69, 197–213.

Greenhalgh, T., Howick, J., & Maskrey, N. (2014). Evidence based medicine: A movement in crisis? *BMJ*, 348, g3725.

Grönberg, H., Adolfsson, J., Aly, M., Nordström, T., Wiklund, P., Brandberg, Y., Thompson, J., Wiklund, F., Lindberg, J., Clements, M., Egevad, L., & Eklund, M. (2017). Prostate cancer screening in men aged 50 to 69 years (STHLM3). A prospective population-based diagnostic study. *Urologic Oncology*, 35(3), 120.

Guirguis-Blake, J.M., Beil, T.L., Senger, C.A., & Coppola, E.L. (2019). Primary care screening for abdominal aortic aneurysm: Updated evidence report and systematic review for the US Preventive Services Task Force. *Journal of the American Medical Association*, 322(22), 2219–2238.

Gulati, R., Feuer, E.J., & Etzioni, R. (2016). Conditions for valid empirical estimates of cancer overdiagnosis in randomized trials and population studies. *American Journal Epidemiology*, 184(2), 140–147.

Guyatt, G., Rennie, D., Meade, M., & Cook, D. (2015). *Users' guides to the medical literature: A manual for evidence-based clinical practice*. McGraw-Hill Professional.

Gyuricza, J.V. (2020). *Psychosocial consequences of labelling in healthy people with mild hypertension: Development of a patient-reported outcome measure*. [Unpublished doctoral dissertation, Faculdade de Medicina, Universidade de São Paulo.]

Gyuricza, J.V., d'Oliveira, A., Machado, L.B.M., & Brodersen, J. (2019). Development of an item pool for a questionnaire on the psychosocial consequences of hypertension labelling. *Journal of Patient-Reported Outcomes*, 4(1), Art. 2.

Haase, C.B., Ajjawi, R., Bearman, M., Brodersen, J.B., Risør, T., & Høyer, K. (2023). Data as symptom: Doctors' responses to patient-provided data in general practice. *Social Studies of Science*, 53(4), 522–544.

Haase, C.B., Bearman, M., Brodersen, J.B., Risør, T., & Høyer, K. (2024). Data driven or data informed? How general practitioners use data to evaluate their own and colleagues' clinical work in clusters. *Sociology of Health & Illness*, 46(5), 948–965.

Haase, C.B., Brodersen, J.B., & Bülow, J. (2022). Sarcopenia: Early prevention or overdiagnosis? *BMJ*, 376, e052592.

Haase, C.B., Gyuricza, J.V., & Brodersen, J. (2019). New hypertension guidance risks overdiagnosis and overtreatment. *British Medical Journal*, 365, l1657.

Haase, C.B., Jensen, A.E., Modin, F.A., Siersma, V., & Brodersen, J.B. (2026). Overdiagnosis in atrial fibrillation screening with wearables. *Scandinavian Journal of Primary Health Care*, 44(1), 2656694.

Hacking, I. (1990). *The taming of chance*. Cambridge University Press.

Hacking, I. (1995). Why multiple personality tells us nothing about the self/mind/person/subject/consciousness. In D. Bakhurst, & C. Sypnowich (Eds.), *The social self* (pp. 159–179). Sage Publications.

Hacking, I. (2002). *Historical Ontology*. Harvard University Press.

Halse, C. (2009). The bio-citizen: Virtue discourses, BMI and responsible citizenship. In J. Wright, & V. Harwood (Eds.), *Biopolitics and the 'obesity epidemic': Governing bodies* (pp. 45–59). Routledge.

Hansen, A.D., Jønsson, A.B.R., & Brodersen, J. (2025). Danish GP trainees' experiences of navigating patient expectations for non-indicated procedures or tests: A qualitative interview study. *Scandinavian Journal of Primary Health Care* [Advance online publication.] https://doi.org/10.1080/02813432.2025.2597784

Hansson, A., Brodersen, J., Reventlow, S., & Pettersson, M. (2012). Opening Pandora's box: The experiences of having an asymptomatic aortic aneurysm under surveillance. *Health, Risk & Society*, 14(4), 341–359.

Haraway, D. (1988). Situated knowledges: The science question in feminism and the privilege of partial perspective. *Feminist Studies*, 14(3), 575–599.

Harris, R.P., Sheridan, S.L., Lewis, C.L., Barclay, C., Vu, M.B., Kistler, C.E., Golin, C.E., DeFrank, J.T., & Brewer, N.T. (2014). The harms of screening: A proposed taxonomy and application to lung cancer screening. *JAMA Internal Medicine*, 174(2), 281–285.

Harris, R.P., Wilt, T.J., & Qaseem, A. (2015). A value framework for cancer screening: Advice for high-value care from the American College of Physicians. *Annals of Internal Medicine*, 162(10), 712–717.

Hart, J.T. (1971). The inverse care law. *Lancet*, *297*(7696), 405–412.

Hartling, O. (2012). Kan sundhedsdyrkelse blive til sundhedisme? Tale ved Vidensråd for Forebyggelse, Dansk Designcenter torsdag den 11. oktober 2012. vidensraad.dk/sites/default/files/vidensraad_for_forebyggelse_ole_hartling_0.pdf

Hastrup, K. (2004a). *Kultur: Det fleksible fællesskab*. Aarhus Universitetsforlag.

Hastrup, K. (2004b). Vidensbegreber og videnskaber: Nye veje til kundskab? In J.J. Bruun, M.L. Hanak, & B.G. Koefoed (Eds.), *Viden og evidens i forebyggelsen* (pp. 10–18). Sundhedsstyrelsen, Viden- og dokumentationsenheden.

Haynes, R.B., Sackett, D.L., Taylor, D.W., Gibson, E.S., & Johnson, A.L. (1978). Increased absenteeism from work after detection and labeling of hypertensive patients. *New England Journal of Medicine*, 299(14), 741–744.

Heleno, B., Thomsen, M.F., Rodrigues, D.S., Jørgensen, K.J., & Brodersen, J. (2013). Quantification of harms in cancer screening trials: Literature review. *BMJ*, 347, f5334.

Heleno, B., Siersma, V., & Brodersen, J. (2018). Estimation of overdiagnosis of lung cancer in low-dose computed tomography screening: A secondary analysis of the Danish Lung Cancer Screening Trial. *JAMA Internal Medicine*, 178(10), 1420–1422.

Henderson, J.T., Webber, E.M., & Sawaya, G.F. (2018). Screening for ovarian cancer: Updated evidence report and systematic review for the US Preventive Services Task Force. *Journal of the American Medical Association*, 319(6), 595–606.

Henriksen, M.J.V., Guassora, A.D., & Brodersen, J. (2015). Preconceptions influence women's perceptions of information on breast cancer screening: A qualitative study. *BioMed Central Research Notes*, 8, 404.

Hermer, L.D., & Brody, H. (2010). Defensive medicine, cost containment, and reform. *Journal of General Internal Medicine*, 25(5), 470–473.

Hestbech, M.S., Siersma, V., Dirksen, A., Pedersen, J.H., & Brodersen, J. (2011). Participation bias in a randomised trial of screening for lung cancer. *Lung Cancer*, 73(3), 325–331.

Hewitson, P., Glasziou, P., Irwig, L., Towler, B., & Watson, E. (2007). Screening for colorectal cancer using the faecal occult blood test, Hemoccult. *Cochrane Database Systematic Reviews*, (1), CD001216.

Hillier, T.A., Pedula, K.L., Ogasawara, K.K., Vesco, K.K., Oshiro, C:E.S., Lubarsky, S.L., & Van Marter, J. (2021). Pragmatic, randomized clinical trial of gestational diabetes screening. *New England Journal Medicine*, 384(10), 895–904.

Hjertholm, P., Fenger-Gron, M., Vestergaard, M., Christensen, M.B., Borre, M., Møller, H., & Vedsted, P. (2015). Variation in general practice prostate-specific antigen testing and prostate cancer outcomes: An ecological study. *International Journal of Cancer*, 136(2), 435–442.

Hoffmann, S.H., Schramm, S., Jarlstrup, N.S., & Christensen, A.I. (2018). *Danskernes rygevaner. Udviklingen fra 1994 til 2017*. Statens Institut for Folkesundhed, SDU.

Hoffmann, T.C., Montori, V.M., & Del Mar, C. (2014). The connection between evidence-based medicine and shared decision making. *JAMA*, *312*(13), 1295–1296.

Hoffmann, T.C., & Del Mar, C. (2015). Patients' expectations of the benefits and harms of treatments, screening, and tests: A systematic review. *JAMA Internal Medicine*, 175(2), 274–286.

Hoffmann, T.C., & Del Mar, C. (2017). Clinicians' expectations of the benefits and harms of treatments, screening, and tests: A systematic review. *JAMA Internal Medicine*, 177(3), 407–419.

Hofmann, B. (2014). Diagnosing overdiagnosis: Conceptual challenges and suggested solutions. *European Journal of Epidemiology*, 29(9), 599–604.

Holme, O., Bretthauer, M., Fretheim, A., Odgaard-Jensen, J., & Hoff, G. (2013). Flexible sigmoidoscopy versus faecal occult blood testing for colorectal cancer screening in asymptomatic individuals. *Cochrane Database of Systematic Reviews*, (9), CD009259.

Hood, L., & Flores, M. (2012). A personal view on systems medicine and the emergence of proactive P4 medicine: Predictive, preventive, personalized and participatory. *New Biotechnology*, 29(6), 613–624.

Hopf, H., Krief, A., Mehta, G., & Matlin, S.A. (2019). Fake science and the knowledge crisis: Ignorance can be fatal. *Royal Society Open Science*, 6(5), 190161.

Hortensius, J., Kars, M.C., Wierenga, W.S., Kleefstra, N., Bilo, H.J., & van der Bijl, J.J. (2012). Perspectives of patients with type 1 or insulin-treated type 2 diabetes on self-monitoring of blood glucose: A qualitative study. *BioMed Central Public Health*, 12(167).

Høyer, K. (2019). *Hvem skal bruge sundhedsdata—og til hvad?* Informations Forlag.

Høyer, K. (2023). *Data paradoxes: The politics of intensified data sourcing in healthcare.* MIT Press.

Huang, K.-L., Wang, S.-Y., Lu, W.-C., Chang, Y.-H., Su, J., & Lu, Y.-T. (2019). Effects of low-dose computed tomography on lung cancer screening: A systematic review, meta-analysis, and trial sequential analysis. *BioMed Central Pulmonary Medicine*, 19(1), 126.

Hueber, S., Biermann, V., Tomandl, J., Warkentin, L., Schedlbauer, A., Tauchmann, H., Klemperer, D., Lehmann, M., Donnachie, E., & Kühlein, T. (2023). Consequences of early thyroid ultrasound on subsequent tests, morbidity and costs: An explorative analysis of routine health data from German ambulatory care. *BMJ Open*, 13(3), e059016.

Hugosson, J., Månsson, M., Wallström, J., Axcrona, U., Carlsson, S.V., Egevad, L., Geterud, K., Khatami, A., Kohestani, K., Pihl, C.G., Socratous, A., Stranne, J., Godtman, R.A., & Hellström, M. (2022). Prostate cancer screening with PSA and MRI followed by targeted biopsy only. *New England Journal of Medicine*, 387(23), 2126–2137.

Hvas, L. (1999). Sygeliggørelse og medikalisering. Forsøg på begrebsafklaring på baggrund af et litteraturstudie. *Ugeskrift for Læger*, 161, 5783–5785.

Hvas, L. (2011). *Syg til det modsatte er bevist.* Politiken.

Hvidt, E.A., Lykkegaard, J., Pedersen, L.B., Pedersen, K.M., Munck, A., & Andersen, M.K. (2017). How is defensive medicine understood and experienced in a primary care setting? A qualitative focus group study among Danish general practitioners. *BMJ Open*, 7(12), e019851.

Ilic, D., Djulbegovic, M., Jung, J.H., Hwang, E.C., Zhou, Q., Cleves, A., Agoritsas, T., & Dahm, P. (2018). Prostate cancer screening with prostate-specific antigen (PSA) test: A systematic review and meta-analysis. *BMJ*, 362, k3519.

Ilic, D., Neuberger, M.M., Djulbegovic, M., & Dahm, P. (2013). Screening for prostate cancer. *Cochrane Database of Systematic Reviews*, 1, Cd004720.

Illich, I. (1976). *Limits to medicine: Medical nemesis, the expropriation of health.* Marion Boyars.

Ingwersen, P., & Larsen, B. (2014). Influence of a performance indicator on Danish research production and citation impact 2000–12. *Scientometrics*, 101, 1325–1344.

Ioannidis, J.P.A. (2018). Screening for diseases: Why, when, and how? *BMJ, 362*, k3359. https://doi.org/10.1136/bmj.k3359

Ioannidis, J.P.A., Stuart, M.E., Brownlee, S., & Strite, S.A. (2017). How to survive the medical misinformation mess. *European Journal of Clinical Investigation*, 47(11), 795–802.

Jacklin, C., Philippou, Y., Brewster, S.F., & Bryant, R.J. (2021). 'More men die with prostate cancer than because of it'—an old adage that still holds true in the 21st century. *Cancer Treatment and Research Communications*, 26, 100225.

Jensen, A., & Stensballe, L.G. (2025). Impact of COVID-19 on testing, positive cases, patient characteristics, and hospital contacts for respiratory syncytial virus, influenza, and pneumococcus in Danish children. *Journal of Infection and Public Health*, 18(2), 102660.

Jensen, A., Andersen, P.K., Andersen, J.S., Greisen, G., & Stensballe, L.G. (2019). Too much? Mortality and health service utilisation among Danish children 1999–2016: A register-based study. *PLoS One*, 14(10), e0224544.

Jensen, A., Jensen, M., Blok, A., Kaltoft, P., Christensen, T., Wier, M., Lind, K.M.H., & Denver, S. (2008). *Mellem skepsis, tvivl og tillid—en sociologisk undersøgelse af lægfolks og eksperters risikoopfattelser i forbindelse med brugen af pesticider.* Fødevareøkonomisk Institut, Københavns Universitet.

Jensen, M.D., Hansen, K.M., Siersma, V., & Brodersen, J. (2021). Using a deliberative poll on breast cancer screening to assess and improve the decision quality of laypeople. *PLoS One*, 16(10), e0258869.

Jensen, M.D., Hansen, K.M., Siersma, V., & Brodersen, J. (2025). Mammography screening: Eliciting the voices of informed citizens. *PLoS One*, 20(1), e0317263.

Jensen, M.D., Siersma, V., Rasmussen, J.F., & Brodersen, J. (2020). Direct and indirect healthcare costs of lung cancer CT screening in Denmark: A registry study. *BMJ Open*, 10(1), e031768.

Jewson, N.D. (1976). The disappearance of the sick-man from medical cosmology, 1770–1870. *Sociology*, 10(2), 225–244.

Jodal, H.C., Helsingen, L.M., Anderson, J.C., Lytvyn, L., Vandvik, P.O., & Emilsson, L. (2019). Colorectal cancer screening with faecal testing, sigmoidoscopy or colonoscopy: A systematic review and network meta-analysis. *BMJ Open*, 9(10), e032773.

Johansson, M., Hansson, A., & Brodersen, J. (2015). Estimating overdiagnosis in screening for abdominal aortic aneurysm: Could a change in smoking habits and lowered aortic diameter tip the balance of screening towards harm? *BMJ*, 350, h825.

Johansson, M., Zahl, P.H., Siersma, V., Jørgensen, K.J., Marklund, B., & Brodersen, J. (2018). Benefits and harms of screening men for abdominal aortic aneurysm in Sweden: A registry-based cohort study. *Lancet*, 391(10138), 2441–2447.

Jønsson, A.B.R. (2014). En familie bliver til. Om kostbehandling som optimeringsproces for familiens socialitet. *Tidsskriftet Antropologi*, 70, 53–72.

Jønsson, A.B.R. (2018). De Usunde: Sundhedsantropologens møde med multisyge ældre på Lolland. *Tidsskriftet Antropologi*, 77, 25–45.

Jønsson, A.B.R. (2024). Medicalization of old age: Experiencing healthism and overdiagnosis in a Nordic welfare state. *Medical Anthropology*, 43(4), 310–323.

Jønsson, A.B.R. (2025). Negotiating normalcy: Epistemic errors in self-diagnosing late-ADHD. *Culture, Medicine and Psychiatry*, 49, 369–391.

Jønsson, A.B.R., & Spalletta, O. (2023). Tuning the self: Revisiting health inequities through the lens of social interaction. *Ethos*, 51(3), 237–254.

Jønsson, A.B.R., Guassora, A.D., & Reventlow, S. (2020). How older men with multimorbidity relate to successful aging. *Journal of Gerontology: Series B Social Sciences*, 75(5), 1104–1112.

Jønsson, A.B.R., Christensen, I.E., Reventlow, S., & Risør, M.B. (2022a). Responsibilities of risk: Living with mental illness during COVID-19. *Medical Anthropology*, 41(3), 302–314.

Jønsson, A.B.R., Brodersen, J., & Kristensen, B. (2022b). Informationens ironi. Patienters frie adgang til sundhedsdata. *Tidsskrift for Forskning i Sygdom og Samfund*, 19(36), 39–57.

Jørgensen, K.J., & Johansson, M. (2018). Drawing conclusions from the VIVA trial. *Lancet*, 391(10133), 1894.

Jørgensen, P., Langhammer, A., Krokstad, S., & Forsmo, S. (2015). Diagnostic labelling influences self-rated health. A prospective cohort study: The HUNT Study, Norway. *Family Practice*, 32(5), 492–499.

Jørgensen, P., Langhammer, A., Krokstad, S., & Forsmo, S. (2017). Mortality in persons with undetected and diagnosed hypertension, type 2 diabetes, and hypothyroidism, compared with persons without corresponding disease—a prospective cohort study; The HUNT Study, Norway. *BioMed Central—Family Practice*, 18(1), 98.

Jørgensen, T., Rotar, O., Juhl, C.B., & Linneberg, A. (2024). WHO Health Evidence Network Synthesis Reports. What is the effectiveness of systematic population-level screening programmes for reducing the burden of cardiovascular diseases? WHO Regional Office for Europe.

Jutel, A. (2009). Sociology of diagnosis: A preliminary review. *Sociology of Health and Illness*, 31(2), 278–299.

Jutel, A. (2011). *Putting a name to it: Diagnosis in contemporary society*. Johns Hopkins University Press.

Juul, F.E., Cross, A.J., Schoen, R.E., Senore, C., Pinsky, P., Miller, E., Segnan, N., Wooldrage, K., Wieszczy-Szczepanik, P., Armaroli, P., Garborg, K.K., Adami, H.O., Hoff, G., Kalager, M., Bretthauer, M., Løberg, M., & Holme, Ø. (2022). 15-year benefits of sigmoidoscopy screening on colorectal cancer incidence and mortality: A pooled analysis of randomized trials. *Annals of Internal Medicine*, 175(11), 1525–1533.

Kainberger, F. (2017). Defensive medicine and overutilization of imaging—an issue of radiation protection. *Wiener klinische Wochenschrift*, 129(5), 157–158.

Kalager, M., Wieszczy, P., Lansdorp-Vogelaar, I., Corley, D.A., Bretthauer, M., & Kaminski, M.F. (2018). Overdiagnosis in colorectal cancer screening: Time to acknowledge a blind spot. *Gastroenterology*, 155(3), 592–595.

Karlsen, R.V., Larsen, S.B., Christensen, J., Brasso, K., Friis, S., Tjønneland, A., & Dalton, S.O. (2013). PSA testing without clinical indication. *Acta Oncologica*, *52*(8), 1609–1614.

Kaufman, S.R., Shim, J.K., & Russ, A.J. (2004). Revisiting the biomedicalization of aging: Clinical trends and ethical challenges. *The Gerontologist*, 44(6), 731–738.

Kernick, D., Chew-Graham, C.A., & O'Flynn, N. (2017). Clinical assessment and management of multimorbidity. *British Journal of General Practice*, *67*(658), 235–236.

Kindt, I.S., Martiny, F.H.J., Gram, E.G., Bie, A.K.L., Jauernik, C.P., Rahbek, O.J., Nielsen, S.B., Siersma, V., Bang, C.W., & Brodersen, J.B. (2023). The risk of bleeding and perforation from sigmoidoscopy or colonoscopy in colorectal cancer screening: A systematic review and meta-analyses. *PLoS One*, 18(10), e0292797.

Kinsinger, L.S., Anderson, C., Kim, J., Larson, M., Chan, S.H., King, H.A., Rice, K.L., Slatore, C.G., Tanner, N.T., Pittman, K., Monte, R.J., McNeil, R.B., Grubber, J.M., Kelley, M.J., Provenzale, D., Datta, S.K., Sperber, N.S., Barnes, L.K., Abbott, D.H., …, & Jackson, G.L. (2017). Implementation of lung cancer screening in the Veterans Health Administration. *JAMA Internal Medicine*, 177(3), 399–406.

Kirmayer, L.J. (1988). Mind and body as metaphors: Hidden values in biomedicine. In M. Lock, & D. Gordon (Eds.), *Biomedicine examined. Culture, illness and healing* (vol. 13, pp. 57–92). Springer.

Kleinman, A. (2006). *What really matters: Living a moral life amidst uncertainty and danger*. Oxford University Press.

Kristensen, B.M., Brodersen, J.B., & Jønsson, A.B.R. (2022). The tyranny of numbers: How e-health record transparency alter patients' perceptions of their health and steer conversations with physicians. *Medicine Anthropology Theory*, 9(2), 1–25.

Kristensen, D.B. (2016). Enquete: Sundhedens univers. *Tidsskrift Antropologi*, (73), 83–87.

Kristensen, D.B., & Ruckenstein, M. (2018). Co-evolving with self-tracking technologies. *New Media & Society*, 20(10), 3624–3640.

Kristensen, D.B., Boye, H., & Askegaard, S. (2011). Leaving the Milky Way! The formation of a consumer counter mythology. *Journal of Consumer Culture*, 11(2), 195–214.

Kristensen, D.B., Lim, M., & Askegaard, S. (2016). Healthism in Denmark: State, market, and the search for a 'moral compass'. *Health*, 20(5), 485–504.

Kristensen, M.A.T., Hølge-Hazelton, B., Waldorff, F.B., & Guassora, A.D. (2017). How general practitioners perceive and assess self-care in patients with multiple chronic conditions: A qualitative study. *BioMed Central Family Practice*, 18(1), 109–118.

Kristensen, M.A.T., Due, T.D., Hølge-Hazelton, B., Guassora, A.D., & Waldorff, F.B. (2018a). 'More constricting than inspiring' – GPs find chronic care programmes of limited clinical utility. A qualitative study. *BJGP Open*, 2(2), bjgpopen18X101591.

Kristensen, M.A.T., Guassora, A.D., Arreskov, A.B., Waldorff, F.B., & Hølge-Hazelton, B. (2018b). 'I've put diabetes completely on the shelf till the mental stuff is in place'. How patients with doctor-assessed impaired self-care perceive disease, self-care, and support from general practitioners. A qualitative study. *Scandinavian Journal of Primary Health Care*, 36(3), 342–351.

Krogsbøll, L.T., Jørgensen, K.J., & Gøtzsche, P.C. (2019). General health checks in adults for reducing morbidity and mortality from disease. *Cochrane Database Systematic Review*, 1, Cd009009.

Krogsgaard, M.R., Brodersen, J., Christensen, K.B., Siersma, V., Kreiner, S., Jensen, J., Hansen, C.F., & Comins, J.D. (2020). What is a PROM and why do we need it? *Scandinavian Journal of Medicine and Science in Sports*, 31(5), 967–971.

Kühlein, T., Macdonald, H., Kramer, B., Johansson, M., Woloshin, S., McCaffery, K., Brodersen, J.B., Copp, T., Jørgensen, K.J., Møller, A., & Scherer, M. (2023). Overdiagnosis and too much medicine in a world of crises. *BMJ, 382*, 1865.

Lafata, J.E., Simpkins, J., Lamerato, L., Poisson, L., Divine, G., & Johnson, C.C. (2004). The economic impact of false-positive cancer screens. *Cancer Epidemiology Biomarkers Prevention*, 13(12), 2126–2132.

Lægemiddelstyrelsen. (2015). *Vejledning til borgere om sundheds-apps og software som medicinsk udstyr*. https://laegemiddelstyrelsen.dk/da/nyheder/2015/faa-styr-paa-sundheds-apps/

Larsen, L.T. (2015). Fra ventelister til frit valg. Neoliberal guvernementalitet i sundhedsvæsenet. *Gjallerhorn*, (20), 17–24.

Larsen, L.T., & Stone, D. (2015). Governing health care through free choice: Neoliberal reforms in Denmark and the United States. *Journal of Health Politics, Policy and Law*, 40(5), 941–970.

Latour, B. (1993). *We have never been modern*. Harvard University Press.

Lauritzen, A.D., Lillholm, M., Lynge, E., Nielsen, M., Karssemeijer, N., & Vejborg, I. (2024). Early indicators of the impact of using AI in mammography screening for breast cancer. *Radiology*, 311(3), e232479.

Li, M., Dal Maso, L., & Vaccarella, S. (2020). Global trends in thyroid cancer incidence and the impact of overdiagnosis. *Lancet Diabetes & Endocrinology*, 8(6), 468–470.

Lin, J., Yang, J., Liang, M., Chen, Y., Huang, W., Wu, L., Chen, X., Vaccarella, S., & Li, M. (2026). Association between Socioeconomic Position and Thyroid Cancer Incidence: A Population-Based Cohort Study in China. *Cancer Epidemiology, Biomarkers & Prevention*, 35(5), 752–761.

Lindberg, L.G., Svendsen, M., Dømgaard, M., & Brodersen, J. (2013). Better safe than sorry: A long-term perspective on experiences with a false-positive screening mammography in Denmark. *Health, Risk & Society*, 15(8), 699–716.

Lindholt, J.S., & Søgaard, R. (2017). Population screening and intervention for vascular disease in Danish men (VIVA), A randomized controlled trial. *Lancet*, 390(10109), 2256–2265.

Lindholt, J.S., Diederichsen, A.C., Rasmussen, L.M., Frost, L., Steffensen, F.H., Lambrechtsen, J., Urbonaviciene, G., Busk, M., Egstrup, K., Kristensen, K.L., Andersen, C.B., & Søgaard, R. (2020). Survival, prevalence, progression and repair of abdominal aortic aneurysms: Results from three randomised controlled screening trials over three decades. *Clinical Epidemiology*, 12, 95–103.

Link, B., & Phelan, J. (1999). The labelling theory of mental disorder (II), The consequences of labeling. In A.V. Horwitz, & T.L. Scheid (Eds.), *A handbook for the study of mental health: Social contexts, theories, and systems* (pp. 361–376). Cambridge University Press.

Link, B., Cullen, T., Struening, E., Elmer, L., Shrout, P.E., & Dohrenwend, B.P. (1989). A modified labeling theory approach to mental disorders: An empirical assessment. *American Sociological Review*, 54(3), 400–423.

Linos, E., & Colditz, G. (2007). Screening programme evaluation applied to airport security. *BMJ*, 335(7633), 1290–1292.

Lock, M. (2001). The tempering of medical anthropology: Troubling natural categories. *Medical Anthropology Quarterly*, 15(4), 478–492.
Lock, M., & Nguyen, V.-K. (2018 [2010]). *An anthropology of biomedicine*. Wiley Blackwell.
Loeb, S., Folkvaljon, Y., Robinson, D., Lissbrant, I.F., Egevad, L., & Stattin, P. (2016). Evaluation of the 2015 Gleason Grade Groups in a nationwide population-based cohort. *European Urology*, 69(6), 1135–1141.
LoTempio, J.E., Jr, Donohue, C.R., Moreno, J.D., Santos Rutschman, A., Sarnoff, J., Sinha, M.S., Stoeger, T., & Contreras, J.L. (2025). Impact of the 23andMe bankruptcy on preserving the public benefit of scientific data. *Nature Genetics*, *57*(12), 2933–2936.
Lou, S., Dahl, K., Risør, M.B., Hvidman, L.E., Thomsen, S.G., Jørgensen, F.S., Olesen, F., Kjærgaard, H., & Kesmodel, U. (2007). En kvalitativ undersøgelse af gravides valg af nakkefoldskanning. *Ugeskrift for Laeger*, 169(10), 914–918.
Lund, K.S., Siersma, V.D., Christensen, K.B., Waldorff, F.B., & Brodersen, J. (2018). Measuring bothersome menopausal symptoms: Development and validation of the MenoScores questionnaire. *Health and Quality of Life Outcomes*, 16(1), Art. nr. 97.
Lund, P.C. (2020). Deconstructing grief: A sociological analysis of Prolonged Grief Disorder. *Social Theory & Health*, 19, 186–200.
Lunde, I.M. (2009). Nocebo: Når forventninger skaber sygdom. In L. Hvas, J. Brodersen, & B. Hovelius (Eds.), *Kan sundhedsvæsenet skabe usundhed? Refleksioner fra almen praksis* (pp. 287–298). Månedsskrift for Praktisk Lægegerning.
Lundh, A., & Bero, L. (2017). The ties that bind. *BMJ*, 356, j176.
Lupton, D. (1994). *Moral threats and dangerous desires: AIDS in the news media*. Taylor & Francis.
Lupton, D. (1995). *The imperative of health: Public health and the regulated body*. Sage Publications.
Lupton, D. (1997). Consumerism, reflexivity and the medical encounter. *Social Science and Medicine*, 45(3), 373–381.
Lupton, D. (2012). M-health and health promotion: The digital cyborg and surveillance society. *Social Theory Health*, 10, 229–244.
Lupton, D. (2013). *Risk*. Routledge.
Lupton, D. (2016). *The quantified self*. Polity Press.
Lupton, D., & Jutel, A. (2015). It's like having a physician in your pocket. *Social Science and Medicine*, 133, 128–135.
Madsen, O.J. (2015). *The therapeutic turn: How psychology altered Western culture*. Routledge.
Madsen, P.V., Jensen, A., Eriksson, F., & Stensballe, L.G. (2024). Pediatric health service utilization at tertiary hospitals in Denmark 2000–2018. *Scientific Reports*, 14(1), 12999.
Malmqvist, J., Siersma, V.D., Hestbech, M.S., Bang, C.W., Nicolaisdóttir, D.R., & Brodersen, J. (2021). Short and long-term psychosocial consequences of participating in a colorectal cancer screening programme: A matched longitudinal study. *BMJ Evidence-Based Medicine*, 27(2), 87–96.
Manning, B.J., Kristmundsson, T., Sonesson, B., & Resch, T. (2009). Abdominal aortic aneurysm diameter: A comparison of ultrasound measurements with those from standard and three-dimensional computed tomography reconstruction. *Journal of Vascular Surgery*, 50(2), 263–268.
Manser, R., Lethaby, A., Irving, L.B., Stone, C., Byrnes, G., Abramson, M.J., & Campbell, D. (2013). Screening for lung cancer. *Cochrane Database of Systematic Reviews*, 6, CD001991.
Marinovich, M.L., & Houssami, N. (2026). AI for enhancing efficiency and effectiveness of population breast cancer screening. *The Lancet*, 407(10527), 471–473.
Marlow, L.A.V., Waller, J., & Wardle, J. (2010). Variation in blame attributions across different cancer types. *Cancer Epidemiology, Biomarkers & Prevention*, 19(7), 1799–1805.

Marquart, J., Chen, E.Y., & Prasad, V. (2018). Estimation of the percentage of US patients with cancer who benefit from genome-driven oncology. *Journal of the American Medical Association Oncology*, 4(8), 1093–1098.

Martins, C.M.S., da Costa Teixeira, A.S., de Azevedo, L.F.R., Sá, L.M.B., Santos, P.A.A.P., do Couto, M.L.G.D., da Costa Pereira, A.M.R., Hespanhol, A.A.O.P., & da Costa Santos, C.M.N. (2017). The effect of a test ordering software intervention on the prescription of unnecessary laboratory tests—a randomized controlled trial. *BMC Medical Informatics and Decision Making*, 17(1), 20.

Martiny, F.H.J., Bie, A.K.L., Jauernik, C.P., Rahbek, O.J., Nielsen, S.B., Gram, E.G., Kindt, I., Siersma, V., Bang, C.W., & Brodersen, J.B. (2024). Deaths and cardiopulmonary events following colorectal cancer screening—A systematic review with meta-analyses. *PLoS One*, 19(3), e0295900.

Matheson, E.M., King, D.E., & Everett, C.J. (2012). Healthy lifestyle habits and mortality in overweight and obese individuals. *Journal of the American Board of Family Medicine*, 25(1), 9–15.

McAfee, T., Davis, K., Alexander, R., Pechacek, T. F., & Bunnell, R. E. (2013). Effect of the first federally funded US antismoking national media campaign. *The Lancet*, 382, 2003–2011.

McCaffery, K.J., & Barratt, A.L. (2004). Assessing psychosocial/quality of life outcomes in screening: How do we do it better? *Journal of Epidemiology and Community Health*, 58(12), 968–970.

McCaffery, K.J., Jansen, J., Scherer, L.D., Thornton, H., Hersch, J., Carter, S.M., Barratt, A., Sheridan, S., Moynihan, R., Waller, J., Brodersen, J., Pickles, K., & Edwards, A. (2016). Walking the tightrope: Communicating overdiagnosis. *BMJ*, *352*, i348.

McCartney, M. (2017). The false promise of preventive medicine. *BMJ*, *358*, j3895. https://doi.org/10.1136/bmj.j3895

Meland, E., & Brodersen, J. (2016). Why several truths can be true. *Scandinavian Journal of Primary Health Care*, 34(3), 282–285.

Merleau-Ponty, M. (1997 [1945]). *Kroppens fænomenologi*. Det lille forlag.

Merrild, C.H., Andersen, R.S., Risør, M.B., & Vedsted, P. (2016). Resisting 'reason': A comparative anthropological study of social differences and resistance toward health promotion and illness prevention in Denmark. *Medical Anthropology Quarterly*, 31(2), 218–236.

Meyer, G. (2000). *De andres viden—frygt og underdanighed I vidensamfundet*. Høst og Søn.

Meyer, G., Folker, A.P., Jørgensen, R.B., von Krauss, M.K., Sandøe, P., & Tveit, G. (2005). The factualization of uncertainty: Risk, politics, and genetically modified crops—a case of rape. *Agriculture and Human Values*, 22(2), 235–242.

Mikkelsen, E.M., Thomsen, M.K., Tybjerg, J., Friis-Hansen, L., Andersen, B., Jørgensen, J.C.R., Baatrup, G., Njor, S.H., Mehnert, F., & Rasmussen, M. (2018). Colonoscopy-related complications in a nationwide immunochemical fecal occult blood test-based colorectal cancer screening program. *Clinical Epidemiology*, 10, 1649–1655.

Mintzes, B., Swandari, S., Fabbri, A., Grundy, Q., Moynihan, R., & Bero, L. (2018). Does industry-sponsored education foster overdiagnosis and overtreatment of depression, osteoporosis and overactive bladder syndrome? An Australian cohort study. *BMJ Open*, 8(2), e019027.

Mogensen, H. O. (2005). Medicalized experience and the active use of biomedicine. In V. Steffen, R. Jenkins, & H. Jessen (Eds.), *Managing uncertainty: Ethnographic studies of illness, risk and the struggle for control* (pp. 225–243). Museum Tusculanum Press.

Møhl, B., & la Cour, P. (2008). Nogle kritiske vinkler på EBM logikken. *Psyke & Logos*, 29(1), 26.

Mol, A. (2000). What diagnostic devices do: The case of blood sugar measurement. *Theoretical Medicine and Bioethics*, 21(1), 9–22.

Mol, A. (2008). *The logic of care: Health and the problem of patient choice*. Routledge.

Montori, V., Montori, J.P., & Montori, V.M. (2025). Reclaiming human care from surveillance capitalism. *BMJ*, 391, r2459.

Mosa, M., Yoo, I., & Sheets, L.A. (2012). A systematic review of healthcare applications for smartphones. *BioMed Central Medical Informatics and Decision Making*, 12, 67.

Moynihan, R. (2010). Who benefits from treating prehypertension? *BMJ*, 341, c4442.

Moynihan, R., & Cassels, A. (2005). *Selling sickness. How drug companies are turning us all into patients*. Allen & Unwin.

Moynihan, R., & Cassels, A. (2005). *Selling sickness*. Nation Books.

Moynihan, R., Nickel, B., Hersch, J., Doust, J., Barratt, A., Beller, E., & McCaffery, K. (2015). What do you think overdiagnosis means? A qualitative analysis of responses from a national community survey of Australians. *BMJ Open*, 5(5), e007436.

Moynihan, R., Brodersen, J., Heath, I., Johannson, M., Kuehlein, T., Minué-Lorenzo, S., Petursson, H., Pizzanelli, M., Reventlow, S., Sigurdsson, J., Stavdal, A., Treadwell, J., & Glasziou, P. (2019). Reforming disease definitions: A new primary care led, people-centred approach. *BMJ Evidence-Based Medicine*, 24(5), 170–173.

Moynihan, R., Johansson, M., Lexchin, J., Macdonald, H., Mintzes, B., Pearson, C., Rodwin, M.A., Stavdal, A., Stegenga, J., Thombs, B.D., Thornton, H., Vandvik, P.O., Wieseler, B., & Godlee, F. (2019). Pathways to independence: Towards producing and using trustworthy evidence. *BMJ, 367*, l6576.

Moynihan, R., Heath, I., & Henry, D. (2002). Selling sickness: The pharmaceutical industry and disease mongering. *BMJ*, 324(7342), 886–891.

Mukai, T.O., Bro, F., Pedersen, K.V., & Vedsted. (2010). Brug af undersøgelse for prostataspecifikt antigen [Use of prostate-specific antigen testing]. *Ugeskrift for Laeger*, 172(9), 696–700.

Mulinari, S., Vilhelmsson, A., Rickard, E., & Ozieranski, P. (2020). Five years of pharmaceutical industry funding of patient organisations in Sweden: Cross-sectional study of companies, patient organisations and drugs. *PLoS One*, 15(6), e0235021.

Muntner, P., Carey, R.M., Gidding, S., Jones, D.W., Taler, S.J., Wright, J.T., & Whelton, P.K. (2017). Potential U.S. population impact of the 2017 American College of Cardiology/American Heart Association high blood pressure guideline. *Journal of the American College of Cardiology*, 71(2), 109–118.

Müskens, J.L.J.M., Kool, R.B., van Dulmen, S.A., & Westert, G.P. (2022). Overuse of diagnostic testing in healthcare. *BMJ Quality & Safety*, 31(1), 54–63.

Navarro, V. (2009). What we mean by social determinants of health. *International Journal of Health Services*, 39(3), 423–441.

Nejstgaard, C.H., Bero, L., Hróbjartsson, A., Jørgensen, A.W., Jørgensen, K.J., Le, M., & Lundh, A. (2020). Association between conflicts of interest and favourable recommendations in clinical guidelines, advisory committee reports, opinion pieces, and narrative reviews: Systematic review. *BMJ*, 371, m4234.

Nexoe, J., Oltarzewska, A.M., & Sawicka-Powierza, J. (2002). Perception of risk information. Similarities and differences between Danish and Polish general practitioners. *Scandinavian Journal of Primary Health Care*, 20(3), 183–187.

Nguyen-Nielsen, M., Møller, H., Tjønneland, A., & Borre, M. (2019). Causes of death in men with prostate cancer: Results from the Danish Prostate Cancer Registry (DAPROCAdata). *Cancer Epidemiology*, 59, 249–257.

Nickel, B., Moynihan, R., Gram, E.G., Copp, T., Taba, M., Shih, P., Heiss, R., Gao, M., & Zadro, J.R. (2025). Social media posts about medical tests with potential for overdiagnosis. *JAMA Network Open*, 8(2): e2461940.

Nielsen, M., & Grøn, L. (2013). Quantify your self! Numbers in ambiguous borderlands of health. *Tidsskrift for Forskning i Sygdom og Samfund*, 10(19). doi: 10.7146/tfss.v10i19.15525.

Nielsen, M., Thomsen, J.L., Primdahl, S., Dyreborg, U., & Andersen, J.A. (1987). Breast cancer and atypia among young and middle-aged women: A study of 110 medicolegal autopsies. *British Journal of Cancer*, 56(6), 814–819.

Nielsen, S.B., Spalletta, O., Toft Kristensen, M.A., & Brodersen, J. (2020). Psychosocial consequences of potential overdiagnosis in prostate cancer a qualitative interview study. *Scandinavian Journal of Primary Health Care*, 38(4), 439–446.

Nielsen, T.H. (2025). Somatic overdiagnosis and hermeneutical injustice. *Erkenntnis*, 91(5), 2297–2315.

Nilsen, S., & Malterud, K. (2017). What happens when the doctor denies a patient's request? A qualitative interview study among general practitioners in Norway. *Scandinavian Journal of Primary Health Care*, 35, 201–207.

Njor, S.H., Friis-Hansen, L., Andersen, B., Søndergaard, B., Linnemann, D., Jørgensen, J.C.R., Roikjær, O., & Rasmussen, M. (2018). Three years of colorectal cancer screening in Denmark. *Cancer Epidemiology*, 57, 39–44.

NORDCAN. https://nordcan.iarc.fr/en

Nørgaard, E. (2005). *Tugt og dannelse: Tre historier fra kulturkampens arena*. Gyldendal.

Nørgaard, M. (2022). Vaks tilskuer opdagede modermærkekræft på bænken under kamp. *DR.dk*. 3. januar. https://www.dr.dk/sporten/ishockey/vaks-tilskuer-opdagede-modermaerkekraeft-paa-baenken-under-nhl-kamp-hun-har-reddet

Øines, M., Helsingen, L.M., Bretthauer, M., & Emilsson, L. (2017). Epidemiology and risk factors of colorectal polyps. *Best Practice & Research Clinical Gastroenterology*, 31(4), 419–424.

Olsen, O., Damhus, C.S., Gram, E.G., Kirkegaard, O., & Brodersen, J.B. (2023). Re: Colorectal cancer incidence and mortality: A pooled analysis of randomized trials—Errors in data? *Annals of Internal Medicine*. https://www.acpjournals.org/doi/10.7326/M22-0835?url_ver=Z39.88-2003&rfr_id=ori:rid:crossref.org&rfr_dat=cr_pub%20%200pubmed#comments-section

Opdal, P.O., Meland, E., & Hjorleifsson, S. (2019). Dilemmas of medical overuse in general practice – A focus group study. *Scandinavian Journal of Primary Health Care*, 37(1), 135–140.

O'Sullivan, S. (2025). *The age of diagnosis*. Hodder & Stoughton.

Ørtenblad, L., Meillier, L., & Jønsson, A.R. (2018). Multi-morbidity: A patient perspective on navigating the health care system and everyday life. *Chronic Illness*, 14(4), 271–282.

Osteoporose-f.dk. (2022). Knogleskørhed. https://www.osteoporose-f.dk/knogleskoerhed

Østerø í Jákupsstovu, J., & Brodersen, J. (2018). Do men with lower urinary tract symptoms have an increased risk of advanced prostate cancer? *BMJ*, 361, k1202.

Østerø, J., Siersma, V., & Brodersen, J. (2014). Breast cancer screening implementation and reassurance. *European Journal of Public Health*, 24(2), 258–263.

Östör, A.G. (1993). Natural history of cervical intraepithelial neoplasia: A critical review. *International Journal of Gynecological Pathology*, 12, 186.

Owens, J. (2020). Relationships between an ADHD diagnosis and future school behaviors among children with mild behavioral problems. *Sociology of Education*, 93(3), 191–214.

Oxlund, B. (2012). Living by numbers: The dynamic interplay of asymptomatic conditions and low cost measurement technologies in the cases of two women in the Danish provinces. *Suomen Antropologi*, 37(3), 42–56.

Paris, J. (2015). *Overdiagnosis in psychiatry: How modern psychiatry lost its way while creating a diagnosis for almost all of life's misfortunes*. Oxford University Press.

Park, S., Oh, C.M., Cho, H., Lee, J.Y., Jung, K.W., Jun, J.K., Won, Y.J., Kong, H.J., Choi, K.S., Lee, Y.J., & Lee, J.S. (2016). Association between screening and the thyroid cancer 'epidemic' in South Korea: Evidence from a nationwide study. *BMJ*, 355, i5745.

Parsons, T. (1951). *The social system*. Free Press.

Pashley, D., Ozieranski, P., & Mulinari, S. (2022). Disclosure of pharmaceutical industry funding of patient organisations in Nordic countries: Can industry self-regulation deliver on its transparency promise? *International Journal of Social Determinants of Health and Health Services*, 52(3), 347–362.

Patel, M.S., Asch, D.A., & Volpp, K.G. (2015). Wearable devices as facilitators, not drivers, of health behavior change. *Journal of American Medical Association*, 313(5), 459–460.

Pathirana, T., Clark, J., & Moynihan, R. (2017). Mapping the drivers of overdiagnosis to potential solutions. *BMJ*, 358, j3879.

PCUK (Prostate Cancer UK). (2024). Faster. Fairer. Better. Reducing prostate cancer inequalities and late diagnosis: The first year plan for Government. https://prostatecanceruk.org

Pedersen, K.M. (2015). *Prioritering i sundhedsvæsenet*. Munksgaard.

Pedersen, L.H., Wahlberg, A., Cordt, M., Schmiegelow, K., Dalton, S.O., & Larsen, H.B. (2020). Parent's perspectives of the pathway to diagnosis of childhood cancer: A matter of diagnostic triage. *BioMed Central Health Services Research*, (20), Art. nr. 969. doi: 10.1186/s12913-020-05821-2.

Pedersen, M.W., Groth, K.A., Mortensen, K.H., Brodersen, J., Gravholt, C.H., & Andersen, N.H. (2019). Clinical and pathophysiological aspects of bicuspid aortic valve disease. *Cardiology in the Young*, 29, 1–10.

Peirson, L., Fitzpatrick-Lewis, D., Ciliska, D., & Warren, R. (2013). Screening for cervical cancer: A systematic review and meta-analysis. *Systematic Reviews*, 2, 35.

Petersen, A., Brodersen, J., & Saxtrup, N. (2021). Sorgdiagnosen på (over)arbejde. In A. Petersen, & S. Brinkmann (Eds.), *Menneskets sorg—et vilkår i forandring* (pp. 361–383). Klim.

Petersen, A., & Lupton, D. (1996). *The new public health: Health and self in the age of risk*. Sage Publications.

Petersen, A. (2019). *Digital health and technological promise: A sociological inquiry*. Routledge.

Petersen, G.B., Damhus, C.S., Jønsson, A.B.R., & Brodersen, J. (2020). The perception gap: How the benefits and harms of cervical cancer screening are understood in information material focusing on informed choice. *Health, Risk & Society*, 22(2), 177–196.

Petrakaki, D., Hilberg, E., & Waring, J. (2018). Between empowerment and self-discipline: Governing patients' conduct through technological self-care. *Social Science & Medicine*, (213), 146–153.

Petryna, A. (2004). Biological citizenship: The science and politics of Chernobyl-exposed populations. *Osiris*, 19, 250–265.

Petursson, H., Sigurdsson, J.A., & Bengtsson, C. (2012). Is the use of cholesterol in mortality risk algorithms in clinical guidelines valid? Ten years prospective data from the Norwegian HUNT 2 study. *Journal of Evaluation in Clinical Practice*, 18(1), 170–171.

Petursson, H., Sigurdsson, J.A., Bengtsson, C., Nilsen, T.I., & Getz, L. (2011). Body configuration as a predictor of mortality: Comparison of five anthropometric measures in a 12 year follow-up of the Norwegian HUNT 2 study. *PLoS One*, 6(10), e26621.

Petursson, H., Getz, L., Sigurdsson, J.A., & Hetlevik, I. (2009). Can individuals with a significant risk for cardiovascular disease be adequately identified by combination of several risk factors? Modelling study based on the Norwegian HUNT 2 population. *Journal of Evaluation in Clinical Practice*, 15(1), 103–109.

Phillips, S.P., Spithoff, S., & Simpson, A. (2022). Artificial intelligence and predictive algorithms in medicine: Promise and problems. *Canadian Family Physician*, 68(8), 570–572.

Pickles, K., Carter, S.M., Rychetnik, L., McCaffery, K., & Entwistle, V.A. (2018). Primary goals, information-giving and men's understanding: A qualitative study of Australian and UK doctors' varied communication about PSA screening. *BMJ Open*, 8(1), e018009.

Piessens, V., Van den Bruel, A., Piessens, A., Van Hecke, A., Brodersen, J.B., Lauwerier, E., Stul, F., De Sutter, A., & Heytens, S. (2025). Do health professionals know about overdiagnosis in screening, and how are they dealing with it? A mixed-methods systematic scoping review. *PLoS One*, 20(2), e0315247.

Pink, S., & Fors, V. (2017). Being in a mediated world: Self-tracking and the mind–body–environment. *Cultural Geography*, 24, 375–388.

Pray, R., & Riskin, S. (2023). The history and faults of the body mass index and where to look next: A literature review. *Cureus*, 15(11), e48230.

Prenosil, G.A., Sari, H., Fürstner, M., Afshar-Oromieh, A., Shi, K., Rominger, A., & Hentschel, M. (2022). Performance characteristics of the Biograph Vision Quadra PET/CT system with a long axial field of view using the NEMA NU 2-2018 standard. *Journal of Nuclear Medicine*, 63(3), 476–484.

Price, N.D., Magis, A.T. Earls, J.C., Glusman, G., Levy, R., Lausted, C., McDonald, D.T., Kusebauch, U., Moss, C.L., Zhou, Y., Qin, S., Moritz, R.L., Brogaard, K., Omenn, G.S., Lovejoy, J.C., & Hood, L. (2017). A wellness study of 108 individuals using personal, dense, dynamic data clouds. *Nature Biotechnology*, 35(8), 747–756.

Prior, L., & Bloor, M. (1993). Why people die: Social representations of death and its causes. *Science as Culture*, 3(3), 346–374.

Prorok, P.C., Wright, P., & Riley, T.R. (2018). Overall and multiphasic findings of the Prostate, Lung, Colorectal and Ovarian (PLCO) Randomized Cancer Screening Trial. *Reviews on Recent Clinical Trials*, 13(4), 257–273.

PwC. (2025). *International research funding systems: A comparative analysis*. https://www.pwc.co.uk/government-public-sector/education/documents/international-research-funding-systems-comparative-analysis-april-2025.pdf

Qaseem, A., Humphrey, L.L., Harris, R., Starkey, M., & Denberg, T.D. (2014). Screening pelvic examination in adult women: A clinical practice guideline from the American College of Physicians. *Annals of Internal Medicine*, 161(1), 67–72.

QS. (2020). Quantified self. Quantifiedself.com

Rabiner, D., Murray, D., Rosen, L., Hardy, K., Skinner, A., & Underwood, M. (2010). Instability in teacher ratings of children's inattentive symptoms: Implications for the assessment of ADHD. *Journal of Developmental & Behavioral Pediatrics*, 31, 175–180.

Rabinow, P. (1996). *Essays on the anthropology of reason*. Princeton University Press.

Raffle, A., & Gray, M. (2007). *Screening: Evidence and practice*. Oxford University Press.

Raffle, A.E., Mackie, A., & Gray, M. (2019). *Screening. Evidence and practice*. Oxford University Press.

Raffle, A.E., Alden, B., Quinn, M., Babb, P.J., & Brett, M.T. (2003). Outcomes of screening to prevent cancer: Analysis of cumulative incidence of cervical abnormality and modelling of cases and deaths prevented. *BMJ*, 326(7395), 901–905.

Rahbek, O., Jauernik, C., Plough, T., & Brodersen, J. (2021). Categories of systematic influences applied to increase cancer screening participation: A literature review and analysis. *European Journal of Public Health*, 31(1), 200–206.

Ransohoff, D.F., & Feinstein, A.R. (1978). Problems of spectrum and bias in evaluating the efficacy of diagnostic tests. *New England Journal of Medicine*, 299(17), 926–930.

Rapp, R. (1998). Refusing prenatal diagnosis: The meanings of bioscience in a multicultural world. *Science, Technology, & Human Values*, 23(1), 45–70.

Rasmussen, J.F., Siersma, V., Malmqvist, J., & Brodersen, J. (2020). Psychosocial consequences of false positives in the Danish Lung Cancer CT Screening Trial: A nested matched cohort study. *BMJ Open*, 10(6), e034682.

Rasmussen, J.F., Siersma, V., Pedersen, J.H., Heleno, B., Saghir, Z., & Brodersen, J. (2014). Healthcare costs in the Dani randomised controlled lung cancer CT-screening trial: A registry study. *Lung Cancer*, 83(3), 347–355.

Rasmussen, J.F., Siersma, V., Pedersen, J.H., & Brodersen, J. (2015). Psychosocial consequences in the Dani randomised controlled lung cancer screening trial (DLCST). *Lung Cancer*, 87(1), 65–72.

Remes, J., Linzer, K., Singhal, S., Dewhurst, M., Dash, P., Woetzel, J., Smit, S., Evers, M., Wilson, M., & Rutter, K.-A. (2020). Prioritizing health: A prescription for prosperity. McKinsey Global Institute.

Reumkens, A., Rondagh, E.J., Bakker, C.M., Winkens, B., Masclee, A.A., & Sanduleanu, S. (2016). Post-colonoscopy complications: A systematic review, time trends, and meta-analysis of population-based studies. *The American Journal of Gastroenterol*, 111(8), 1092–1101.

Reventlow, S., Hvas, L., & Malterud, K. (2006). Making the invisible body visible. Bone scans, osteoporosis and women's bodily experiences. *Social Science and Medicine*, 62, 2720–2731.

Riboe, D.G., Dogan, T.S., & Brodersen, J. (2012). Potential biases in colorectal cancer screening using faecal occult blood test. *Journal of Evaluation in Clinical Practice*, 19(2), 311–316.

Ries, N.M., & Jansen, J. (2021). Physicians' views and experiences of defensive medicine: An international review of empirical research. *Health Policy*, 125(5), 634–642.

Risør, M.B. (2005). Introduktion: Sundhedsfremme og forebyggelse. *Tidsskrift for Forskning i Sygdom og Samfund*, 2(3). doi: 10.7146/tfss.v2i3.465.

Rødbro, K.V., & Jervelund, S.S. (2025). The effect of displaying laboratory test prices on physicians' ordering behaviour: A systematic review of European studies. *European Journal of Health Economics*, 26(8), 1459–1467.

Rogers, W.A., & Mintzker, Y. (2016). Getting clearer on overdiagnosis. *Journal of Evaluation in Clinical Practice*, 22(4), 580–587.

Rolfe, A., & Burton, C. (2013). Reassurance after diagnostic testing with a low pretest probability of serious disease: Systematic review and meta-analysis. *Journal of the American Medical Association Internal Medicine*, 173(6), 407–416.

Romains, J. (1941 [1923]). *Knock eller Medicinens Triumf. Komedie i tre Akter*. Overs. af Ole Vinding.

Ropers, F.G., Barratt, A., Wilt, T., Nicholls, S., Taylor-Phillips, S., Kramer, B.S., Esserman, L., Norris, S.L., Gibson, L.M., Harris, R.P., Carter, S.M., Jacklyn, G., & Jørgensen, K.J. (2021). Health screening needs independent regular re-evaluation. *BMJ*, 374, n2049.

Rose, G. (1985). Sick individuals and sick populations. *International Journal of Epidemiology*, 14(1), 32–38.

Rose, N., & Novas, C. (2004). Biological citizenship. In A. Ong, & S. Collier (Eds.), *Global anthropology* (pp. 439–463). Blackwell.

Rose, N. (2007). *The politics of life itself: Biomedicine, power and subjectivity in the twenty first century*. Princeton University Press.

Rose, S.L., Highland, J., Karafa, M.T., & Joffe, S. (2017). Patient advocacy organizations, industry funding, and conflicts of interest. *JAMA Internal Medicine*, *177*(3), 344–350.

Røssell, E-L., Bo, A., Grønborg, T.K., Kristiansen, I.S., Borgquist, S., Scherer, L.D., & Støvring, H. (2023). Danish women want to participate in a hypothetical breast cancer screening with harms and no reduction in mortality: A cross-sectional survey. *Medical Decision Making*, 43(4), 403–416.

Rowan, K., McAlpine, D.D., & Blewett, L.A. (2013). Access and cost barriers to mental health care, by insurance status, 1999–2010. *Health Affairs* (Millwood), 32(10), 1723–1730.

Rozing, M.P., Jønsson, A., Køster-Rasmussen, R., Due, T.D., Brodersen, J., Bissenbakker, K.H., Siersma, V., Mercer, S.W., Guassora, A.D., Kjellberg, J., Kjellberg, P.K., Nielsen, M.H., Christensen, I., Bardram, J.E., Martiny, F., Møller, A., & Reventlow, S. (2021). The SOFIA pilot trial: A cluster-randomized trial of coordinated, co-produced care to reduce mortality and improve quality of life in people with severe mental illness in the general practice setting. *Pilot and Feasibility Studies*, 7(1), 168.

Rubeis, G. (2023). Liquid health. Medicine in the age of surveillance capitalism. *Social Science & Medicine*, 322, 115810.

Rutherford, V., & Pickup, I. (2015). Negotiating liminality in higher education: Formal and informal dimensions of the student experience as facilitators of quality. In A. Curaj, L. Matei, R. Pricopie, J. Salmi, & P. Scottet (Eds.), *The European higher education area* (pp. 35–52). Springer.

Ryborg, A.B. (2011). Madmagi: At spise sig ud af en adfærdsforstyrrelse. *Tidsskrift for Forskning i Sygdom og Samfund*, 8(14). doi: 10.7146/tfss.v8i14.5420.

Rychetnik, L., Carter, S.M., Abelson, J., Thornton, H., Barratt, A., Entwistle, V.A., Mackenzie, G., Salkeld, G., & Glasziou, P. (2013). Enhancing citizen engagement in cancer screening through deliberative democracy. *Journal of the National Cancer Institute*, 105(6), 380–386.

Saghir, Z., Dirksen, A., Ashraf, H., Bach, K.S., Brodersen, J., Clementsen, P.F., Døssing, M., Hansen, H., Kofoed, K.F., Larsen, K.R., Mortensen, J., Rasmussen, J.F., Seersholm, N., Skov, B.G., Thorsen, H., Tønnesen, P., & Pedersen, J.H. (2012). CT screening for lung cancer brings forward early disease: The randomised Danish Lung Cancer Screening Trial: Status after five annual screening rounds with low-dose CT. *Thorax*, 67(4), 296–301.

Sah, S., Elias, P., & Ariely, D. (2013). Investigation momentum: The relentless pursuit to resolve uncertainty. *Journal of American Medical Association Internal Medicine*, 173(10), 932–933.

Sand, C.D., Rahbek, K. Willadsen, T.G., & Jønsson, A.R. (2021). Prioritizing social identities: Patients' perspective on living with multimorbidity. *Journal of Multimorbidity and Comorbidity*, 11. doi: 10.1177/26335565211009375.

Sanders, S., Barratt, A., Buchbinder, R., Doust, J., Kazda, L., Jones, M., Glasziou, P., & Bell, K. (2024). Evidence for overdiagnosis in noncancer conditions was assessed: A metaepidemiological study using the 'Fair Umpire' framework. *Journal of Clinical Epidemiology*, 165, 111215.

Santhouse, A. (2025). *No more normal: Mental health in an age of overdiagnosis*. Granta Books.

Saxtrup, N., & Petersen, A. (2018). Who owns the diagnosis? The doctor's tool on the move. *Bibliotek for Læger*, 210, 116–133.

Scheff, T.J. (1966). *Being mentally ill: A sociological theory. Observations*. Weidenfeld & Nicolson.

Scheper-Hughes, N. (1992). *Death without weeping. The violence of everyday life in Brazil*. University of California Press.

Schilling, F.H., Spix, C., Berthold, F., Erttmann, R., Fehse, N., Hero, B., Klein, G., Sander, J., Schwarz, K., Treuner, J., Zorn, U., & Michaelis, J. (2002). Neuroblastoma screening at one year of age. *New England Journal of Medicine*, 346(14), 1047–1053.

Schneider, U.V., Forsberg, M.W., Leineweber, T.D., Jensen, C.B., Ghathian, K., Agergaard, C.N., Mortensen, K.K., Cohen, A., Jørgensen, C.S., Larsen, H., Hansen, M.B., Saleme, U., Koch, A., Kirkby, N.S., Kallemose, T., Schaadt, M.L., Jensen, F.H., Jørgensen, R.L., Ma, C.M.G., ... & Lisby, J.G. (2022). A nationwide analytical and clinical evaluation of 44 rapid antigen tests for SARS-CoV-2 compared to RT-qPCR. *Journal of Clinical Virology*, 153, 105214.

Schröder, F.H., Hugosson, J., Roobol, M.J., Tammela, T.L., Ciatto, S., Nelen, V., Kwiatkowski, M., Lujan, M., Lilja, H., Zappa, M., Denis, L.J., Recker, F., Berenguer, A., Määttänen, L., Bangma, C.H., Aus, G., Villers, A., Rebillard, X., van der Kwast, T., Blijenberg, B.G., Moss, S.M., de Koning, H.J., & Auvinen, A. (2009). Screening and prostate-cancer mortality in a randomized European study. *New England Journal of Medicine*, 360(13), 1320–1328.

Shiga, T., Wajima, Z., Apfel, C.C., Inoue, T., & Ohe, Y. (2006). Diagnostic accuracy of transesophageal echocardiography, helical computed tomography, and magnetic resonance imaging for suspected thoracic aortic dissection: Systematic review and meta-analysis. *Archives of Internal Medicine*, 166(13), 1350–1356.

Shorter, E. (1985). *Doctor's and their patients: A social history*. Simon & Schuster.

Sigurdsson, J.A., Getz, L., Sjonell, G., Vainiomaki, P., & Brodersen, J. (2013). Marginal public health gain of screening for colorectal cancer: Modelling study, based on WHO and national databases in the Nordic countries. *Journal of Evaluation in Clinical Practice*, 19(2), 400–407.

Simmel, G., & Hughes, E. (1949). The sociology of sociability. *American Journal of Sociology*, 55(3), 254–261.

Sjørslev, I. (2017). *Sandhed og genre. Videnskabsteori i antropologi og kulturanalyse*. Samfundslitteratur.

Skolbekken, J.A. (1996). Risiko som begrep og utfordring i helsevesenet. *Tidsskrift for den Norske Laegeforening*, 116(22), 2673–2676.

Skrabanek, P. (1994). *The death of humane medicine and the rise of coercive healthism*. Social Affairs Unit.

Slovic, P., Finucane, M.L., Peters, E., & MacGregor, D.G. (2004). Risk as analysis and risk as feelings: Some thoughts about affect, reason, risk, and rationality. *Risk Analysis*, 24, 311–322.

Smith, G.J.D., & Vonthethoff, B. (2017). Health by numbers? Exploring the practice and experience of datafied health. *Health Sociology Review*, 26(1), 6–21.

Smith, J. (2022, January 2). The hockey manager who beat cancer and became a fan favorite. *The New York Times*. https://www.nytimes.com/2022/01/02/sports/hockey/canucks-cancer-manager-fan.html

Smith, S.M., Fahey, T., Smucny, J., & Becker, L.A. (2017). Antibiotics for acute bronchitis. *Cochrane Database of Systematic Reviews*, 6, Cd000245.

Smokefree Sweden. (2026). European Parliament declares Sweden smoke-free. https://smokefreesweden.org/2026/06/02/european-parliament-declares-sweden-smoke-free/

Sørensen, T.I.A., Sandbæk, A., & Pedersen, B.K. (2013). *Skal overvægtige voksne tabe sig? Rapport*. Vidensråd for Forebyggelse.

Spence, D. (2016). Bad medicine: The worried hell. *British Journal of General Practice*, 66(651), 526.

Speyer, H., Nørgaard, H., Birk, M., Karlsen, M., Jakobsen, A.S., Pedersen, K., Hjorthøj, C., Pisinger, C., Gluud, C., Mors, O., Krogh, J., & Nordentoft, M. (2016). The CHANGE trial: No superiority of lifestyle coaching plus care coordination plus treatment as usual compared to treatment as usual alone in reducing risk of cardiovascular disease in adults with schizophrenia spectrum disorders and abdominal obesity. *World Psychiatry*, 15(2), 155–165.

SSI. (2022). *Sygdomme der indgår i screeningen*. Screening af nyfødte. nyfoedte.ssi.dk/medfoedte-sygdomme/sygdomme-der-screenes-for

Starfield, B., Hyde, J., Gérvas, J., & Heath, I. (2008). The concept of prevention: A good idea gone astray? *Journal of Epidemiology and Community Health*, 62(7), 580–583.

Steffen, V., & Meldgaard, M.B.A. (2007). Afveje-om normalitet og afvigelse. I V. Steffen (Ed.), *Sundhedens veje -grundbog i sundhedsantropologi* (pp. 155–176). Hans Reitzels Forlag.

Steffen, V. (2005). Challenging control. In V. Steffen, R. Jenkins, & H. Jessen (Eds.), *Managing uncertainty. Ethnographic studies of illness, risk and the struggle for control* (pp. 11–21). Museum Tusculanum Press.

Steffen, V., Jenkins, R., & Jessen, H. (Eds.). (2005). *Managing uncertainty. Ethnographic studies of illness, risk and the struggle for control*. Museum Tusculanum Press.

Strathern, M. (2000). The tyranny of transparency. *British Educational Research Journal*, 26(3), 309–321.

Stull, D., Starling, R., & Haas, G. (1999). Becoming a patient with heart failure. *Heart & Lung*, 28(4), 284–292.

Svendsen, J.H., Diederichsen, S.Z., Højberg, S., Krieger, D.W., Graff, C., Kronborg, C., Olesen, M.S., Nielsen, J.B., Holst, A.G., Brandes, A., Haugan, K.J., & Køber, L. (2021). Implantable loop recorder detection of atrial fibrillation to prevent stroke (The LOOP Study), A randomised controlled trial. *Lancet*, 398(10310), 1507–1516.

Svensjö, S., Björck, M., Gurtelschmid, M., Djavani, G.K., Hellberg, A., & Wanhainen, A. (2011). Low prevalence of abdominal aortic aneurysm among 65-year-old Swedish men indicates a change in the epidemiology of the disease. *Circulation*, 124(10), 1118–1123.

Tabor, A., Vestergaard, C.H., & Lidegaard, O. (2009). Fetal loss rate after chorionic villus sampling and amniocentesis: An 11-year national registry study. *Ultrasound in Obstetrics and Gynecology*, 34(1), 19–24.

Tabor, A., Hornnes, P.J., & Ottesen, B.S. (1997). UL-scanning for ovariecancer. *Ugeskrift for Læger*, 159(10), 1461–1463.

Taylor, C. (1989). *Sources of the self: The making of the modern identity*. Harvard University Press.

Team National Lung Screening Trial Research. (2019). Lung cancer incidence and mortality with extended follow-up in the National Lung Screening Trial. *Journal of Thoracic Oncology*, 14(10), 1732–1742.

Teknologirådet. (2011). *Test dig selv!* tekno.dk/project/test-dig-selv-2/

Temkin, S.M., Miller, E.A., & Samimi, G. (2017 [1990]). Outcomes from ovarian cancer screening in the PLCO trial: Histologic heterogeneity impacts detection, overdiagnosis and survival. *European Journal of Cancer*, 87, 182–188.

Thomas, E.T., Del Mar, C., Glasziou, P., Wright, G., Barratt, A., & Bell, K.J.L. (2017). Prevalence of incidental breast cancer and precursor lesions in autopsy studies: A systematic review and meta-analysis. *BMC Cancer*, 17(1), 808.

Thomas, P.R., Shaw, J.C., Ashton, H.A., Kay, D.N., & Scott, R.A. (1994). Accuracy of ultrasound in a screening programme for abdominal aortic aneurysms. *Journal of Medical Screening*, 1(1), 3–6.

Thompson, S.G., Ashton, H.A., Gao, L., Buxton, M.J., & Scott, R.A. (2012). Final follow-up of the Multicentre Aneurysm Screening Study (MASS) randomized trial of abdominal aortic aneurysm screening. *British Journal of Surgery*, 99(12), 1649–1656.

Thorgaard, K., Nissen, M., & Jensen, U.J. (2010). Viden, virkning og virke. Forslag til forselser i sundhedspraksis. In K. Thorgaard, M. Nissen, & U.J. Jensen (Eds.), *Viden, virkning og virke: Forslag til forseelser i sundhedspraksis* (pp. 7–16). Roskilde Universitetsforlag.

Tilma, A. (2020). Tarmkræftscreeningens veje—og især vildveje. *Ugeskriftet*, 16.

Timmermans, S., & Buchbinder, M. (2010). Patients-in-waiting: Living between sickness and health in the genomics era. *Journal of Health and Social Behavior*, 51(4), 408–423.

Topol, E.J. (2019). High-performance medicine. *Nature Medicine*, *25*(1), 44–56.

Tørring, M.L., Frydenberg, M., Hansen, R.P., Olesen, F., Hamilton, W., & Vedsted, P. (2011). Time to diagnosis and mortality in colorectal cancer. *British Journal of Cancer*, *104*(6), 934–940.

Tsou, J. (2007). Hacking on the looping effects of psychiatric classifications: What is an interactive and indifferent kind? *International Studies in the Philosophy of Science*, 21(3), 329–344.

Tsoukas, H. (1997). The tyranny of light: The temptations and the paradoxes of the information society. *Futures*, 29(9), 827–843.

Tulloch, J., & Lupton, D. (2005). *Risk and everyday life*. Sage Publications.

Turner, V.W. (1967). *The forest of symbols: Aspects of Ndembu ritual*. Cornell University Press.

Turner, V.W. (1974). *Dramas, fields, and metaphors: Symbolic action in human society*. Cornell University Press.

Turner, V.W. (1981 [1969]). *The ritual process: Structure and anti-structure*. Aldine Publishing Company.

UK National Screening Committee. (2025). https://nationalscreening.blog.gov.uk/2025/11/28/uk-nsc-opens-consultation-on-draft-prostate-cancer-screening-recommendation/

USPSTF. (2018). Screening for prostate cancer: US Preventive Services Task Force Recommendation Statement. *JAMA*, 319(18), 1901–1913.

Vaccarella, S., Franceschi, S., Bray, F., Wild, C.P., Plummer, M., & Dal Maso, L. (2016). Worldwide thyroid-cancer epidemic? The increasing impact of overdiagnosis. *New England Journal of Medicine*, 375(7), 614–617.

Vaccarella, S., Li, M., Bray, F., Kvale, R., Serraino, D., Lorenzoni, V., Auvinen, A., & Dal Maso, L. (2024). Prostate cancer incidence and mortality in Europe and implications for screening activities: Population based study. *BMJ*, 386, e077738.

Vallgårda, S. (2005). Hvad er sundhedsfremme? En analyse af begrebet og styringsmetoderne. *Tidsskrift for Forskning i Sygdom og Samfund*, 2(3). doi: 10.7146/tfss.v2i3.466.

Van Der Geest, S., Whyte, S., & Hardon, A. (1996). The anthropology of pharmaceuticals: A biographical approach. *Annual Review of Anthropology*, 25, 153–178.

van der Kamp, J., Betten, A.W., & Krabbenborg, L. (2022). In their own words: A narrative analysis of illness memoirs written by men with prostate cancer. *Sociology of Health & Illness*, 44, 236–252.

Van Gennep, A. (1960). *The rites of passage*. Routledge.

Venekamp, R.P., Sanders, S.L., Glasziou, P.P., Del Mar, C.B., & Rovers, M.M. (2015). Antibiotics for acute otitis media in children. *Cochrane Database Systematic Reviews*, 6, Cd000219.

Vinther, J.L., Jørgensen, T., & Borglykke, A. (2013). Need to combine individual strategies with population-level strategies in the prevention of coronary heart disease. *Danish Medical Journal*, 60(10), A4726.

Vleugels, J.L.A., Hazewinkel, Y., Fockens, P., & Dekker, E. (2017). Natural history of diminutive and small colorectal polyps: A systematic literature review. *Gastrointestinal Endoscopy*, 85(6), 1169–1176.

Vogt, H., Green, S., & Brodersen, J. (2018). Precision medicine in the clouds. *Nature Biotechnology*, 36(8), 678–680. [Author correction: *Nature Biotechnology*, 36(10), 1016.]

Vogt, H., Green, S., Ekstrøm, C.T., & Brodersen, J. (2019). How precision medicine and screening with big data could increase overdiagnosis. *BMJ*, 366, l5270.

von Euler-Chelpin, M., Olsen, A.H., Njor, S., Jensen, A., Vejborg, I., Schwartz, W., & Lynge, E. (2008). Does educational level determine screening participation? *European Journal of Cancer Prevention*, 17(3), 273–278.

Voss, T., Krag, M., Martiny, F., Heleno, B., Jørgensen, K.J., & Brodersen, J.B. (2023). Quantification of overdiagnosis in randomised trials of cancer screening: An overview and re-analysis of systematic reviews. *Cancer Epidemiology*, 84, 102352.

Wahlberg, A., & Rose, N. (2015). The governmentalization of living: Calculating global health. *Economy and Society*, 44(1), 60–90.

Wahlberg, A. (2007). Measuring progress: Calculating the life of nations. *Distinktion: Scandinavian Journal of Social Theory*, 14, 65–82.

Walshe, J., Elphinstone, B., Nicol, D., & Taylor, M. (2024). A systematic literature review of the 'commercialisation effect' on public attitudes towards biobank and genomic data repositories. *Public Understanding of Science (Bristol, England)*, *33*(5), 548–567. https://doi.org/10.1177/09636625241230864

Wang, D., Wright, J.M., Adams, S.P., Cundiff, D.K., Gueyffier, F., Grenet, G., & Ambasta, A. (2025). Pharmacotherapy for mild hypertension. *Cochrane Database of Systematic Reviews*, 9(9), Cd006742.

Weeldreyer, N.R., De Guzman, J.C., Paterson, C., Allen, J.D., Gaesser, G.A., & Angadi, S.S. (2025). Cardiorespiratory fitness, body mass index and mortality: A systematic review and meta-analysis. *British Journal of Sports Medicine*, 59(5), 339–346.

Wegwarth, O., Schwartz, L.M., Woloshin, S., Gaissmaier, W., & Gigerenzer, G. (2012). Do physicians understand cancer screening statistics? A national survey of primary care physicians in the United States. *Annals of Internal Medicine*, 156(5), 340–349.

Weil, J.G., & Hawker, J.I. (1997). Positive findings of mammography may lead to suicide. *BMJ*, 314(7082), 754–755.

Welch, H.G. (2006). *Should I be tested for cancer? Maybe not and here's why*. University of California Press.

Welch, H.G., & Black, W.C. (2010). Overdiagnosis in cancer. *Journal of the National Cancer Institute*, 102(9), 605–613.
Welch, H.G., & Dey, T. (2023). Testing whether cancer screening saves lives: Implications for randomized clinical trials of multicancer screening. *JAMA Internal Medicine*, 183(11), 1255–1258.
Welch, H.G., & Fisher, E.S. (2017). Income and cancer overdiagnosis. *New England Journal of Medicine*, *376*(23), 2208–2209.
Welch, H.G., Woloshin, S., Schwartz, L.M., Gordis, L., Gøtzsche, P.C., Harris, R., Kramer, B.S., & Ransohoff, D.F. (2007). Overstating the evidence for lung cancer screening: The International Early Lung Cancer Action Program (I-ELCAP) study. *Archives of Internal Medicine*, 167(21), 2289–2295.
Welch, H.G., Schwartz, L., & Woloshin, S. (2011). *Overdiagnosed. Making people sick in the pursuit of health*. Beacon Press.
Weller, D., Vedsted, P., Rubin, G., Walter, F.M., Emery, J., Scott, S., Campbell, C., Andersen, R.S., Hamilton, W., Olesen, F., Rose, P., Nafees, S., van Rijswijk, E., Hiom, S., Muth, C., Beyer, M., & Neal, R.D. (2012). The Aarhus statement: Improving design and reporting of studies on early cancer diagnosis. *British Journal of Cancer*, 106(7), 1262–1267.
Whyte, S. (2005). Uncertain undertakings: Practicing health care in the subjunctive mood. In V. Steffen, R. Jenkins, & H. Jessen (Eds.), *Managing uncertainty. Ethnographic studies of illness, risk and the struggle for control* (pp. 245–264). Museum Tusculanum Press.
Whyte, S.R. (1997). *Questioning misfortune: The pragmatics of uncertainty in Eastern Uganda*. Cambridge University Press.
Whyte, S.R. (2009). Health identities and subjectivities: The ethnographic challenge. *Medical Anthropology Quarterly*, 16(2), 6–15.
Widding, J.L., Stroomberg, H.V., Dalton, S.O., Brasso, K., Røder, A., & Larsen, S.B. (2025). The association between lower urinary tract symptoms and urinary tract infections, and subsequent prostate cancer workup: A nationwide population-based case–control study. *British Journal of Cancer*, 134(3), 486–492.
Winsløw, A.E., Brodersen, J.B., Hori, M., & Jervelund, S.S. (2026). Lung cancer screening in the Nordic countries: Approaching implementation ahead of the evidence. *Scandinavian Journal of Public Health*, Feb 24, 14034948261422102.
Woloshin, S., & Kramer, B. (2021). Overdiagnosis: It's official. *BMJ*, 375, n2854.
Woloshin, S., & Schwartz, L.M. (2011). Communicating data about the benefits and harms of treatment: A randomized trial. *Annals of Internal Medicine*, 155(2), 87–96.
Woloshin, S., Patel, N., & Kesselheim, A.S. (2020). False negative tests for SARS-CoV-2 infection—challenges and implications. *New England Journal of Medicine*, 383(6), e38.
Woods, W.G., Gao, R.N., Shuster, J.J. Robison, L.L., Bernstein, M., Weitzman, S., Bunin, G., Levy, I., Brossard, J., Dougherty, G., Tuchman, M., & Lemieux, B. (2002). Screening of infants and mortality due to neuroblastoma. *New England Journal of Medicine*, 346(14), 1041–1046.
World Health Organization. (2022). *Screening programmes: A short guide. Increase effectiveness, maximize benefits and minimize harm*. WHO Regional Office for Europe. https://iris.who.int/server/api/core/bitstreams/b3922afd-3ff9-4bf3-9254-fa6b3f2b6023/content
World Health Organization. (2023). *Regulatory considerations on artificial intelligence for health*. WHO.
World Health Organization. (2025). *Artificial intelligence is reshaping health systems: State of readiness across the WHO European Region*. WHO Regional Office for Europe.
World Health Organization. (2026). Obesity—overview. https://www.who.int/health-topics/obesity#tab=tab_1 (accessed 19 June 2026)
Wyatt-Walter, A. (1996). Adam Smith and the liberal tradition in international relations. *Review of International Studies*, 22(1), 5–28.

Yavchitz, A., Boutron, I., Bafeta, A., Marroun, I., Charles, P., Mantz, J., & Ravand, P. (2012). Misrepresentation of randomized controlled trials. *PLoS Medicine*, *9*(9), e1001308. https://doi.org/10.1371/journal.pmed.1001308

Yoder, P.S. (1997). Negotiating relevance: Belief, knowledge and practice in international health projects. *Medical Anthropology Quarterly*, 11(2), 131–146.

Yoder, S.D. (2002). Individual responsibility for health: Decision, not discovery. *Hastings Center Report*, 32(2), 22–31.

Yudkin, J.S., & Montori, V.M. (2014). The epidemic of pre-diabetes: The medicine and the politics. *BMJ*, 349, g4485.

Zicari, R.V., Ahmed, S., Amann, J., Braun, S.A., Brodersen, J., Bruneault, F., Brusseau, J., Campano, E., Coffee, M., Dengel, A., Düdder, B., Gallucci, A., Gilbert, T.K., Gottfrois, P., Goffi, E., Haase, C.B., Hagendorff, T., Hickman, E., Hildt, E., . . ., & Wurth, R. (2021a). Co-design of a trustworthy AI system in healthcare: Deep learning based skin lesion classifier. *Frontiers in Human Dynamics*, 3, 2021.

Zicari, R.V., Brodersen, J., Brusseau, J., Düdder, B., Eichhorn, T., Ivanov, T., Kararigas, G., Kringen, P., McCullough, M., Möslein, F., Mushtaq, N., Roig, G., Stürtz, N., Tolle, K., Tithi, J.J., van Halem, I., & Westerlundet, M. (2021b). Z-Inspection®: A process to assess trustworthy AI. *IEEE Transactions on Technology and Society*, 2(2), 83–97.

Zoega, H., Furu, K., Halldorsson, M., Thomsen, P.H., Sourander, A., & Martikainen, J.E. (2011). Use of ADHD drugs in the Nordic countries: A population-based comparison study. *Acta Psychiatrica Scandinavica*, 123(5), 360–367.

Zola, I.K. (1975). Medicine as an institution of social control. In: C. Cox, & A. Mead (Eds.), *A sociology of medical practice* (pp. 223–241). Collier–Macmillan.

Zorzela, L., Loke, J.P., Ioannidis, Y.K., Golder, S., Santaguida, P., Altman, D.G., Moher, D., Vohra, S. (2016). PRISMA harms checklist: Improving harms reporting in systematic reviews. *BMJ*, 352, i157. doi: 10.1136/bmj.i157

Index

For the benefit of digital users, indexed terms that span two pages (e.g., 52–53) may, on occasion, appear on only one of those pages.

Tables, figures, and boxes are indicated by an italic *t*, *f*, and *b* following the page number.

The manufacturer's authorised representative in the EU for product safety is Oxford University Press España S.A. of El Parque Empresarial San Fernando de Henares, Avenida de Castilla, 2 - 28830 Madrid (www.oup.es/en or product.safety@oup.com). OUP España S.A. also acts as importer into Spain of products made by the manufacturer.
Printed and bound by CPI Group (UK) Ltd, Croydon, CR0 4YY
03/09/2026
02209091-0002